The Diabetic and Nursing Care

The Diabetic
and Nursing Care

Dorothy R. Blevins
Associate Professor of Nursing
Kent State University
Kent, Ohio

McGraw-Hill Book Company

New York   St. Louis   San Francisco   Auckland   Bogotá   Düsseldorf
Johannesburg   London   Madrid   Mexico   Montreal   New Delhi
Panama   Paris   São Paulo   Singapore   Sydney   Tokyo   Toronto

Library of Congress Cataloging in Publication Data

Main entry under title:

The Diabetic and nursing care.

    Includes index.
    1. Diabetes—Nursing. I. Blevins, Dorothy R.
[DNLM: 1. Diabetes mellitus—Nursing texts. WY155
D536]
RC 660.D56   616.4'62   78-24724
ISBN 0-07-005902-0

THE DIABETIC AND NURSING CARE

1 2 3 4 5 6 7 8 9 0 DODO 7 8 3 2 1 0 9

This book was set in Times Roman by Bi-Comp, Incorporated.
The editors were Laura A. Dysart and Moira Lerner;
the cover was designed by Saiki & Sprung Design;
the production supervisor was Jeanne Selzam.
The drawings were done by ANCO/Boston.
R. R. Donnelley & Sons Company was printer and binder.

To Marie Rennie and
Bob, Lynne, Bill, and Jim

Contents

List of Contributors

MARY ADAMS, R.N., Ph.D.
Associate Professor of Public Health
Nursing, Case Western Reserve Univer-
sity; Associate in Nursing, University
Hospitals of Cleveland; Research Asso-
ciate, School of Medicine, Cleveland,
Ohio

DOROTHY BLEVINS, R.N., M.S.N.
Associate Professor of Nursing, Kent
State University, Kent, Ohio; Guest
Lecturer at Cleveland Diabetes Associa-
tion, Cleveland, Ohio

VIOLET A. BRECKBILL, R.N., Ph.D.
Associate Professor of Nursing and In-
structor in Biology, Case Western Re-
serve University; Associate in Nursing,
University Hospitals of Cleveland,
Cleveland, Ohio

KAREN BUDD, R.N., M.S.N.
Assistant Clinical Professor, Case
Western University; Nurse Clinician in
High-Risk Pregnancy, Maternity-Gyne-
cological Nursing, University Hospitals
of Cleveland, Cleveland, Ohio

MARY ANN CASTON, R.N., M.S.N.
Instructor in Gerontological Nursing,
Case Western Reserve University; As-
sociate in Nursing, Cleveland, Ohio

ANAS A. EL ATTAR, M.D., M.Sc.,
D.Sc.
Works Physician of Jones and Laughlin
Steel Corporation; Adjunct Assistant
Clinical Professor of Occupational Medi-
cine, Graduate School of Public Health,
University of Pittsburgh, Pittsburgh,
Pennsylvania

CAROL E. HARTMAN, R.N., M.S.N.
Staff Nurse, Pettis Memorial Veterans
Administration Hospital, Loma Linda,
California; Formerly Assistant Professor
of Medical-Surgical Nursing, Case
Western Reserve University, Cleveland,
Ohio

ELLEN H. KING, R.N., M.N.
Doctoral Student, Texas Women's Uni-
versity; Formerly Assistant Professor of
Pediatric Nursing, Case Western Re-
serve University; Associate in Nursing,
University Hospitals of Cleveland,
Cleveland, Ohio

JANICE N. NEVILLE, R.D., D.Sc.
Professor and Chairman in Nutrition,
Case Western Reserve University,
Cleveland, Ohio

ANTOINETTE T. RAGUCCI, R.N.,
Ph.D.
Associate Professor of Medical-Surgical
Nursing, Case Western Reserve Univer-
sity; Associate in Nursing, University
Hospitals of Cleveland, Cleveland, Ohio

MARTI SACHSE, Pharm.D.
Assistant Professor of Clinical Phar-
macy, University of Colorado School of
Pharmacy, Denver, Colorado

BETSY A. SCHENK, R.N., M.S.N.
Lecturer in Gerontological Nursing,
Case Western Reserve University;
Nurse Clinician, Rehabilitation, High-
land View Hospital, Cleveland, Ohio

SHIRLEY O. WOOD, R.N., M.S.N.
Assistant Clinical Professor of Mater-
nity Nursing and Maternity Nurse
Educator, Cleveland Regional Perinatal
Network, Cleveland, Ohio

MAY L. WYKLE, R.N., M.S.N.
Associate Professor of Psychiatric Nursing, Case Western Reserve University;
Associate in Nursing, University Hospitals of Cleveland, Cleveland, Ohio

Preface

This book was written to provide students and practitioners of nursing with a reference text for care of individuals with diabetes mellitus. Nurses who teach, counsel, and provide care to persons with this chronic illness contribute significant effort to improving the well-being of individuals, families, and communities. While much remains to be learned about the disease and its treatment, the health behaviors of people, and the best ways in which people can be assisted in their quest for health, much is known that can guide nursing practice.

It is said that over 10,000,000 persons in the United States are affected by diabetes mellitus (half of them unaware) and that many known diabetic persons are receiving inadequate health care. Diverse factors influence the extent to which nurses can effectively implement roles of teaching, counseling and care giving with diabetic persons: some of these are related to the resources and constraints in particular health care settings, some are related to the utilization of nurses in the health care delivery system, and some are related to the knowledge held by nurses and the expertise with which they practice.

The first part of the book reflects the wide scope of knowledge that underlies nursing practice; thus, chapters deal with cultural and social dimensions of nursing care of diabetic persons, with the diabetic individual's personal adjustment to chronic illness, with physiological alterations that occur in diabetes mellitus, with diagnosis, and with management by hypoglycemic agents and by nutrition. Authors with specialized knowledge were selected from the fields of anthropology, mental health, physiology, medicine, pharmacology, and nutrition so that both scope and depth of knowledge would be presented. Each of these authors discusses those facts, principles, and theories that seem most relevant to the care of diabetic people.

The disease of diabetes mellitus is complex, involving multihormonal and metabolic derangements and degenerative changes in blood vessels and nerves. Furthermore, the disease and the physical and behavioral responses of diabetic persons to current treatment modalities and to recommendations for preventive health care practices are greatly influenced by such variables as age, level of growth and development, and the psychosocial/cultural milieu in which each diabetic lives. Education and counseling about self-care practices are emphasized throughout; in particular, Chapter 2 includes discussion of principles and methods of counseling; and Chapter 9 reviews the elements of an educational program.

In the second part of the book, authors describe the nursing care requirements specific to hospitalized adults, children and adolescents, pregnant women, and the elderly. Each contributor shares experience gained through working with diabetic persons and their families; with nursing students and practitioners of nursing; and in the development of assessment guides, standards of care, audit criteria, and strategies for nursing interventions.

It is the hope of the authors that the book will contribute to the knowledge of nurses and the effectiveness with which they practice. While some programs of health maintenance are involving nurses in ambulatory care, and while a small number of nurses specialize in teaching or in the delivery of primary health care, currently most interactions between nurses and diabetic persons occur when the latter are sick or recuperating. It is true that the majority of nurses presently practice within the secondary health care system and as generalists in nursing. If there is a bias to this book, it is the belief that knowledgeable nurses capable of implementing the roles of care giver, teacher, and counselor can have a significant impact upon the well-being of diabetic people and their families.

ACKNOWLEDGMENTS

Several persons merit recognition for their wise counsel and for special kinds of assistance—in particular, Mrs. Carol Mitten, formerly a nurse clinician in diabetes mellitus, who provided encouragement throughout the project and reviewed much of the manuscript; Dr. Harvey Rodman, who allowed us to use unpublished material of his in Chapter 2; and Dr. Saul Genuth, who reviewed parts of the manuscript.

The editorial staff of McGraw-Hill Book Company provided welcome guidance to the novice editor. Gratitude is especially extended to Mr. Orville Haberman, Ms. Laura Dysart, and Ms. Moira Lerner.

We sincerely thank Mrs. Geraldine Mink for editorial assistance, and Mrs. Sandi Williams, Mrs. Sandra Payne, and Mrs. Barbara Selwyn for their assistance in typing the final manuscript.

Dorothy R. Blevins

Chapter 1

An Overview

Dorothy R. Blevins

A "state of well-being" was the definition of *health* derived by the World Health Organization and the common goal toward which health professionals endeavor; *optimal well-being* is the term more frequently used to describe health care goals in a less utopian manner. This term acknowledges the imperfect and transitional nature of knowledge about health and its nurturance, the inadequacies of societal resources for the promotion of health, and the multiple variables that affect the extent to which individuals, groups, and communities can achieve health.

While current knowledge about the health-seeking behavior of human beings is limited and much is yet to be learned about the best and most efficient ways to support and assist humans in their quest for well-being, much can be learned about the extent to which health has been achieved in American society by the study of the diabetic subpopulation.

Diabetes mellitus, a chronic illness with components of hormonal imbalance and alterations in blood vessels and nerves, has a marked impact on the well-being of individuals, groups, and communities. It is responsible for considerable amounts of "sickness" care needed by people in the United States, and increasing attention is being paid to the maintenance of health in diabetic people who are ambulatory and not feeling ill. Desired health care

1

outcomes are frequently specified as avoidance of preventable complications and adjustment of the individual in life roles. These outcomes are influenced by a person's behavior when she or he is not in contact with the health care system. Besides skilled and compassionate sickness care, people with this disease need assistance with learning how to prevent complications and how to adjust to chronic illness.

DIABETES MELLITUS: INFLUENCE ON HEALTH

All levels of wellness and illness can now be identified in the diabetic subpopulation, which includes people of diverse ages, races, socioeconomic, political, and geographic groups, and both sexes. Once, acute illness and rapid death occurred with diabetes mellitus. However, complex and multiple facets of the nature of diabetes mellitus and its treatment have been discovered since Areteus the Cappadocian described the disease around 150 A.D.:

> Diabetes is a wonderful affliction a melting down of the flesh into urine. The patients never stop making water. The flow is incessant as if from the opening of aqueducts. The fluid does not remain in the body, but uses the man's body as a ladder, whereby to leave it.[1]

This description of overt diabetes mellitus, weight loss, and polyuria remains accurate today. In addition, fatigue, polyphagia, and polydipsia are found when there is hyperglycemia, osmotic diuresis, and negative caloric balance. Insulin deficit resulting in changes in metabolism of carbohydrate, fat, and protein may be absolute—as in insulin-dependent diabetes mellitus—or may be relative—as in insulin-independent diabetes mellitus. Often people with the first type are thin, young at the age of onset, and need daily injections of insulin, while those with the second type are older at the time of onset, are frequently obese, and need to reduce caloric intake and weight if they are to maintain normal blood glucose levels.

Increasingly, the term *prediabetic* is used to define in retrospect the period of life prior to the development of detectable, or overt, diabetes mellitus, or to depict the person who is known to be genetically predisposed to the disease. There is increasing evidence of early changes in capillary basement membranes in the genetically predisposed person—perhaps before the onset of signs of hyperglycemia. This knowledge has influenced the evolving definition of diabetes mellitus to include vascular and neurologic changes as part of the underlying disease process. The presence of diabetes mellitus is considered a risk factor in atherosclerosis and hypertension and their sequelae: stroke, renal disease, cardiomyopathy, and peripheral arterial disease. While some illness and deaths still occur from acute hormonal disorders of the disease, increasing morbidity and mortality occur when there are chronic complications resulting from alterations in large and small blood vessels and nerve cells.

Increasing numbers in the United States population are developing diabetes mellitus. Steinke and Soeldner suggest the following reasons for this:

Increasing numbers of aged people
Increasing life expectancy
Increasing numbers of children who have inherited the disease
Increasing incidence of obesity
The wider use of detection drives for diabetes mellitus[2]

Impact of Illness

Much of what is known about the impact of diabetes mellitus on individuals, families, and communities is derived from epidemiological studies. The following statistics are from the Report of the National Commission on Diabetes.

There are marked differences in the extent to which diabetes mellitus is present in various segments of American society. Incidence and prevalence are related to factors of age, sex, race, and income. People with the highest risk of developing diabetes mellitus are those who are aged, women, poor, and nonwhite. Of the 10 million people estimated to be diabetic, the majority are adult, while 90,000 are juvenile. As age advances, the frequency with which diabetes mellitus is reported increases. At all ages more women than men and more nonwhite than white people report diabetes. In addition, the highest rates of prevalence and incidence are found in people reporting family incomes of less than $5000 per year.

In 1973, 38,000 deaths were reported with diabetes mellitus noted as the underlying cause. It has been estimated that if the contributory effect of this disease on other underlying causes was reported on death certificates, over 300,000 people could be expected to die annually from diabetes mellitus; and diabetes mellitus would rank as the third greatest cause of death. Fifty percent of juvenile diabetics die as a result of renal disease, while those with older-onset diabetes die most frequently from cardiovascular disease.[3]

Illness of the newly diagnosed and younger diabetic is often related to acute disorders of hormonal imbalance and that illness of older diabetics and those with longer duration of the disease tend to be related to long-term complications affecting the kidneys, eyes, heart, blood vessels, and nerves. In one study, 14 percent of hospital admissions of diabetics were due to ketoacidosis or coma; in patients aged 1 to 19, 65 percent of admissions were due to ketoacidosis; in patients aged 20 to 34, that statistic dropped to 40 percent.[4] Ketoacidosis is responsible for death rates of 5 to 13 percent of patients hospitalized for ketoacidosis.[5] The National Commission on Diabetes estimates that the increased risk in diabetic people over nondiabetic people of blindness is 25 times; for renal disease, 17 times; for gangrene, 30 times; and for heart attacks or strokes, 2 times.[6] In the Health Interview Survey of 1973, known diabetics reported an average of 14.5 days of activity restriction because of their disease; 5.8 days of this restriction were because of bed confinement.[7]

In Chapter 4, Breckbill reviews current knowledge about physiological alterations that occur in diabetes mellitus. In Chapter 5, El Attar discusses diagnostic aspects and the initial planning of treatment. Current modalities of management by nutritional modifications and by pharmacologic agents are discussed in Chapters 6 and 7 by Neville and Sachse, respectively.

Psychosocial Impact

A commonly stated goal of care is to enable people with diabetes mellitus to live full and active lives. If optimal well-being of the individual is the focus in health care, attention to the diabetic person's adjustment to the environment is the concern of health care professionals. Not only is the biological state different from the norm and from the patient's past, often orientation to life and life-style of the newly diagnosed diabetic require major changes. Becoming a diabetic can be viewed as a process of changing identity, as well as changing patterns of behavior, in order to regain and maintain health. Much attention has been given to the difficulty with which young patients with insulin-dependent diabetes mellitus and their families incorporate therapeutic measures and adjust to the disease. Two other areas of adjustment that are of concern are (1) changing the eating patterns of older and obese diabetics, and (2) helping diabetics and their families cope when long-term complications bring disability and anticipation of death.

ADJUSTMENT AND CONTROL OF THE DISEASE

There is evidence that incorporating strict regimens of therapy exact a heavy toll on some insulin-dependent diabetic patients and families. The literature is full of references helping people and their families in adjusting to the diagnosis and the chronic illness, to perceptions of differentness, to restrictive regimens, and to difficult decisions about career choice, employment, marriage, and child rearing.

A commonly held view is that insulin-dependent diabetes and its related therapeutic measures pose a threat to psychosocial well-being. Some research findings support this view, while others do not. For example, in 1967, Swift, Seidman, and Stein reported more emotional disturbances, including manifest and latent anxiety, among diabetic children than among nondiabetic children in a control group.[8] In contrast, Simond reported that no greater frequency of psychiatric disorders was found in diabetic children under good control than in a comparable group of nondiabetic children. However, mild depression and anxiety were found more frequently in those children who were not in good control of their diabetes.[9] Krosnick, in writing about psychiatric aspects of diabetes, stated that anxiety is the most striking personality trait of diabetic children.[10] Pinkerton and Pless, in a review of studies of coping with chronic illness, pointed out recurrent findings that home and family influence the coping abilities of diabetic children, and that there is lack of clear-cut evidence between diabetic control and illness variables.[11] Krosnick points out, "There are many diabetics, both children and adults alike, who accept the diagnosis, the restrictions, the responsibilities and the potential dangers of diabetes in a healthy, mature and admirable way.''[12]

While all physicians would agree that therapy should control blood glucose levels in the *direction* of normal, debate does exist over whether control at levels approximating those of normal is the best policy. There is little doubt that close control of blood glucose levels in insulin-dependent people requires effort, a structured existence, and regularity of daily life. Proponents of close control cite the values of normal growth and development, the delay or amelioration of vascular complications, and the beneficial effect of self-discipline in promoting a mature, self-controlled, productive adult.[13] Schmitt reviewed arguments for a less rigorous regimen with an unmeasured diet and stated that too rigorous control may result in physical harm, e.g., increased risk of repeated hypoglycemia, epilepsy, mental deterioration, and acquired and permanent neuromotor deficits. This author also discusses emotional harm that may follow when food is restricted, becomes the focus of parent-child conflict, and evokes stress in parents and children.[14] He cited Knowles' study of 108 juvenile diabetics who were followed for 10 years and treated with an unmeasured diet. No differences were found in the incidence of degenerative complications in these subjects and those treated with measured diets reported in other studies.[15]

Control of Obesity

Control of blood glucose levels in obese and insulin-independent diabetics is closely related to caloric intake and weight control. Less rigor, structure, and regularity are needed in their daily lives chiefly because they do not need to regulate food and activity to balance the effect of previously injected insulin. However, weight reduction and regulation of caloric intake are important if blood glucose levels are to be controlled. While, in the past, there has been much pessimism about the ability of patients to achieve weight loss, recently reports of obesity control in adult-onset diabetics have been encouraging.[16]

Disability and Death

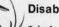

Little is found in the literature related to the adjustment processes of those diabetics who are manifesting the long-term complications of diabetes and suffering loss and grief. True, one can find references to assisting the disabled or dying in the literature of other fields, e.g., rehabilitation and thanatology. However, several factors may account for this seeming lack of attention in diabetes literature: (1) the slow recognition that insulin was not a panacea, (2) the view of diabetes as primarily a hormonal imbalance, and (3) the "shifting" of the disabled or dying diabetic to other fields and other disease conditions (e.g., renal disease, cardiovascular disease).

This brief overview presents some of the dimensions of adjustment of diabetic patients and their families to diabetes as a chronic disease. Indeed, the concerns involved in patient and family adjustment to diabetes mellitus, its treatment, and its potential impact on well-being are multifaceted.

CHANGING THROUGH LEARNING

One way in which people can increase the level of their well-being is to engage in learning, an active process that can be guided by others. Bigge defined *learning* as "an enduring change in insights, behavior, perception or motivation, or a combination of these."[17] The Task Force on Consumer Health Education listed a set of six activities that comprise *consumer health education:*

1 Inform people about health, illness, disability, and ways in which they can improve and protect their own health, including more efficient use of the delivery system
2 Motivate people to want to change to more healthful practices
3 Help them to learn the necessary skills to adopt and maintain healthful practices and life-styles
4 Foster teaching and communication skills in all those engaged in educating consumers about health
5 Advocate changes in the environment that will facilitate healthful conditions and healthful behavior
6 Add to knowledge through research and evaluation concerning the most effective ways of achieving these objectives[18]

Consumer health education was defined as a field of interest to many diverse disciplines including those in health care professions, education, communications, and the new "consumerism."

Consumer health education, as defined above, is broader in scope than that traditionally identified as patient education. *Patient education* implies the transmission of selected knowledge, skills, and attitudes to people with particular diseases or conditions. It often focuses on those prescribed measures which patients are asked to incorporate into their lives. That the diabetic person should be educated about diabetes and its management has been given wide acceptance by health care providers. In the past, this disease was often described as unique because of the necessity for patients to be involved in their own therapy. The National Commission on Diabetes has reaffirmed the key nature of education in the treatment of diabetes and has identified six problems of patient education:

1 Diabetic patients do not receive adequate education as part of their initial treatment or home management.
2 Inadequate education of the diabetic patient compounds the psychological problems and seriously affects the life-style of the individual.
3 People with diabetes who also have physical complications receive inadequate education.
4 People with diabetes who also have language difficulties and special ethnic needs fail to receive adequate education.
5 People with diabetes who also have learning disabilities fail to receive adequate education.
6 Needs of the person with diabetes at different ages (e.g., infant, child,

adolescent, young adult, aged) are not adequately recognized and provided for.[19]

Some evidence suggests that more preventive health measures occur when individuals perceive themselves at risk, vulnerable to specific and serious health problems, and able to influence their own health in some way.[20] Both acute and chronic complications of diabetes mellitus place individuals at grave risk, and educational programs for these people should emphasize both the measures by which patients can influence their own well-being and the rationale for such measures.

Teaching about two acute complications is a central feature of diabetic education. One, ketoacidosis (characterized by metabolic acidosis and severe dehydration), is more likely to occur in insulin-dependent diabetics, although it may occur in insulin-independent diabetics as well. Stress, infection, or failure to take adequate amounts of insulin may precipitate this condition. In contrast, hypoglycemia (reaction to insulin), occurs in the diabetic when excessive insulin is present in relation to food intake and activity. Thus hypoglycemia occurs only in those taking insulin or hypoglycemic agents; its onset is very rapid and can easily be treated by ingestion or intravenous infusion of glucose. Death can result from either of these conditions if they are untreated. The well-educated patient can prevent both conditions to a large extent.

Increasingly, more openness about and disclosure of potential and probable long-term complications are being suggested by specialists in diabetes.[21] Current knowledge and skills are not as successful in preventing and treating these conditions as they are in the acute disorders. However, there is strong belief that the reduction of certain risk factors may delay the onset or ameliorate the severity of some of these complications, e.g., close control of blood glucose levels, weight control, avoidance of smoking, and inclusion of planned and regular exercise. Since it is not possible to determine which people with diabetes mellitus will be free of these complications, preventive measures are recommended to all.

It is true that anxiety and fear in diabetic people and their families may be related to perceptions of vulnerability for both acute and chronic complications. Support is necessary to assist these people in dealing with their concerns, experiencing their abilities to live with the disease, and incorporating therapeutic and preventive measures into their daily lives.

NURSING AND DIABETIC PATIENTS AND FAMILIES

"Start where the patient is" is a long-hallowed phrase in nursing which focuses on people, their perceptions and concerns about health, their behaviors related to health, and those facets of their existence which affect well-being. Nurses who wish to influence the movement of others toward health should understand not only disease processes and treatment but also health behaviors of people; they should be concerned with the sociocultural milieu in which people interact, the factors which influence their decision making and practices involved in health care.

Self-Care

Backsheider applied concepts of self-care as developed by Orem and the Nursing Development Conference Group to diabetic patient education. She stressed the importance of assessing the ongoing self-care practices of the person and determining those changes in self-care practices which need to be made. She asked two important questions:

1 Which dimensions of the therapeutic plan of care might involve the patient, and in what ways?
2 What are the capabilities of the patient in relation to those required by the plan of care?[22]

A well-educated diabetic patient is able to monitor and perceive alterations in health status, incorporate prescribed measures into his or her life-style with comfort and competence, and make knowledgeable choices about basic aspects of living. Knowing about the disease and its treatment is not sufficient; acting on knowledge is necessary if the patient is to be effective in the management of the disease.

In Chapter 2, Ragucci reviews concepts from behavioral science and the multiple sociocultural factors that affect health behavior and often lead to patient acceptance or rejection of the efforts of health care professionals. Nurses should attend to these factors and the emotional responses of patients and families to the diagnosis and impact of chronic disease. In Chapter 3, Wykle presents concepts of mental health and the ways in which nurses can facilitate adaptation of patients and families. Both these writers underscore the importance of focusing on patient and family concerns. In Chapter 9, Hartman reviews principles of teaching and learning and discusses the many alternative methods that nurses may use to teach. Other authors include health education as an integral part of the services nurses provide.

The view presented in this book is that education is achieved most effectively when learning and teaching are focused on choices that are perceived as necessary in daily life by the patient and his or her family. Engaging the attention and commitment of the learner(s) is a prerequisite for teaching, and guidance through the learning process is a major function of the teacher. More effective and efficient educational programs can be implemented when the learner(s) has imput into the content and methods by which learning occurs.

Multiple forces affect the ability of individual nurses and groups of nurses to practice in a manner that reflects a holistic approach to those served and nurtures those behaviors most likely to foster optimal health. Evolving systems in nursing of health-status assessment that reflect the multiple dimensions of human well-being, standards of nursing performance, and quality assurance programs not only reaffirm nursing's holistic and humane approach to human health, but also its commitment to excellence of practice. Such systems hold promise in assisting nurses in delineating universal, rather than situationally determined, functions and roles.

It is the thesis of this book that three traditional nursing roles are particularly applicable to diabetic individuals and groups: care giver, educator, and counselor. Nurses provide significant services when they care for the ill, teach patients how to manage the disease within their daily lives, and foster the inner strengths and adaptive abilities of people with a chronic illness. It is the hope of the authors of this book that it will contribute to the knowledge and expertise of nurses who carry out these three roles.

REFERENCES

1 Laufer, I. J., and Kadeson, H. *Diabetes Explained: A Layman's Guide* (New York: Dutton, 1976), pp. 24–25.
2 Steinke, J., and Soeldner, J. S. Diabetes mellitus, G. W. Thorn et al. (eds.), *Harrison's Principles of Internal Medicine,* 8th ed. (New York: McGraw-Hill, 1975), p. 564.
3 *Report of the National Commission on Diabetes to the Congress of the United States,* vols. I and III, DHEW publication no. (NIH)76-1018, 1975.
4 Ibid.
5 Ibid.
6 Ibid.
7 Ibid.
8 Swift, C. R., Seidman, F. L., and Stein, H. Adjustment problems in juvenile diabetes, *Psychol. Med.,* **29:**555, 1967.
9 Simond, J. F. Psychiatric states of diabetic youth matched with a control group, *Diabetes,* **26:**921–925, 1977.
10 Krosnick, A. Psychiatric aspects of diabetes, in Ellenberg, M. and Rifkin, H. (eds.), *Diabetes Mellitus: Theory and Practice* (New York: McGraw-Hill, 1970), p. 923.
11 Pless, I. B., and Pinkerton, P. *Chronic Childhood Disorders: Promoting Patterns of Adjustment.* (London: Henry Kimpton Publication, 1975).
12 Krosnick. Op. cit., p. 922.
13 Guthrie, D. W., and Guthrie, R. A. *Nursing Management of Diabetes Mellitus.* (St. Louis: Mosby, 1977), pp. 26–29.
14 Schmitt, B. D. The unmeasured diabetic diet, *Clin. Pediatr. (Phila.),* **14:**72–73, 1975.
15 Knowles, H. C., et al. The course of juvenile diabetes treated with unmeasured diet, *Diabetes,* **14:**249, 1965.
16 Davidson, J. K. Educating diabetic patients about diet therapy, *International Diabetes Federation Bulletin,* **20**(2):3–7, 1975.
17 Bigge, M. L. *Learning Theories for Teachers,* 2d ed. (New York: Harper & Row, 1971), p. 11.
18 Somers, A. R. *Promoting Health Consumer Education and National Policy,* Part III: Summary and Recommendations, Aspen Systems Corporation, Germantown, Maryland, 1976.
19 *Report of the National Commission on Diabetes.* Loc. cit.
20 Pender, N. J. A conceptual model for preventive health behavior, *Nurs. Outlook,* **23:**385–390, 1975.
21 Duncan, T. The editors speak, *Diabetes Forecast,* **30:**2, 1977.
22 Backsheider, J. E. Self-care in diabetes, *Am. J. Public Health,* **64:**1138–1146, 1974.

Chapter 2

Cultural and Social Dimensions of the Nursing Care of Persons with Diabetes Mellitus

Antoinette T. Ragucci

Actions directed toward the maintenance of health, prevention of disease, and amelioration of symptoms associated with illness are part of the cultural inventory of all human groups. The forms and functions of a people's preventive and healing practices vary according to its social structure—primitive or complex, urban or rural, industrialized or traditional. However, despite the wide variations in cultural health caring and curing practices, health maintenance, illness, and death are the universals of the human condition.

The diversity of human responses to events associated with illness and death and the adaptive arrangements that must be made by individuals and groups have been the subject of study in the behavioral, medical, and nursing sciences. Consonant with the aim of this chapter, it is notable that few studies derived from these disciplines have specifically focused upon the social and cultural determinants or dimensions of health-seeking behaviors of people with diabetes. A review of the nursing literature, in particular, showed a dearth of research designed to take into account the interrelationship of social and cultural variables and diabetes mellitus. Quint, a nurse-sociologist, has been one of the first in nursing to break ground in the research of the meaning of becoming a diabetic (juvenile) within the social structure of the family. On the basis of her findings, Quint concluded that the present health system is neither well organized nor prepared to guide children and their families when the diagnosis of a chronic illness marks the transition of a person from "normal" to "non-normal" by ordinary social standards and cultural definitions.[1] Looking at her own study in a larger context in an attempt to develop a theory of chronicity for nursing, Quint stated that the clustering of social, psychological, and cultural variables into recognizable patterns will permit identification of critical points during the process of socialization in the role of diabetic.

The purpose of this chapter is to examine the interconnections between a chronic disease entity which affects a human being's biological integrity and some social and cultural variables which need to be taken into account in planning nursing interventions on behalf of the diabetic patient and his or her significant others. Those readers who wish prescriptions for counseling, teaching, or managing diabetics in terms of their illness will be disappointed. The state of knowledge about the health-seeking behavior of human beings and about effective means of influencing their health care practices is imperfect. "Start where the patient is" may still be the most valid direction one can give to nurses. This chapter will explore the meaning of that aphorism by examining some sociocultural concepts developed by anthropologists and sociologists for their relevance to nursing.

The study of the nursing care of the diabetic patient from the perspective of cultural beliefs, values, and social roles will serve to increase our understanding of the human condition and the diversity of human responses under conditions of adversity. The quotation that follows is an appropriate introduction to the task. The substitution of the word *nursing* for the words *anthropology* and *medical anthropology* wherever these occur conveys the intention of this chapter.

> Health and disease are fundamentally connected with reproduction, quality, preservation, and loss of life. In view of the significance of these phenomena for human society, it is not surprising that an anthropological study of health and the occurrence and means of coping with disease can involve one deeply in the manner in which people perceive their world, in the characteristics of human social systems and in social values. In this perspective medical anthropology is not only a way of viewing the states of health and disease in society, but a way of viewing society itself. . . .[2]

A person who becomes sick is faced with an entirely new set of cultural and social expectations. Different patterns of behavior are assumed. These behaviors are determined by the social and cultural context in which the person exists, namely, the family, community, and health care institutions. The cultural variables that will be examined in this chapter include the physical anthropology and epidemiology of diabetes mellitus and cultural beliefs and values as determinants of health-seeking behaviors. The social determinants of a diabetic person's health-seeking behavior will be analyzed in terms of the "sick role," a concept which serves to link ego to *alter,* i.e., the individual to others in the social system. The emphasis will be placed upon the nurse-patient reciprocal role relationship, a dimension largely neglected by Parsons in the seminal paper on the sick role published in 1967[3] and in the review of the concept in 1975.[4] Theoretical constructs and methodological approaches from anthropology and sociology will be examined for their usefulness and relevance in developing the social and cultural dimensions of the art and science of nursing as it relates to the care of the person with diabetes mellitus.

PHYSICAL ANTHROPOLOGY: CULTURE CHANGE AND DIABETES MELLITUS

The interrelationship between society and culture and the biochemical and pathophysiologic attributes of diabetes mellitus cannot be ignored in planning nursing interventions directed at preventive and therapeutic aspects of the illness. Understanding of the epidemiology of diabetes mellitus and a recognition of its cultural, social, and ecological correlates will facilitate the nurse's identification of individuals or populations who are at risk. Although conclusive evidence about cause-and-effect relationships is lacking, nursing actions may be directed toward change or prevention of those conditions believed to be predisposing factors of diabetes mellitus.

Demographic and Cultural Variability in the Incidence of Diabetes

The etiologic factors in diabetes mellitus are still poorly understood. Some epidemiological and genetic evidence suggests that viruses may be involved in causing at least one type of diabetes.[5] Genetic determinants are assumed to play an important role in the incidence of diabetes among certain cultural groups. The high incidence of obesity among some populations appears to have a positive correlation with the prevalence of the disorder.[6] Economic deprivation is associated with an increased incidence of diabetes,[7] and diabetes itself may intensify economic deprivation because of the increased costs of carrying out prescribed medical and dietary regimes, as well as the probability of work disruption resulting from sickness, absenteeism, or disability arising out of diabetic complications. Changes in specific components of a cultural group's diet and activity pattern have also been identified as leading to the expression of diabetes.[8,9] Sexual and racial differences have been identified as correlates of diabetes. Statistics show that diabetic death rates for women in the United States are higher than for men. The crude diabetes death rate for the years 1968 to 1973 was 15 per 100,000 for males and 21 per 100,000 for females. Racial differentials become apparent when the trends of diabetes deaths for whites and nonwhites are compared. The trend for whites moved steadily upward during the 1930s, but beginning in 1940 the rate leveled off and varied little over the next 34 years. However, although the trend for nonwhites was the same during the aforementioned period, their rates rose steadily between 1957 and 1967. The pattern for nonwhites was lower than that for whites during most of the century, but the patterns showed a change during the 1960s. Now the rate for nonwhites is the higher of the two, 23 per 100,000 versus 17 to 18 per 100,000 for whites.[10] Other demographic contrasts relative to the diabetic death rate (age-adjusted) are the state and regional differentials found within the United States. Alaska has the lowest incidence of deaths, Delaware the highest. Age-adjusted death rates were higher in the Eastern and Central states and lower in the Mountain and Pacific states.

The reasons for the observed differences between regions, states, race, and sex groups are not completely understood. One may assume that differences in social class, cultural customs, and life-styles may account in part for the differences. Study of the temporal and spatial distributions of diabetes mellitus and intensive studies of specific subcultural groups have contributed to a potentially etiologically significant understanding of the interrelationship between diabetes and population characteristics. The findings from intensive studies of American Indian tribal groups and other American subcultural groups are providing data about the natural history of the disease. Wide variations in the frequency of diabetes have been found to exist between Caucasians (11 per 1000) and pure-blooded Hawaiian workers on the island of Oahu (78 per 1000).[11] Rates among southwestern American Indian adults who attended the Public Health Service Hospital in Phoenix during the years 1959 to 1964 ranged from 10 per 1000 for the Navaho to 450 per 1000 for the Pima. The latter tribe has been the subject of intensive study of the interrelationship of pathophysiologic, nutritional, and cultural variables. The Pima Indians provide an ideal model for comparisons that are directed at gaining insight in the marked ethnic variability which has been found among population groups. The findings of hyperinsulinemia in the Pima, for example, suggest that the operative mechanism for the maintenance of hyperglycemia is not always due to impaired insulin production, storage, release, or distribution but may be due to target resistance to glucose acceptance and utilization in the presence of "normal" insulin levels.[12-14]

The findings of comparative studies of various populations suggest a general correlation between obesity and prevalence of diabetes within certain ethnic groups. However, when the clinical form of the disease and the customary diet are compared in different populations, no clear relationships are discernible.[15] For example, although the diet of the Navaho Indian is similar to that of the Pennsylvania Amish in terms of fat and carbohydrate intake, both ketosis and vascular complications are rare in the Navaho but common in the Amish, whose diet represents a variant of a western European type. Both the Japanese and Ceylonese consume a diet low in fat and carbohydrates. The form of diabetic complications for these cultural groups is similar to that found in the Navaho. Both the Pima and Alabama Coushatta Indians consume diets high in animal fats and carbohydrates. Ketoacidosis is rare in these tribes, but vascular complications are fairly common.[16] The Natal Indian and Negro groups of South Africa have similar diets, at least in terms of total fat and carbohydrates, but ketosis is rare in the Natal Indian and common in the South African black. The reverse holds for vascular complications.[17]

A detailed dietary survey was carried out to determine whether there was an association between dietary intake of selected nutrients, change in customary diets, and the prevalence of diabetes mellitus among Pima and Papago Indian women.[18] There were few significant differences between diabetic and nondiabetic women with respect to 18 nutrients. Diabetic women reported a significantly lower total carbohydrate and sucrose intake than the nondiabetic women. The two most widely used foods in the Pima diet are beans and tortillas which are prepared from wheat flour rather than corn. These foods, along with chili peppers, were eaten by most families on a regular basis.[19]

Culture Change and Diabetes

The data pertaining to geographical and cultural differentials in the incidence of diabetes and pathological complications raise questions concerning the nature of human adaptation to a changing environment, i.e., the movement from a rural to an urban environment or the change from a less complex to a more technologically complex one. The increased incidence of diabetes in peoples undergoing culture change has led some to refer to diabetes as a disease of civilization.[20] Neel postulated that the diabetic gene had at one time functioned to enhance survival.[21] Neel's theory of diabetes as a "thrifty genotype" holds that in prehistoric times the prediabetic individual was better equipped to adapt to the environment. The gene or genes responsible for diabetes mellitus allowed for gaining extra pounds during times of relative plenty and, therefore, enhanced survival during times of famine. Since human dependence on nature, i.e., the hunting of game and the gathering of foods, has been lessened and the feast-and-famine cycle that was common in a more primitive or rural environment no longer exists, the diabetic gene, once an aid to survival, has become a liability.

Prosnitz and Mandell studied all diabetic patients of Navaho and Hopi origin who were seen at a hospital over a 2-year period.[22] Most patients consumed diets high in saturated fats and carbohydrates (candy and soda pop). Of the 69 patients hospitalized, one-half had complications, but the hypertension and renal disease were generally mild. Some correlates of the incidence of rare vascular disease were suggested. These were low incidence of smokers, lack of urban stress, physical exercise, regular and long sleeping habits, and heredity. Prosnitz and Mandell hypothesized that it is possible that the disease entity is not the same for Indian and western European populations.

Precise changes and the impact of culture change on food patterns and dietary habits cannot be determined until other significant environmental factors have been adequately studied. These include composition of diets, available food supplies and the effect of increasing urbanization, with its resultant change in energy expenditure, and the quality and quantity of health care programs. The increased psychological stress to which individuals in the city are subjected and changes in exercise patterns are environmental factors that might be operative in the etiology of diabetes mellitus. Cohen et al., Campbell, and Schaefer believed that the composition of diet influences the expression of diabetes in humans undergoing culture change.[23-25] Settled Yemenite immigrants (born and/or living in Israel for more than 25 years) had a higher incidence of diabetes than the recent immigrant of less than 10 years. In Yemen carbohydrate consumption consisted mainly of starches, but in Israel sucrose accounted for 20 percent of the carbohydrate intake.[26] Increased intake of sugar appeared to be the most salient feature of the diets of urban Natal Indians and Zulus in South Africa as compared with their rural counterparts.[27] Campbell concluded that dietary factors have played a major role in the high rate of diabetes in these two groups.

Recent reports of the incidence of diabetes mellitus among the Eskimos reveal three times as many cases among the natives as in the prior 10-year period.[28] More new cases were discovered in one group of Eskimos living in the Canadian western Arctic than occurred in Eskimo groups in all Canada in the recent past. The change in customary diet to the Western high-sugar diet has occurred within the past 20 years. Following G. D. Campbell's rule that the marked increase in diabetes morbidity in various populations follows by about 20 years the acceptance of a westernized diet, Schaefer predicted that an increase in the incidence of diabetes mellitus in central and eastern Canadian Eskimos will follow that of the western Eskimos.* The western Arctic Eskimo diet had changed from one that consisted primarily of fish, seaweed, and clams to one that included a high intake of sugar with frequent daily intakes of soda pop and candy.

In the present state of medical knowledge the nature-nurture debate, i.e., the debate over the degree to which biology or heredity and culture interact or determine the etiology and symptomatology of diabetes, is an important yet controversial issue. According to MacDonald, the investigations which have been conducted suggest the expression of diabetes is influenced more by environmental factors than by ethnic or cultural considerations.[30] Comparability in survey methods, standardized diagnostic criteria, and improved accuracy in laboratory methods could give valuable clues to the significance of the interaction between hereditary and environmental factors.

NURSING'S CONTRIBUTION TO THE STUDY OF DIABETIC HEALTH-SEEKING BEHAVIORS

Cross-cultural studies and intensive field research of within-group variations in the incidence and expression of diabetes would be important steps toward answering questions pertaining to the prevention and treatment of diabetes and the prevention of complications. At present there are no ethnographic or descriptive studies relating subcultural group beliefs and practices about health to

---

* The low diabetic rate for Eskimos can be partly explained by the relatively young age distribution. In Greenland only one definite case was found among 4249 surveyed.[29]

the incidence of diabetes. Nurses, by virtue of their contacts with patients in hospitals, homes, and community health facilities, are in an enviable position to observe and document the social and cultural correlates of health-seeking behaviors of people in general and the diabetic in particular.

In the American urban setting, ethnic enclaves, in particular, provide study populations that would facilitate the comparative study of within-group and between-group differences and similarities in cultural belief systems and in folk or lay person health and caring (preventive) and curing practices as these relate to diabetes. A focus on identification of cultural variables would facilitate the contributions of nurses to the medical anthropology or ethnomedical variables associated with the disease category diabetes mellitus.

CULTURAL DIMENSIONS OF THE NURSING CARE OF THE DIABETIC PATIENT

An effective therapeutic nursing plan for a diabetic patient requires knowledge and understanding of subcultural or ethnic beliefs and values as they interact with other features of the social structure. This section will discuss some concepts and analytic approaches that may be useful for nurses in the assessment of a cultural or ethnic group's health care needs.

Cultural phenomena are those objects or events which are patterned and arranged into a system whose different parts are interrelated to form values, beliefs, and symbolic systems. Some categories of culture are technology, beliefs, values, and symbols associated with religion, medicine, nursing, politics, and so on. *Culture* is variously defined as the ways of life or designs for living common at any one time to all humanity, the ways of living peculiar to groups or societies between which there is a greater or lesser degree of interaction, the patterns of behavior peculiar to a group, and the special ways of behaving characteristic of the segments of a large and complexly organized society. The notion of diversity is implicit in the notion of culture. Culture is conceptualized as a historically derived system of "explicit and implicit designs for living which tend to be shared by all or specifically designated members of a group."[31] Culture is learned behavior that is transmitted from generation to generation.

Culture may be studied according to large national or regional units or at a smaller unit of analysis, e.g., tribe, village, or urban ethnic enclave. Subcultures, or subdivisions of a national culture, are composed of factorable social sets such as class, status, ethnic background, region, and religion. For example, analysis at the regional level requires specification of subcultural and social class groups. A study of food habits in the South revealed, for example, differences at the cultural and social level of five major groups: white owners, white sharecroppers, black owners, black sharecroppers, and wage laborers.[32]

Ethnic groups make for diversity within a national culture. An ethnic group is a social group within a larger cultural or social system that claims or is accorded a special status because of a complex of traits it exhibits or is believed to have. These traits are diverse and variable and include language, religion, skin pigment, and national or geographic origins of members or their forebears.[33]

It is important to note for this discussion that assessment of the cultural determinants of health-seeking behaviors requires a careful delineation of both idiosyncratic and cultural variables. The nurse must question whether the belief or behavior expressed is of cultural origin, i.e., patterned and generalizable to the group or idiosyncratic and applicable only to an individual. It is notable, too, that intragroup variations must be taken into account when one assesses the functional or dysfunctional aspects of cultural beliefs and value systems in health-seeking behavior. For example, a person's age, sex, place in the social structure (social class), and education tend to stimulate a wide range of variations within a cultural group.

In America, analysis of the cultural systems of urban ethnic groups, in particular, requires a specification of generation (i.e., foreign-born, first-generation, or native); rural or urban origin; and literary and language skills. For example, findings of a study of cultural change in health beliefs and practices of three generations of Italian-American women residents of an urban enclave revealed convergence and divergence in beliefs and customs not only between generations but also within generations. The differences in customs and beliefs were a function of education, age at marriage, experiential variables, and the state of the medical art and science at the time the women attained maturity.[34]

Lay Referral Systems

The articulation of diabetic people with health care delivery systems—formal or informal, professional or nonprofessional—requires assessment by the nurse. The designation *lay, folk,* or *popular medicine* is used to differentiate lay people's beliefs and practices from those of medical specialists or professionals. The original meaning of *folk medicine* was intended to convey the notion that "folk" knowledge was that common to or possessed by most people as distinguished from specialized knowledge possessed by the educated few, i.e., professionals.[34,35]

The constructs *illness referral systems* or *lay referral systems* provide an analytic unit for differentiation of professional and consumer roles within cultural health belief and action systems. Weaver, summarizing the definitions of a number of investigators and theorists, defined a medical system as being comprised of the "whole complex of a people's beliefs, attitudes, practices and roles associated with concepts of health and disease and with patterns of diagnoses and treatment."[36]

Conceptualizations about health maintenance and patterns of treatment have meaning only when the totality of social, structural, and group actions is taken into account. An illness referral system is conceptualized as a subsystem of the medical system, which includes all health actors and their potential and actual behaviors in illness situations. According to Weaver, an illness situation begins with an individual's perception of an altered state of health and proceeds to validation of the illness condition by a person or persons in the referral system, followed by therapeutic interventions or terminated in death.

Weaver's construct bears similarity to Friedson's conceptualization of the lay referral system as a "variable lay culture and a network of personal influence along which the patient travels on his way to the physician."[37,38] Two variants of the illness referral system are identified: an extended system and a truncated form.[39] The former is found most often among certain indigenous and lower socioeconomic cultural groups. The truncated version is one in which individuals participate directly with the professional health care giver. Weaver identifies four distinct phases within the illness referral model which are differentially used by traditional and acculturated Spanish Americans. The typical traditional Spanish American patient using the extended system would progress through the following phases: the "self-addressed" phase, or self-perception of change in health status; the kinship phase, in which consultants are members of the patient's own social group; the community phase, in which friends, neighbors, and other influential community members are sought for help and advice in making a diagnosis and prescribing therapy; and a folk specialist phase, which is reached when culturally recognized practitioners are consulted.[40]

Weaver's model of the referral system of the Spanish Americans of the southern Rocky Mountains is similar to that which was found by this author to be operating in an ethnic enclave in an Eastern city. The "home medical specialist" in the Spanish American community who treated minor ailments within the home or neighborhood had functions analogous to those of the "therapeutic women" and "lay medical specialists" in the Eastern ethnic community. The therapeutic women prescribed traditional or folk treatments for emotional or physical dysfunctions of elderly Italian immigrants (first generation). The lay medical specialists were American born, i.e., second generation. Acting in the role of mediators between the traditional culture and the modern health care system, the lay medical specialist had internalized a large amount of modern medical knowledge. Through their function as translators for those women who lacked language skills in English, this category of lay healers had gained skills and knowledge that enabled them to make differential diagnoses when consulted by kin or neighbors. They exhibited a wide repertoire of knowledge about the rationale of dietary, medical, and treatment prescriptions and were available for interpretation of a number of ailments, including those associated with diabetes.[41]

It is reasonable to assume that other cultural or subcultural groups have social networks and pathways to medical and health care similar to those just identified. It would appear that lay health care givers have a positive function within the community. Nurses working within the acute care setting and in the community might consider seeking out and including lay medical specialists in the home nursing care plan for diabetic people of traditional cultures.

How can the nurse identify the alternate medical or healing systems that function in urban and rural communities? There are several sources of information: personal interviews with patients and their visitors within the natural setting of the health care agency; physicians and nurses of ethnic origin, particularly those who minister to the needs of people from their own ethnic groups; and the content of local or ethnic newspapers. For example, Hostetler has noted that concerns about illness and the sick are subjects of major interest in every Amish community.[42] News items in the weekly newspaper *The Budget* reflect the attitudes and interests of the Amish people from a number of communities in the United States and Canada. The news media cover actions directed toward diagnosis and treatment of illness. A content analysis of *The Budget* revealed that the Amish are extremely health conscious.[43] Advertisements in ethnic newspapers may give clues about the group's use of folk healers or spiritualists who may be consulted for diagnosis, i.e., divination, of illness and treatment by traditional methods. The assessment of health-seeking behaviors outside the conventional medical model requires the specification of whether this is patterned or idiosyncratic behavior. In any event, the nurse must make some judgment about the consequences of using alternate medical systems for individual health care. In most cases, both systems, the modern or "scientific" and the folk or traditional, are used.

The articulation for comparative purposes of lay referral and modern medical systems has not received much attention. The reason for this may be the general disregard and condescending attitude toward folk or lay people's health beliefs and practices held by health professionals. Folk health practices and lay interventions are variously perceived by health professionals as "quaint," irrelevant, or scientifically unproved. Yet cultural and individual beliefs about the etiology of illness, to a greater or lesser degree, do determine what actions people will take for the amelioration of symptoms or the prevention of disease or illness. The identification of the medical lag or discrepancy between lay and professional knowledge must be undertaken and nursing care actions directed toward closing the gap. This may be brought about by the application and modification by nursing of the ethnoscientific approach that has been developed within the field of cultural anthropology. Some salient features of this approach will be presented briefly.

Ethnoscience and Ethnomedicine

Cultural anthropologists use ethnographies as the chief analytic instruments for making valid cross-cultural comparisons aimed at the development of theory. An *ethnography* or *monograph* is a descriptive account of a specific group's technology (including medical practices), customary behavior, social structure, belief and value systems, and their interrelationships. The goal of an ethnographer is "to grasp the native's point of view, his relation to life, . . . *his* vision of *his* world."[44] Ethnographies are used not only to describe distinctive features of a specific culture but also to identify similarities and differences between cultures. Cross-cultural comparisons facilitate the identification of distinctive cultural features or responses and features that hold for more than one culture or are universal. Identification of universal responses allows for generalizations that hold for all peoples; distinctive or salient cultural responses are unique to a group and must be taken into account when health care services are implemented.

The ethnographic approach is a naturalistic, comparative approach in which human behavior, beliefs, and values are explored "against or within the context of other behaviors and attitudes of the individuals making up the life of the community."[45] Ethnoscience, a relatively recent development in ethnographic methodology, is referred to as the "new ethnography." The essential difference from the "old ethnography," which focused on holistic cultural descriptions, is the emphasis on intensive study of specific cultural domains, i.e., botany, history, medicine.

Ethnoscience refers to the system of cognition typical of a given culture.[46] The suffix *science* is not used in the usual sense. It refers to classification or taxonomy. For example, *ethnomedicine* is that division of ethnoscience which deals with *folk* or lay people's classifications and/or definitions of health and illness phenomena. The intent is to discover the lay person's model for perceiving, relating, interpreting, and classifying data about health and illness. The techniques are directed toward identifying folk or lay person's categories without the imposition of a priori categories derived from the modern medical model.

The use of an ethnoscientific or ethnomedical approach provides a systematic method by which the discrepancy between professional and lay knowledge may be assessed and nursing interventions implemented to decrease the knowledge or cultural gap. Most studies using this approach have been carried out for domains other than health and medicine, e.g., folk classifications of kinship, color categories, etc. A number of ethnomedical studies have been carried out with indigenous or non-Western cultures. Although diabetes mellitus has not been subjected to intensive analysis, it would appear that there are several specific domains by which more knowledge and understanding of the folk or lay person's classificatory system may be obtained. These include ethnophysiology and ethnoanatomy, people's understanding of the anatomy and physiology of the pancreas, the functions of insulin, etc.; ethnomedicine, people's beliefs about the etiology, treatment, and prevention of diabetes; ethnogenetics, people's theories and beliefs about the hereditary transmission of disease traits in general and diabetes in particular.

It would seem reasonable to propose that an ethnomedical study of diabetes is an appropriate task for nursing. A compilation of descriptive accounts of patient responses to diabetes would provide nursing with ethnographies that would take into account the interrelationship of diabetes mellitus and the social and cultural dimensions. Although nurses have not yet addressed this task, it is notable that there is a source from which the profession can draw for a beginning study of diabetes from the lay person's perspective. Nursing care studies of diabetic patients published over a period of years in nursing journals give excellent descriptive accounts or ethnographies of the socialization of specific patients in the role of diabetic. These nursing care studies may provide the focal point for a compilation of a number of ethnographies of diabetic patients from different ethnic and social groups.

Another source for a beginning study of patients' or lay people's classifications and perceptions of diabetes mellitus, the ethnomedicine of diabetes, is the recorded testimony of a number of diabetics and their significant others compiled by the National Commission on Diabetes.[47] The author noted that the experiential accounts, definitions, and perceptions of patients with diabetes mellitus, expressed in their own words, showed both variance from and congruency with health professionals' definitions of the disease. An analysis of these first-person accounts would help health professionals identify the culturally relevant language lay people use in talking about diabetes. Nurses may then use this language to communicate information to patients. In addition, nurses can develop interview schedules for eliciting questions in the persons' own languages for the intensive study of the ethnomedicine of diabetes. In this way, the a priori categories of the professional are avoided. More knowledge about the diversity in conceptualization of the etiology and treatment of diabetes on the part of lay people would give clues or predictors of health-seeking behaviors. People's beliefs and values about staying well and getting well do determine the actions they take toward these goals.

Beliefs about Food

Much of the treatment of diabetes mellitus is dependent on the patient's *actions in relation to food*. Many cultural and social variables determine the patient's ability to learn and to modify patterns of eating.

Ideas associated with prescribed and proscribed foods are found in a number of religious and cultural groups. The ritualistic use of food by people of the Jewish and Moslem religions is well known. The social uses of food may conflict with medical prescriptions that place restrictions on amounts and times of eating. Classification systems may also direct the choices and combinations of food, with value placed on those believed to be most conducive to health. For example, elderly Italian immigrants in an Italian American enclave classified foods according to a wet-dry polarity. Maintenance of the body in a proper state required a balanced dietary regimen of wet foods (boiled greens, soups, etc.) and dry foods (pasta, bread, potatoes, etc.). Eating too many foods in the dry category was believed to be particularly harmful to hospitalized patients or to those who were ailing.[48] A hot-cold classification system plays a central role in the Puerto Rican culture.[49] To enhance compliance with dietary regimens, attention must be paid to the system of classification developed over time and transmitted to group members.

Other beliefs about food and health have been identified in groups of diabetics. A study of elderly black patients attending a diabetic clinic revealed that a weight-reduction program was unsuccessful. The elderly associated being thin with illness and believed they felt better when they were fat.[50]

Unlike the case of the Canadian Eskimos referred to earlier, food customs and preferences may show little change from generation to generation or during transition from a rural to an urban milieu. Food habits are among those first learned and therefore last to change. In addition, the cultural and social meanings of food restrictions require understanding. A study of cultural change in health concepts and customs of three generations in an ethnic enclave revealed that noncompliance of the elderly with prescribed medical regimens was more common in diet than in medicine or physical therapy. Among the elderly women in the community, the term *diet* had a connotation of extreme dietary limitation. In addition, adherence to a diabetic diet meant the curtailment of the valued social activities associated with hospitality, neighbor and kin visiting patterns, and reciprocal exchanges of food.[51]

Empirical observations have revealed another area of misunderstanding among lay people of the label *dietetic* on prepared foods. Unless the small print is read, *dietetic* is interpreted by many lay people to mean the food substance may be consumed in unlimited quantities.

Social class and educational variables influence a people's understanding of the therapeutic plan of care. Experience at the Duke Medical Center Diabetic Clinic indicated that exchange lists in the present form could be used only by literate patients with average or above average comprehension.[52] For those who had problems in comprehension, graphic or concrete representations of food and exchange lists were devised. In addition, familiar foods, or the culturally relevant foods, were used as illustrations.

Lay people may identify or define foods according to their morphologic or concrete qualities. Abstract notions or concepts such as the calorie may not be understood. For example, some patients may curtail or limit the use of foods with a distinctively sweet taste while continuing to consume foods with a tart taste, e.g., grapefruits or lemons, in unlimited quantities. The lay person's interpretation is that since grapefruits and lemons do not possess the concrete quality of sweetness, these may be used without restriction because of the association of diabetes with sugar and the need to curtail "sweet things."

Evaluation of patients' language and literary skills in their own or adopted cultures must be carried out with sensitivity, tact, and respect. Patients who have difficulty in understanding spoken or written communications are particularly handicapped if they do not disclose their deficits because of shame and the contemporary societal stigma attached to illiteracy.

Bilingual educational materials that are literal translations of the English without consideration of cultural variations in food habits and preferences will meet with something less than success. An exchange list for Mexican Americans should ideally include tortilla and beans; for blacks of rural origin, the "soul" foods.

Other predictors of noncompliance with prescribed diet are lack of basic knowledge of the principles of food exchange, low socioeconomic class, and ethnic background. Feldman reports the findings of the 1968 Diabetes Supplement of the National Health Survey.[53] One-half the diabetic population was making no effort to follow a diet. Of the group not following a diet, 50 percent were not given a diet and 50 percent received a dietary prescription but did not follow it. One significant finding was that some patients could not afford the foods prescribed. Fruits and vegetables comprise a large portion of the budget in terms of cost. Carbohydrate-rich foods are generally the least-expensive items found in the market.

Perpetuation of certain cultural stereotypes may result in the underserving of members of some groups. Dr. George Ham, for example, cautions against the perpetuation of the widely held belief that people of Asian origin don't have problems, that "they have made it [in America and] they take care of their own."[54] There is a lack of health education materials for Asian Americans, a group that underutilizes public services, including those for diabetics. Little research information is available about the 2 million Asian Americans, of whom 1 out of 20 is potentially diabetic.

Stigma and Pollution

A subtle area of inquiry about the relationship of cultural or lay belief systems and diabetes mellitus is that associated with the concepts of stigma and pollution. Lay definitions of the inheritance of diabetes are often expressed as the "passing on" of "bad blood." Families or individuals are then perceived as stigmatized. Although diabetes may present no visible signs, diabetics may view themselves as discreditable or discredited under certain circumstances. The writer recalls the concern of a newly diagnosed juvenile diabetic when he was being taught how to inject insulin both at home and at school. He feared that his classmates would think he was a "junkie" because he carried a syringe. An 8-year-old girl wore long-sleeved dresses even during the summer to hide the needle marks on her upper arm. She, too, feared that disclosure of diabetes would mark her transition from the category Goffman termed "discreditable" to that of "discredited."[55] Thus she would, according to Goffman, be placed in the situation of the individual who is disqualified from full social acceptance. A person's social identity may be "spoiled" or stigmatized by other outward signs. Some diabetics refuse to wear the Medic Alert Foundation International bracelet because it calls attention to their deviance from normal. Many diabetics fear the occurrence of insulin reactions in public places because uninformed onlookers apply the label "fit" to these seizures. This term is linked with epilepsy, one of the oldest diseases perceived as stigmatizing.

The writer has encountered some lay people who conceptualize diabetes as a "dirty" disease. Some cultural groups and individuals have elaborated themes associated with pollution and its polar opposite, pure or clean. Highly complex rituals and customs of avoidance to protect groups and individuals from potentially polluting substances or people have been described in a number of primitive and developed societies. The Hindu caste system of India has developed the most intricate rules for behaviors that conform to or infringe on the maintenance of purity. However, vestiges of pollution beliefs similar to those of the Indians may be discovered in all social and cultural groups. The notion that contact with human emissions is polluting or "dirty" is basic to all human groups. Thus nurses should not be surprised that some diabetics report that they, or a family member, feel a sense of disgust about testing urine and handling the equipment that has come in contact with this body excretion. Diabetics and family members may need assistance in devising ways to conceal and store equipment hygienically and to accomplish this basic task in a discreet manner.

Religion and Magic as Coping Mechanisms

An important area for consideration in planning nursing assessments and interventions is the function of religious and magical beliefs in human attempts to cope with the adversities of illness. Of particular interest would be the degree of fatalism expressed by cultural value orientations about humanity's ability to control diabetes. Fatalism connotes a resignation to fate, destiny, or God's will. An assumption underlying the concept is that calamitous events such as illness and accidents are preordained and the individual is rendered powerless in the face of these events. An essentially passive, dependent mode of coping is used. Fatalism is an attribute traditionally identified as the response to adversity of peasants and peoples in lower socioeconomic classes.[56,57] Yet fatalistic beliefs about diabetes are not limited to lay people. Diabetes, despite technological advances in insulin and dietary knowledge, is an illness about which there is widespread resignation, even among experts, because of inadequacy of present therapy.[58] One of the major conclusions of a study by the National Commission on Diabetes was that even with the best of medical care, the complications of diabetes are inevitable.[59] If fatalistic beliefs are held by health professionals, then one might ask what is the response of the diabetic person to the present state of the art and science of healing in diabetes. In the absence of research concerning the relationship of fatalism and diabetes, the concept will be examined in terms of its effect on compliance with medical and nursing plans of care.

When viewed from the negative point of view, individuals or groups exhibiting a high degree of fatalism would be less apt to take positive health actions. However, given the nature of the complications of diabetes, a fatalistic orientation might help a person accept the inevitable or come to terms with the illness. Resignation to God's will or fate or destiny may better be viewed as one stage in the illness process rather than as an all-pervading response to illness events. The testimony given by juvenile diabetics and their parents to the National Commission revealed resignation and a sense of despair.[60] These were not irrational reactions on the part of the diabetics, given the knowledge of the expected outcome of the juvenile form of the disease. Most respondents, however, expressed faith that science would find a cure.

If a sense of rational mastery over the disease is lacking, then one would expect that diabetics would look to sources other than science for a cure. Beliefs in miraculous cures may lead some diabetics to join healing cults or seek the services of faith healers. The use of these alternate healing systems as adjuncts to or complements of the professional health care system may and often does have a positive effect. However, hope for cure may be so strong that these people will affiliate with groups who claim to use magical means to transcend natural laws. A United Press International news item, dated August 27, 1973, appeared in newspapers across the nation and announced that a young diabetic boy's insulin had been discontinued after a faith-healing ceremony. His parents and members of the religious sect to which he belonged awaited his resurrection. Thus the use of magic as a means of coping is not limited to peoples of relatively underdeveloped technology.

Brosman proposes a novel nursing intervention that can be used for those subcultural groups who exhibit a high degree of fatalism in response to the threatening events associated with diabetes.[61] She stressed to Puerto Rican diabetic patients that it was God's will, or fate, that brought the nurse in contact with them. In this way, she was able to decrease alienation and social and cultural distance between health care giver and recipient. Compliance with the nursing plan of care was enhanced.

The question nurses must ask in the assessment of nursing needs is, What are the consequences of a religious belief or cultural value in motivating a patient and/or group to seek help for health care problems. A question that might be asked of people of all religious faiths is, To whom do you pray? Among Catholics of diverse ethnicity, "specialist" saints may be petitioned for their healing powers. Among some Catholic patients, St. Rocco and St. Lucy may be asked to mediate in bringing about a cure or amelioration of two complications associated with diabetes: delayed healing of wounds and blindness. St. Rocco is believed to have special powers for healing wounds, and St. Lucy is a patron of vision.

The nurse may reinforce the resources of faith and hope by encouraging prayer and by showing respect for those symbols associated with religion. Religious symbols include prayer cards, amulets such as religious medals and good luck charms, etc. Eliciting information about the specific hope objects and resources used by peoples of diverse cultures and incorporating these into the nursing care plan have not received much emphasis in nursing. It would appear that the incorporation of these strategies into the therapeutic plan of care would serve to decrease the social and cultural distance that may be built into the professional nurse–diabetic patient role relationship.

SOCIAL DIMENSIONS IN NURSING CARE OF THE DIABETIC PATIENT

Diabetes is a chronic illness of unknown etiology for which there is no known cure. For the insulin-dependent diabetic, therapy is based on a regimen that requires careful daily balance of food intake, exercise, and insulin replacement in order to prevent insulin overdose and ketoacidosis. The diabetic, or family member responsible for care if the individual is a child, is faced with the need for making critical decisions about the adjustment and regulation of therapy independent of a physician or health care professional. Since there is no agreement on the fundamental disturbance in diabetes, the relationship between the degree of control of the metabolic dysfunctions and later complications of the disease is uncertain. In addition, despite a history of compliance with prescribed medical regimens and adequate control of blood sugar levels by the juvenile diabetic, the onset of retinal, renal, and neurologic pathology is inevitable.[62] As a result of controversy and disagreement among experts as to the degree of control of the diabetic condition, uncertainty and ambiguity are prevalent. This uncertainty is transmitted to the lay people who are attempting to cope with the problems of adaptation to a new diagnosis or to the long-standing complications of diabetes at an individual or family level. Differing opinions about the modes of therapy by medical experts tend to diffuse to the lay person's level. The uncertainty is compounded by comparison of the relative merits of various modes of therapy (for example, the "strict" diet versus the "free" diet) within the circle of kin, relatives, and friends. Uncertainty or doubts arising from the current state of the art of medical control of diabetes will have an effect on adherence to prescribed therapy.

Nurse and Patient Relationships

Compliance and noncompliance in the management of the diabetic state require an understanding by the nurse of such contextual variables as intrafamilial and extrafamilial role relationships. Parsons' concept of the sick role, originally explicated for illnesses of acute onset and later modified to take into account chronic illnesses, provides a point of departure by means of which the role of the nurse may be articulated with respect to the role sets presented by the diabetic patient and/or family.[63,64] Parsons defined *health* as the state of optimum capacity of an individual for the effective performance of the roles and tasks for which he or she has been socialized. *Illness,* on the other hand, is seen as a disturbance of an individual's ability to carry out valued tasks or perform socially defined roles. According to Parsons, the social role of being sick is defined by three criteria: it is accepted by the self and others that the illness is not the person's fault; the individual is exempted from ordinary daily role obligations and expectations; and the individual seeks competent professional help. The individual is obliged not only to seek competent help, but also to comply with the prescribed medical therapy. Implicit in Parsons' conceptualization is the recognition of the asymmetry of roles that characterizes the patient–health professional relationship. This asymmetry is characterized by such traits as dependence, dominance, unequal knowledge base, and status differentials. The individual is expected to show "motivatedness" to get well, to work hard to relinquish the dependent role. Illness is seen as a particularly undesirable state because it poses a threat to such dominant American values as activism, achievement, mastery over nature, and progress. In addition, illness is viewed as an impairment of the sick person's integration into solidary relationships with others in several contexts: the family, work and school settings, etc.

In the original and subsequent articles by Parsons, the sick role is analyzed almost wholly from the perspective of a physician-patient reciprocal dyad. The dimensions of the nurse-patient role relationship have neither been sufficiently explored nor analyzed. An analysis of the nursing tasks and functions that are directed toward helping the diabetic and significant others adapt to the illness state would reveal some differences between the role expectations of the physician and those of the professional nurse. The major difference arises out of the fact that the goals of nursing are primarily to reduce the role asymmetry, characterized by dependence, and to reduce the knowledge of information gap between patient and health professional.

Interventions directed toward meeting the health care needs of the diabetic are those which ideally will close the gap between professional and lay knowledge. Thus the asymmetric relationship that Parsons posits as an attribute of the patient-physician dyad would not hold for the patient-nurse dyad. Nursing interventions would be those directed toward assumption by the patient of increasing control and responsibility in the tasks associated with personal hygiene, care of teeth and extremities, selection of a diet to meet nutritional needs, and the administration of insulin. Diabetics require knowledge so that they can make *independent* daily decisions about the modification of dietary intake and the regulation of insulin dosage according to urine tests or situational variables, e.g., nausea or vomiting. The major task of nursing is to transmit to diabetic patients and significant others as much professional knowledge as needed to ensure independence in accomplishing the tasks associated with maintaining health and well-being.

The effective professional management of the diabetic sick role has as the end product the weaning of patients from dependence on physicians or nurses in order to expedite reentry into the usual social and career roles. Diabetics and family members need help in assuming the functions usually associated with clinical specialists in order to cope with events associated with hypoglycemic or hyperglycemic reactions. Teachers and coworkers in particular need explanations of the pathology underlying hypoglycemic symptoms and explanations about the underlying mechanisms of the sometimes erratic or bizarre behavior caused by insulin overdose. Knowledge of the symptoms of insulin reaction by lay people in general would prevent interpretation of insulin shocks as "fits," a pejorative term used by some lay people.

In general, the knowledge base of the diabetic about daily management of the illness should approximate that of the professional. The identified task of nursing to decrease the discrepancy between professional and lay information about the diabetic condition requires that nurses have an adequate knowledge base. The degree to which this ideal has been achieved is open to question.

Krall stated that every diabetic must have the knowledge and skill of the paramedic.[65] Benoliel observed that parents of the juvenile diabetic, and the mother, in particular, must assume the role of clinician around the clock to ensure adequate monitoring of the diabetic condition.[66]

The state of the art and science of the nursing care dimensions of diabetes mellitus is a cause for concern. The paucity of research concerning the social and cultural correlates of diabetes mellitus has been mentioned. At a more basic level, there is some evidence that nursing students upon graduation have not acquired the basic skills and knowledge required for the task. Feustel investigated nursing students' knowledge of diabetes mellitus to determine whether students ($N = 144$) about to graduate from baccalaureate programs knew enough about diabetes mellitus to be able to teach patients and their families.[67] The findings indicated that the graduating students were not prepared to do diabetic teaching. Although it is hazardous to generalize from one study in one region of the country, the implications are clear. Etzwiler evaluated the knowledge of diabetes among nurses and dietitions. From his findings he concluded that patients' lack of knowledge about diabetes could result from the inadequate knowledge of those teaching them.[68,69]

Professional Roles and Relationships

Parsons' sick role construct has some value in explaining the structure of role relationships. How a person defines his or her role vis-à-vis others does have consequences for that person and others in the management of an acute illness. However, a different analytic model is required for insight into an understanding of the chronic illness diabetes. Nurses must look to their profession for assistance in the development of such a model.

The self-care model developed by Orem and explicated by Backscheider and Allison would appear to include those elements which would enhance symmetry in the nurse-patient (and/or family) role relationship.[70-72] Self-care, as conceptualized by Orem, is comprised of those health care actions an individual would perform for herself or himself on a continuing basis. Two broad categories of care action requirements have been identified: universal and health-deviation self-care. *Universal* self-care activities include those related to health and personal hygiene, such as rest, exercise, elimination, eating, and sleeping. *Health-deviation* self-care activities are those actions required because of illness, disease, or injury. The basic assumption underlying the self-care model is that patients outside of health care institutions are responsible for managing their own health care on a continuing basis. Since health care personnel are expected to assist only when patients have inadequate knowledge or limited skills, the patient's potential for assuming independence is enhanced. Nursing is viewed as the health service most responsible for assisting patients and/or family members in overcoming self-care limitations and deficits. This model for nursing care is useful in reduction of the role asymmetry within the nursing process and in distinguishing nursing's unique function and contribution from those of other health professionals.

Intrafamily Role Relationships

How the illness of one member of a family affects other members and the relationships among them is a question that has been explored by various disciplines. Research of the social-structural correlates of diabetes mellitus is limited. Hill's formulation of the impact of illness on family functioning is particularly relevant to an understanding of the adjustment and adaptation that must take place within family structures when one member is diagnosed as diabetic. In the periods of crisis caused by the diagnosis, the family's structure is often modified and the ability of family members to perform their usual roles may be reduced or altered.[73] The family finds itself in a state of disequilibrium and goes through a "roller coaster" pattern until a new equilibrium is achieved. This new equilibrium results from the readjustment of the power and role relationships within the system and will be characterized by either a higher or lower level of family functioning than existed prior to the onset of the illness crisis.[74,75] A family crisis revolving around the newly diagnosed diabetic child, for example, may disrupt family balance severely before a new equilibrium is established. Disruption in meal patterns, changes in the spacing of meals, supervision of eating, on-time administration of medicines, and the need to alter basic life-styles are some of the variables that may introduce structural or family stress. Parental response may take the form of blame and recrimination of one member of the partnership. This may be the case particularly if there is a history of diabetes in one or the other family line. Coupled with the use of these projective mechanisms, feelings of guilt may be expressed.

Crain et al. tested the hypothesis that there is a greater degree of marital integration, less marital conflict, and greater agreement on how to react to the child among parents of the nondiabetic child as compared with parents of the diabetic child.[76] It was found that the parents of diabetic children had a significantly lower goal consensus score than the parents of nondiabetic children, and that the amount of role tension was significantly greater among parents of diabetic children. Mothers of diabetic children reported more marital conflict as compared with mothers whose children were not diabetic. While arguments between parents on how to react to the child's actions was greater among parents of nondiabetic children, the differences between the two groups for this last variable were not statistically significant.

A variable identified by Crain et al. as operative in the perpetuation of crisis states within families with a diabetic child was the nature of diabetes itself. It is controllable but not curable. Control is dependent on the modification of eating habits, restriction of certain foods that have a high value in the American youth culture, and adherence to regular medication and exercise regimens that are especially difficult for children. The illness is chronic and long-lasting; the diabetic condition must be taken into account not only on a daily basis but for allocations of small time units within a 24-h period. Family decisions about vacations, or even a picnic to a distant park, require preplanning and scheduling that will take into account the always unrelenting schedule for meals and insulin administration.

Benoliel used total family interviewing as a research strategy in the study of the social meaning of diabetes within a family constellation.[77] In this way, both siblings of diabetics and parents contributed to the investigation, which focused on the meaning of being diabetic and the management of social visibility of diabetes at different time points in the transition from preadolescence to adulthood, transfer of responsibility for care from physician to family member(s), and the effects of diabetes and its treatment on the enactment of social roles by the diabetic person.

Benoliel identified four styles by which parents functioned as agents for their child's diabetic treatment: the protective, the adaptive, the manipulative, and the abdicative. These styles were differentiated on two bases, namely, the emphasis given to the supervision of a child's activity and the delegation of responsibility for the specific tasks associated with treatment.

The *protective* style of diabetes care management perpetuated the assumed major responsibility of the parent for performing diabetic procedures and maintaining control over the child's time and activity away from home. The *adaptive* style placed emphasis on assumption by the child of more responsibility in the performance of diabetic procedures and fostered age-graded control over time and activities. The *manipulative* style was characterized by the manner used in the performance of procedures, and usually one or more tasks or requirements of the diabetic role become a source of tension and strain between the parent(s) and child. The pattern of supervision was characterized by inconsistency. The parent whose style was *abdicative* was involved only peripherally in management of the diabetic regimen and supervision of the child's activities.

Within-family variations of parental styles were found. These differences were more or less related to tension in family relationships. However, differences in one parent's coping style could act to counterbalance the other spouse's tendencies toward protective or manipulative mechanisms. For example, the adaptive style assumed by one parent could serve to counterbalance or minimize the overprotective or manipulative style of the partner. The development of a diabetic subculture was identified with some family constellations. This subculture was characterized by "recurring crisis events," in which the diabetes persisted as a source of tension and strain. Conditions of living were such that three of the young people studied were using a type of diabetic role performance that was keeping them in a consistent state of poor diabetic control. On the basis of these findings, Benoliel concluded that the effects of the daily social interaction on diabetic role identity suggest that basic family themes and parental styles create a learning field that can facilitate or inhibit a young diabetic's choice of compliance or noncompliance with medically prescribed care practices. She postulated that the young diabetic's sense of self-esteem is directly related to the emotional climate that exists within his or her primary groups. Moral judgments about worth are conveyed mainly through the expressive processes used by parents and, to a lesser degree, siblings.

Benoliel used the method of participant observation as an adjunct to total family interviewing. These techniques can be modified and used as primary assessment tools by nurses in the practice setting. The typology of parental styles provides an additional analytic measure by which nurses can predict or assess with greater precision the consequences of different family styles in the management of diabetes. Use of typologies in conjunction with naturalistic observational techniques would also contribute to a compilation of nursing ethnographies of people's responses to diabetes mellitus.

Occupational Roles*

If *health* is sociologically defined as a state of optimum capacity for effective performance of valued tasks and roles, then a person's work role and employment and career opportunities require assessment.[78] Knowledge of the problems diabetics face in obtaining employment will enable nurses to structure patients' expectations about available employment and career roles. In this section, the findings of some studies will be reviewed in order to place in perspective current employment practices and areas· that may be problematic for diabetics in assuming or resuming work and career roles.

Diabetics have long been subjected to unwarranted discrimination when seeking employment. The federal government did not employ known diabetics in any capacity prior to 1941. Interpretation of the findings of a number of studies about employment practices is open to question because of the relatively low proportion of replies to survey questionnaires. Brandaleone and Friedman studied the work experiences of over 3500 employees of an urban transit company during a 5-year period.[79] Forty were known diabetics. The absence rate of diabetics and nondiabetics was the same, except for two diabetics who had prolonged absences. The findings revealed the effect a small number of diabetics can have on the overall employment record. The employment experience for diabetics was less favorable than for nondiabetics because of two diabetic employees who had long periods of disability. When these two were omitted from the sample, the performance of diabetic workers was equal to that of nondiabetics.

The Committee on Employment of the American Diabetes Association mailed questionnaires to 434 business and industrial concerns in the United States.[80] Of the 127 companies that responded, 88 (69 percent) employed known diabetics, and 31 (25 percent) did not. Eight companies did not answer the question about employment practices. Seventy-two companies (56 percent) stated that while they did not employ known diabetics, they did continue to keep in their employ workers who developed diabetes after they were hired. Forty-three percent of the responding companies did not answer the question designed to elicit responses about company practices for continuing employment of a worker diagnosed as diabetic after being hired.

Tetrich and Colwell surveyed 500 members of the Central States Society of Industrialized Physicians.[81] Replies were received from 169 physicians (33.4 percent). Seventy-five responded affirmatively to the question, Do you recommend for employment a known diabetic certified by his private physician as being in good control? Fifteen percent of the physicians who responded stated that a positive urine test for glucose automatically disqualified an applicant for employment.

In summarizing the findings of a number of studies, Rodman concluded that employers' objections to the hiring of diabetics may be influenced by the

* The author acknowledges the assistance of Harvey Rodman, M.D., in the preparation of this section.

following concerns: excess absenteeism may result in poor job performance; excess injuries or disabilities due to accidents would result from the diabetic state; on-the-job insulin reactions would cause job disruption or injury; and diabetic employees may have adverse effects on group medical insurance rates.[82]

An early study of absenteeism at a company employing diabetics revealed that absenteeism among diabetics was less than that of other employees.[83] The diabetics were absent once for every 102 working days; the controls showed one absence for every 53 working days. Sickness and absenteeism of 90 diabetic employees in a large refinery and chemical plant were not significantly high when compared with nondiabetic employees.[84] The 1957 report of the American Diabetes Association Committee on Employment concerning the companies employing diabetics revealed that 94 percent reported their experience with diabetic employees to be satisfactory with respect to the variables of reliability and absenteeism. A 1971 survey of industrial physicians revealed that 81.9 percent of diabetic employees were considered no worse than those who did not have diabetes with respect to reliability or absenteeism; 5.6 percent were considered better than those who did not have diabetes for these two variables.[85]

Pell and D'Alonzo followed 622 diabetics and 626 controls matched by sex, location, and occupation who worked for the du Pont Company.[86] As a group, the diabetics had more bouts of illness, almost twice as many days of disability, and, when ill, were disabled over longer periods of time. However, 72 percent of the diabetics had either no absences or one absence during the period of a year, and only 6 percent had more than three illness events in the 1-year period. Based on these findings, it was concluded that the problems of excess sickness absenteeism in diabetics and nondiabetics arise from a minority of workers. Absenteeism for the care and management of diabetes occurred in only 7 percent of the diabetics. It was notable that absenteeism for the care and management of diabetes was strikingly high among younger production workers with severe cases. The median days of disability were not different among production workers taking insulin and those on diets alone or on diets and oral agents. Among salaried workers, the median days of disability did not vary significantly between diabetics and controls.

Nasr et al. studied 213 known diabetics and a control population at a Ford Motor Company plant.[87] Sickness absence among white diabetic employees was twice that of the control population—an average of 8.78 days for white diabetics and 3.88 for white nondiabetics. Among black diabetic employees sickness absence was three times greater than the control group—an average of 11.5 days for black diabetics and 3.46 for black nondiabetics. Although absences were more frequent and longer for diabetics than for nondiabetics, 73.5 percent of diabetics had fewer than five absences during the year of study.

A more recent study of work absenteeism in workers employed in a manufacturing and chemical plant revealed that 1.4 percent of the total work force was diabetic.[88] Ninety percent of the diabetic study group became diabetic after they were hired. Absentee rates of the diabetic group (6.3 days annually) were compared with absentee rates of the nondiabetic group and controlled for age. In every age group the absentee rate of diabetics was less than that of nondiabetics. This study is biased, however, in that only one laborer is included in the sample. The majority in the sample were drawn from officials and managers, professionals, technicians, and craft workers.

The data on absenteeism remain inconclusive and controversial. Controls for social class, race, type of job (i.e., salaried versus production workers), and age may yield information that will lead to more valid conclusions. However, the findings show that the risk of hiring a diabetic job applicant needs to be determined on an individual basis. The probability of poor attendance is no higher for the majority of diabetics than it is for nondiabetics.

Injuries   Pell and D'Alonzo compared the frequency of dispensary visits for a variety of injuries and minor complaints (colds, headaches, etc.) between diabetics and controls.[89] The findings show no significant differences between the two groups. Records of minor injuries were available for 384 diabetics and 382 controls. For a 1-year period, the diabetic group experienced 82 injuries, or 21.4 per 100 persons; the control group had 78 injuries, a rate of 20.4 per 100. Many minor injuries were not reported by employees. However, one would expect that the diabetic employee would be more likely to report an injury than would a nondiabetic. If this is true, then the rate of minor injuries may actually be lower for diabetics. The Pell and D'Alonzo study is the only study that examined the comparative incidence of injuries, and it clearly demonstrated that diabetics were no more susceptible to injury than nondiabetics.[90]

Insulin Reactions   Little or no data are available that deal with the question of on-the-job insulin reactions. Pell and D'Alonzo's survey of 408 diabetics employed by a major American company reported 25 absences related to the care and management of diabetes. Four absences were for "insulin shock."[91] Copplestone's survey of 88 diabetics attending a clinic over a 5-year period revealed that 36 of the employed group were being treated with insulin and 28 of these experienced reactions outside the hospital. Reactions were severe and involved unconsciousness in eight cases.[92] The Copplestone series did not reveal an excess of industrial accidents among diabetics.

Mills et al. studied the socioeconomic problems of 60 insulin-dependent individuals. Mild hypoglycemia was accepted as a nuisance, but severe hypoglycemia was a terrifying experience for the individuals, family members, and friends.[93] Diabetics reported concern with the appearance of posthypoglycemic irritability, violence, simulation of drunkenness, and accidents while in the hypoglycemic state. The subjects experienced fears related to the disruption of family life, lessening of job opportunities, cancellation of driving licenses, and pervasive feelings of anxiety if hypoglycemia was not controlled. No data were given concerning the social problems encountered on the job because of hypoglycemic reactions. Fifty percent of the subjects had suffered a severe hypoglycemic episode in the 12 months preceding the study; only seven of them had never undergone a disabling insulin reaction. Thirteen of these insulin-dependent individuals cited hypoglycemia as their worst problem, while 20 of the 60 subjects stated that injections were the worst problem.

Industrial and plant physicians differ in their opinions of whether insulin-dependent diabetics should be restricted from situations in which hypoglycemic episodes might endanger them or their coworkers. Rodman's report of the literature makes the case that many of the restrictions placed on diabetic employment because of the possibility of insulin reactions are without basis in fact. The diabetic is not in the same category as the epileptic, in whom complete unconsciousness is likely to occur rapidly.

> Most diabetics understand or are capable of learning the mechanics of their condition. . . . They know the time of day in which insulin reactions are likely to occur. They know how to treat reactions and carry food with them. Most important of all, they usually have sufficient warning to take remedial measures before their consciousness becomes clouded. This applies to most patients who have even severe reactions.[94]

Some medical authorities advise diabetics concerning the need for reorganization of their daily activities, anticipation of situations likely to produce hypoglycemia, and acceptance of some degree of glycosuria and raised blood sugar as an aid in prevention of insulin reaction and its disruption of activities.

Chronic Complications and Work Role   Chronic complications, particularly those of the eye and foot, might force a change of employment or incapacitate the patient from performing a usual work role. Many diabetics fear failing vision.[95] Kantrow's study of the first 100 diabetics referred for vocational and counseling services revealed that 22 had diabetic complications; 8 had more than one complication. Of this group of 22, 13 had problems with vision, 9 with peripheral vascular disease, 7 with peripheral neuropathy, 5 with heart disease, and 2 with kidney disease.[96] Peripheral neuropathy and consequent sensory impairment make it difficult to learn braille and the use of the cane. It has been estimated that approximately 6 percent of all diabetics are unable to read newsprint with glasses, even when there is an attempt at maximal correction.[97]

One may conclude that too much emphasis has been placed on the potential problems of insulin reactions and too little on chronic complications of diabetes as the chief limiting aspects of employment.

Insurance   Most states have passed second injury laws that provide protection for the employer and restrict the penalties incurred should a physically handicapped employee suffer a subsequent industrial injury. The basic features of most of the second injury laws are (1) injured employees are compensated for all the disability they suffer as a result of an industrial injury; (2) employers are encouraged to employ the physically handicapped; (3) if a physically handi-capped employee should incur a subsequent industrial injury, the employer would not be penalized by the imposition of a greater liability than would be the case if the employee did not have a preexisting physical impairment; and (4) the employer is entitled to limited liability and the loss is cushioned by a second injury fund and not charged solely to the employer's insurance.

There is an age differential in attitudes toward employment of diabetic workers. Reports of experiences by juvenile diabetics reveal no consistent policy regarding employment. Large and small concerns, private companies and civil service systems alike, have employed juvenile diabetics or refused them employment.[98] Some department stores employ diabetics, others will not. Similar conditions exist among insurance companies and accounting, banking, and engineering firms. Eighteen of the forty-one diabetics reported in the Kantrow survey as rejected for employment subsequently concealed their diabetes when applying for work. Sixteen of the twenty-six who had never been re-jected for employment stated that they concealed their diabetes. Various sub-terfuges were used to obtain employment, e.g., false answers to questions and substitute urine specimens. The practice of concealment was found to be much less prevalent among professional workers when compared with office and unskilled workers. As a result of the survey, the New York Diabetic Associa-tion has established vocational and counseling services to help adolescents and young adults in areas of social, economic, and emotional adjustment.[99]

The adult-onset diabetic who has had the opportunity to succeed on the job has experienced little change in his or her employment status after diagnosis of diabetes. The American Diabetes Association Committee on Employment sur-vey reported that 56 percent of the companies said they would not hire a diabetic but would continue to keep a person who developed diabetes while employed.[100] Young people with diabetes, however, must demonstrate their value as workers.

Based on the review of relevant literature on employment practices and employee work experiences, discrimination against diabetic people solely on the basis of diagnosis is unwarranted. Emphasis should be placed on individual attitude, aptitude, educational experience, degree of control of diabetes, and the demands of the job or career. The majority of diabetics have adapted to their condition and the demands of daily living.[101]

SUMMARY

This writer has proposed that the major task of nursing is to transmit to diabetic patients and significant others as much professional knowledge as needed to ensure independence in maintaining health and well being.

This chapter identifies concepts, approaches, and theories that are relevant to an analysis of the social and cultural components underlying the care of people with diabetes mellitus. These include the physical anthropology of dia-betes mellitus, the nature of professional and lay social relationships considered within the context of the sick role and self-care concepts, the ethnomedical aspects of cultural belief and value systems, the lay referral system, and family and work roles.

REFERENCES

1 Quint, J. C. Some thoughts on a theory of chronicity, *Proceedings: First Nursing Theory Conference, University of Kansas Medical Center*, 1969, pp. 58–67.
2 Lieban, R. W. The field of medical anthropology, in D. Landy (ed.), *Culture, Disease and Healing* (New York: Macmillan, 1977).
3 Parsons, T. Definitions of health and illness in the light of American values and social structure, in E. G. Jaco (ed.), *Patients, Physicians and Illness* (New York: Free Press, 1967), pp. 165–187.
4 Parsons, T. The sick role and the role of the physician reconsidered, *Milbank Mem. Fund Q.*, **53**:257–277, Summer 1975.
5 Maugh, T. H. Diabetes: model systems indicate virus a cause, *Science*, **188**:436–438, 1976.
6 Reid, J. M., et al. Nutrient intake of Pima Indian women: relationship to diabetes mellitus and gallbladder disease, *A. J. Clin. Nutr.*, **24**:1281–1289, 1971.
7 Davidson, J. K. Diabetes in socioeconomically deprived neighborhoods, in *Diabetes Mellitus: Diagnosis and Treatment* (New York: American Diabetes Association, 1971), pp. 207–210.
8 Neel, J. V. Diabetes mellitus: a thrifty genotype rendered detrimental by progress? *A. J. Hum. Genet.*, **14**:353–362, 1962.
9 Schaefer, O. When the Eskimo comes to town, *Nutrition Today*, **6**:8–16, 1971.
10 U.S. Department of Health, Education and Welfare. *Report of the National Commission on Diabetes*, vol. 3, NIH-76-1019, 1975.
11 Sloan, N. R. Ethnic distribution of diabetes mellitus in Hawaii, *J.A.M.A.*, **183**:123, 1963.
12 Genuth, S. M., et al. Hyperinsulinism in obese diabetic Pima Indians, *Metabolism*, **16**:1010, 1967.
13 Remoin, D. L. Ethnic variability in glucose tolerance and insulin secretion, *Arch. Intern. Med.*, **124**:695–700, 1969.
14 Smith, R. L. Cardiovascular-renal deaths among Navajos. *Public Health Reports*, **72**:33–38, 1951.
15 Remoin. Loc. cit.
16 Johnson, J. E., and McNutt, C. W. Diabetes mellitus in an American Indian population isolate, *Tex. Rep. Biol. Med.*, **22**:110, 1964.
17 Remoin. Loc. cit.
18 Reid et al. Loc. cit.
19 *Report of National Commission on Diabetes*, vol. 3, p. 19.
20 Judkins, R., and Lieberman, L. Specialist reports—biomedicine and nutrition, *Med. Anthropol. Newsletter*, **6**:14–17, 1974.
21 Neel. Loc. cit.
22 Prosnitz, L. R., and Mandell, G. L. Diabetes mellitus among Navajo and Hopi Indians: the lack of vascular complications, *A. J. Med. Sci.*, **253**:700, 1967.
23 Cohen, A. M., Bauly, S., and Pozanski, R. Change of diet of Yemenite Jews in relation to diabetes and ischaemic heart disease, *Lancet*, **2**:1399, 1961.
24 Campbell, G. D. Diabetes in Asians and Africans in and around Durban, *S. Afr. Med. J.*, **37**:1195, 1963.

25 Schaefer. Loc. cit.
26 Cohen, A. M. Prevalence of diabetes among different ethnic Jewish groups in Israel, *Metabolism,* **10**:50, 1961.
27 Campbell. Loc. cit.
28 Schaefer. Loc. cit.
29 MacDonald, G. W. The epidemiology of disease, in M. Ellenberg and H. Rifkin (eds.), *Diabetes Mellitus: Theory and Practice* (New York: McGraw-Hill, 1970).
30 Ibid.
31 Kluckhohn, C., and Kelly, W. The concept of culture, in R. Linton (ed.), *The Science of Man in the World Crisis* (New York: Columbia Univ. Press, 1945), pp. 78–106.
32 Cassel, J. Social and cultural implications of food and food habits, *Am. J. Public Health,* **47**:732–740, 1957.
33 Gould, J., and Kalb, W. L. (eds.). *A Dictionary of Social Sciences* (New York: UNESCO, Free Press, 1969).
34 Redfield, R. *Peasant Society and Culture* (Chicago: Univ. of Chicago Press, 1956; Phoenix Books, 1965).
35 Redfield, R., and Freidson, E. *Patients' Views of Medical Practice* (New York: Russell Sage, 1961).
36 Weaver, T. The use of hypothetical situations in a study of Spanish-American illness referral system, *Hum. Organ.,* **29**:140–154, 1970.
37 Freidson, E. Client control and medical practice, *Am. J. Sociol.,* **65**:374–382, 1960.
38 Freidson. 1961. Loc. cit.
39 Freidson, E. Client control and medical practice.
40 Weaver. Loc. cit.
41 Ragucci, A. T. Generational continuity and change in concepts of health, curing practices and ritual expressions of the women of an Italian-American enclave, unpublished Ph.D. dissertation, Boston University, 1971.
42 Hostetler, J. A. Folk medicine and sympathy healing among the Amish, in W. D. Hand (ed.), *American Folk Medicine: A Symposium* (Univ. of California Press, 1976).
43 Hostetler, J. A. Folk and scientific medicine in Amish society, *Hum. Organ.,* **271,** Winter 1963–1964.
44 Malinowski, B. *Argonauts of the Southern Pacific* (New York: Dutton, 1954; originally published in 1922).
45 Arensberg, C., and Kimball, S. T. *Culture and Community* (New York: Harcourt, Brace & World, 1965).
46 Sturtevant, W. C. Studies in ethnoscience, *Am. Anthropol.* **66**:99–131, 1964.
47 *Report of the National Commission on Diabetes,* vols. 1–5.
48 Ragucci. Loc. cit.
49 Harwood, A. The hot-cold theory of disease, *J.A.M.A.,* **216**:1153–1158, 1971.
50 Anderson, R. S., Gunter, L. M., and Kennedy, E. J. Evaluation of clinical, cultural and psychosomatic influences in the teaching and management of diabetic patients: a study of medically indigent Negro patients, *Am. J. Med. Sci.,* **245**:682–690, 1963.
51 Ragucci. Loc. cit.
52 Feldman, J. M. Diet principles and applications, in M. Ellenberg and H. Rifkin (eds.), *Diabetes Mellitus: Theory and Practice* (New York: McGraw-Hill, 1970).
53 Ibid.
54 *Report of the National Commission on Diabetes,* vol. 2, p. 215.

55 Goffman, E. *Stigma* (Englewood Cliffs, N. J.: Prentice-Hall, 1963).
56 Kluckhohn, F., and Strodtbeck, F. *Variations in Value Orientations* (Evanston, Ill.: Row, Peterson, 1961).
57 Milio, N. Values, social class and community health, *Nurs. Res.,* **16:**26–31, 1967.
58 Maugh. Loc. cit.
59 Maugh. Loc. cit.
60 *Report of the National Commission on Diabetes,* vol. 2, part 2.
61 Brosman, J. A proposed diabetic educational program for Puerto Ricans in New York City, in P. Brink (ed.), *Transcultural Nursing* (Englewood Cliffs, N.J.: Prentice-Hall, 1976), pp. 263–275.
62 Maugh. Loc. cit.
63 Parsons, T., and Fox, R. Illness, therapy and the modern urban American family, *J. Soc. Iss.,* **8:**2–3, 31–44, 1952.
64 Parsons, T., and Shils, E. (eds.). *Toward a General Theory of Action* (New York: Harper & Row, Harper Torchbooks, 1962).
65 *Report of the National Commission on Diabetes,* vol. 2.
66 Benoliel, J. Q. The developing diabetic identity: a study of family influence, in Marjorie V. Batey (ed.), *Communicating Nursing Research: Methodological Issues* (Boulder, Colorado: Western Interstate Commission for Higher Education, 1970).
67 Feustel, D. E. Nursing student's knowledge about diabetes mellitus, *Nurs. Res.,* **25:**4–7, 1976.
68 Etzwiler, D. D., and Sines, L. K. Juvenile diabetes and its management, *J.A.M.A.,* **181:**304–308, 1962.
69 Etzwiler, D. D. What the juvenile diabetic knows about his disease, *Pediatrics,* **29:**135–141, 1962.
70 Orem, D. E. *Nursing: Concepts of Practice* (New York: McGraw-Hill, 1971).
71 Backscheider, J. Self care requirements, *Am. J. Public Health,* **64:**1138–1146, 1974.
72 Allison, S. E. A framework for nursing action in a nurse conducted diabetic management clinic, *J. Nurs. Admin.,* **3:**53–60, 1973.
73 Hill, R. Social stresses on the family, *Soc. Casework,* **39:**139–150, 1958.
74 Crain, A. J., Sussman, M., and Weil, W. B. Effects of a diabetic child on marital integration and related measures of family functioning, *J. Health Hum. Behav.,* **7:**122–127, 1966.
75 Hill, 1958. Loc. cit.
76 Crain et al. Loc. cit.
77 Benoliel. Loc. cit.
78 Parsons, 1967. Loc. cit.
79 Brandaleone, H., and Friedman, G. J. Diabetes in industry, *Diabetes,* **2:**448–453, 1953.
80 Committee on Employment of the American Diabetes Association, *Diabetes,* **6:**550, 1957.
81 Tetrich, L., and Colwell, J. A. Employment of the diabetic subject, *J. Occup. Med.,* **13:**380–383, 1971.
82 Rodman, H. Employment of the diabetic, unpublished paper, University Hospitals, Cleveland, Ohio, 1976.
83 Beardwood, J. T. Industry's role in the employment of diabetics, *Ind. Med. Surg.,* **19:**271–274, 1950.

84 Weaver, N. K., and Perret, J. T. The diabetic in industry, *Standard Oil Co. Med. Bull.* **18**:304–316, 1958.

85 Tetrich, and Colwell. Loc. cit.

86 Pell, S., and D'Alonzo, C. A. Diabetes mellitus in an employed population, *J.A.M.A.*, **172**:1000–1006, 1960; and Sickness absenteeism in employed diabetics, *Am. J. Public Health*, **57**:253, 1967.

87 Nasr, A. N. M., Block, D. L., and Magnuson, H. J. Absenteeism experience in a group of employed diabetics, *J. Occup. Med.*, **8**:621–625, 1966.

88 Moore, R. H. Work absenteeism in diabetics, *Diabetes*, **23**:957–961, 1974.

89 Pell, S., and D'Alonzo, C. A. Sickness and injury experience of employed diabetics, *Diabetes*, **9**:303–310, 1960.

90 Rodman. Loc. cit.

91 Pell and D'Alonzo, Sickness and injury experience of employed diabetics. Loc. cit.

92 Copplestone, J. F. Employment of diabetics, *Br. J. Ind. Med.*, **16**:170, 1959.

93 Mills, J. W., Saunders, K., and Martin, F. I. R. Socioeconomic problems of insulin dependent diabetes, *Med. J. Aust.*, **2**:1040–1044, 1973.

94 Rodman. Loc. cit.

95 Mills et al. Loc. cit.

96 Kantrow, A. H. A vocational and counseling service for diabetics, *Diabetes*, **12**:454–457, 1963.

97 Rodman. Loc. cit.

98 Kantrow, A. H. Employment experiences of juvenile diabetes, *Diabetes*, **10**:476–481, 1961.

99 Kantrow, A. H. 1963. Loc. cit.

100 Committee on Employment of the American Diabetes Association. Loc. cit.

101 Friedman, G. J. Employability of diabetic persons, *N. Y. State J. Med.*, **66**:1662–1669, 1966.

Personal Adjustment of the Diabetic Individual

May L. Wykle

Personal adjustment to diabetes refers to an individual's total response and continuous adaptation to a chronic illness. The term *adjustment* implies an alteration so as to make fit, regulate, restructure, or become suited to a new predicament. This definition indicates a change in the previous status quo of the individual which calls forth subsequent behavioral changes. Thus the diabetic individual is faced with a new stress and challenge to see how smoothly the self system can integrate the necessary changes in life-style that chronic illness management requires. For the person with diabetes, personal adjustment includes not only understanding reactions and responses to living with a chronic disease but also adapting to an illness known for its serious complications and exacerbations.

The psychosocial impact of the diagnosis of diabetes is often overwhelming, although individual reactions to the disease are determined by a variety of factors. Knowledge of the disease, past and present associations with diabetic people, age of onset, maturity, and available support systems are a few factors that influence individual response. In spite of these factors, there are certain predictable responses based on general knowledge of behavioral reactions to crisis situations that the diabetic person may display. Individuals respond to their own social image of diabetes as an illness according to whatever knowledge they have from past experience. For most, diabetes is thought of as a chronic illness that imposes restrictions on the normal activities of daily living. Feelings are related to loss of normalcy and fear of living with a restricted diet, susceptibility to infection, injections, and physical changes that may include impaired circulation, loss of limbs, and eventual blindness.

The psychosocial impact of diabetes is often far-reaching, affecting the individual, the family, and friends. Furthermore, the emotional response to diabetes may in turn affect an individual's physical responses to the disease. Psychological stress has been thought to produce and accentuate diabetic symptoms. Humans have long been aware of the relationship between psyche and soma, and diabetes may be an example of an illness that is further aggravated by failure of personal adjustment to the disease. This belief alone underscores the importance of accurate assessment of an individual's emotional reaction to the illness and appropriately planned nursing interventions to reduce stress and foster optimum personal adjustment.

Snyder and Wilson suggest that "the greater one's repertoire of responses to stress, the more realistic they are likely to be, and the more they enable the release of appropriate emotion, the stronger is one's adaptive ability."[1] These authors present a model of assessment of psychological status. It has relevance for nurses appraising diabetic responses to stress. Ten elements are considered:

1 Coping and defense mechanisms
2 Interpersonal relationships
3 Motivation and life-style
4 Thought processes and verbal behavior
5 Nonverbal behavior
6 Awareness and handling of feelings
7 Support systems
8 Talents, strengths, and assets
9 Physical health
10 The interview and self of the nurse

BEHAVIORAL REACTIONS TO DIABETES MELLITUS

The word *diabetes* has individualized meaning to patients, yet it is commonly known to be a disease that is often devastating, costly, pleasure limiting, and, if not properly treated, fraught with crises along a downhill course leading to eventual loss of life. With this general view of the illness in mind, and despite some highly individualized responses that patients may have, behavioral reactions to diabetes are somewhat predictable. Nurses having a thorough understanding of the predictable behavior will be able to help patients adjust optimally.

In order to plan appropriate interventions for the diabetic patient, the nurse should have a thorough understanding of behavioral reactions to chronic illness and use interviewing skills to assess the patient's initial response to a diagnosis of diabetes mellitus.

Adaptation to a chronic illness is a *normal process*, and intervention is designed to prevent maladaptation. The initial impact of the illness may be one of shock and disbelief. One young school teacher remarked, "I was devastated! I could see it [diabetes] ruining my whole life and career plans!" Often the initial reaction manifests itself as an overwhelming increase in anxiety. The anxiety may be of such intensity as to cause feelings of panic and an inability to comprehend or plan. A real threat to the self-concept exists, but the threat may also be blown out of proportion to the eminent danger. Nurses may observe an increase in patient physiological activity, such as pacing, fidgeting, and an increased urge to urinate, as well as evidences of disturbance in the cognitive processes.

Concept of Body Image

The normal process of adaptation to a chronic illness can be considered in terms of the individual's body image concept. Body image is a social creation basic to identity that includes both the conscious and unconscious thoughts and perceptions one has about body makeup. The concept of body image includes both physical and emotional characteristics which are slowly learned in the process of growth and development. Self-exploration and interaction with others contribute to the developing self system, which reflects a sense of "me," how I feel, look, and behave, and also how I believe others see me. The concept of body image includes beliefs about tasks the individual knows she or he can and cannot do.

The notion of body image, however, can be disturbed and threatened by illness. The nature of the threat depends on the personal value and meaning of the part of the body affected and the understanding of how the disease affects body functioning.

A diagnosis of diabetes may not always produce a sudden dramatic upheaval or a crisis situation in a patient, but the potential for a crisis situation does exist.

Crisis Theory

One frame of reference for nurses to use in their planning strategy for the newly diagnosed diabetic is a crisis theory framework. All crises require a sudden restructuring of both physiological and psychological integration. It will be helpful to the reader to review Shontz's framework of crisis theory, which can be used as a tool for planning intervention strategies.

Shontz refers to three crisis reaction stages: the preimpact phase, the impact phase, and the postimpact phase.[2] For the diabetic, the preimpact phase may begin with the first symptoms or signs of disturbance. Noted are complaints of "not feeling well," and although the individual continues to function, complaints of weight loss, fatigue, thirst, and other early signs of diabetes are voiced.

A 60-year-old man was hospitalized for a severe urinary infection. Six months prior to his admission he had symptoms of weight loss, increased urination, increased thirst, and fatigue. He had paid little attention to these symptoms as a health threat, but once he was confronted with the diagnosis, he could clearly recall these events.

Shontz refers to these early symptoms of an illness as the prelude, the worry stage. Usually this prelude stage ends when the individual realizes that ordinary coping mechanisms (denial) are no longer working. The prelude stage is transitional and the tension level is much higher than normal. Of course the more knowledge a person has about diabetes, its symptoms, and onset, the more sensitive that individual is to cues or the more he or she can rationalize the symptoms present. Realistically, the preimpact stage ends with the diagnosis. For the asymptomatic diabetic, the preimpact stage may coincide with the diagnosis.

The impact stage, according to Shontz, is intense, pervasive, and relatively brief; the overriding emotional state is one of despair. The impact or encounter phase is the stage of shock. This is most evident if the event comes without any warning. In shock, there is a feeling of depersonalization, of numbness, of nothingness. The individual feels as though struck by a thunderbolt. Shontz speaks of the experience as "cognitive flooding." In their description of this phase, patients speak of seeing their lives pass before them. This encounter stage is the experience most readily described in a crisis state. Panic is easily recognized, since the person experiences disorganization and feelings of helplessness. Later this experience is relived, and patients can learn to manage future crisis situations by reviewing this phase.

In the postimpact phase, emotions are too intense to be withstood for a long period. Therefore the patient uses a type of avoidance, the extreme form of which is denial. The patient may actually refuse to admit to the existence of the illness or the implications of the situation, or she or he may become passive and display an increased focus on symptoms.

Acknowledgment is the final phase of adaptation to an illness. This phase is longest in duration and involves appraisal and reappraisal of status. It includes a succession of limited reencounters with the crisis, each producing a reevaluation of progress toward stable reorganization. Shontz recognizes these phases as normal reactions to illness. Maladaptation may occur in any of them.

While it is important to realize that reactions to diabetes can be assessed within a crisis theory framework, it is just as important to realize that reactions vary and may never approach the crisis stage. Nurses need to be aware of the possible emotional reactions to diabetes and utilize such knowledge in their interventions. Moreover, because of the chronicity of diabetes, patients may experience a number of crises. Planned interventions to assist the patient in an initial crisis therefore better prepare that individual for future adjustments.

Stages of Anxiety

The diabetic patient may vacillate among several stages of anxiety. Peplau describes four stages of anxiety: mild, moderate, severe, and panic.[3] These stages are characterized by different behaviors which the nurse can assess to determine the patient's immediate needs. Anxiety can be reduced by others since it is communicated empathically. Therefore nurses must be aware of their own level of anxiety as well as the patient's need for help in reducing his or her anxiety to a mild or moderate stage. In these first two stages (mild, moderate), cognitive processes are more likely to function within reality and there is less scattering of thoughts.

In the severe and panic stages of anxiety, the diabetic patient requires firm direction and support from the nurse. For example, the nurse may sit with the patient, because another's presence is often reassuring. The nurse should allow the patient to talk about what he or she feels and respond simply to the questions asked. Recognition of feelings and the offer of support are often more crucial than providing technical answers to questions. The patient may need help in recognizing some feelings as anxiety. If the patient is hospitalized, the nurse may reduce anxiety simply by answering lights promptly and scheduling visits at frequent intervals.

The level of anxiety engendered in the diabetic patient and its manifestations will depend on the individual's emotional maturity, understanding of diabetes, level of self-esteem, past illness experience, use of coping mechanisms, and support system, as well as his or her physiological status.

Coping Mechanisms

Denial   Denial is a coping mechanism frequently used by patients; it salvages the ego and allows a temporary retreat from the line of fire. Health professionals are all aware of the power of this defense in reducing overwhelming anxiety in patients, so much so, in fact, that sometimes noncompliance with the prescribed treatment regime appears. One task of assessment is to determine when denial is useful and when it is not useful.

The use of denial may be particularly evident in diabetics with mild symptoms who "cheat" on their diets without suffering any obvious consequences. These individuals may say to themselves, "The tests were wrong, probably the lab got the reports mixed up," or "I know I'll grow out of it." One diabetic man I know spends a great part of his time practicing "reflexology." He believes that he is able to stimulate his pancreas to produce insulin, and he actually reduces his insulin intake according to the amount of time spent on this exercise. If this man could follow his diet and insulin prescription, his use of denial would not be so hazardous.

Denial may be even more operative in the individual who is familiar with diabetes and is aware of the disease course and possible outcomes. Such individuals, in making comparisons with other diabetic patients, will claim that they are not like that person who is indeed in "bad shape." Patients who feel little alteration or change of sensation in their bodies as a result of diabetes find it much easier to use denial. Nurses must be alert to this phenomenon, recognize the symptoms, and help the patient in accepting the illness by teaching self-observation. It is extremely difficult to accept a diagnosis of diabetes when one is regulated by diet, has no perceived symptoms, and is not on insulin or medications.

Denial may be partial or complete. Partial denial allows the individual to admit having diabetes, but only to a few select people, while hoping that it will magically disappear. It is in partial denial that the patient tests to see if the diagnosis is true. The individual may skip insulin for a day and not follow the prescribed diet. Recently I was approached by a woman who wanted to tell me that she had not taken her insulin that morning and, furthermore, that she found it quite difficult keeping to her prescribed dietary regime. She was overweight, and as she chatted she revealed some sophisticated knowledge about her illness, stating that she knew she could get herself "in trouble." It was obvious that this woman intellectualized and operated on partial denial of the consequences of her illness.

For a period of time, denial seemed to fall into ill repute among health professionals and was thought of as a truly negative aspect of patient care. There was a push to confront patients directly with their diagnosis and its consequences so that denial would not interfere with the treatment regime. This approach has been reconsidered, since there is evidence that a direct attack on an individual's denial does not always work and in fact may serve to increase fear and resistance. If the individual gets enough support, reassurance, and education, he or she will be able to give up denial and face reality. Thoughts of lifelong dietary restrictions and social deprivations may be so overwhelming that the patient needs denial in order to regroup. The diabetic treatment regime should be presented with emphasis placed on the normal aspects of adjustment. If denial (a normal coping mechanism used by everyone) can be useful to a patient in the face of overwhelming anxiety, then it is appropriate to support this use of denial. However, if denial becomes detrimental to the patient's progress or adherence to a treatment regime, then its use must be reevaluated and appropriate assistance given. The task of nurses is to make the assessment that determines when denial is not useful.

Denial works well for patients who have been independent and think of themselves as strong self-made individuals or for those who view sickness as a sign of weakness. Nursing interventions should be made so that the patient who needs to deny also gains some awareness of the seriousness of the disease and its management and enough understanding and acceptance so as to participate in his or her own health care. Recognition on the part of the nurse of when patients are or are not using denial appropriately can greatly enhance the patient's adjustment.

Aggression—Turned Outward　　As with any chronic illness, the diabetic may become discouraged, especially when denial begins to lift and the full impact of the illness and its effects are realized. The patient often becomes irritable, cross, or angry and voices resentment at being at this point and time in life and suffering from a chronic illness. This event is similar to the stage of anger described by Kubler-Ross and labeled, "Why me?"[4] One diabetic patient stated that she did not deserve such a misfortune. She had thought that she could stand anything except the thought of taking insulin the rest of her life and giving up ''sweets.'' The anxiety felt is often turned into aggressive feelings and behavior which is then directed toward those around the individual.

Aggression turned outward may take the form of insults, sarcastic remarks, or failure to comply with the treatment regime. The individual may refuse to administer his or her own medications. Such patients may resent the loss they are experiencing and project their anger to staff and family members by becoming demanding. It is imperative that the nurse accept this hostility without retaliation. This is possible only when the nurse understands the dynamics of this behavior. The patient need not be made to feel guilty for such actions. Nurses can help by anticipating demands. Anger reaction is a part of the acknowledgment stage of crisis. Patients may require firm limit setting and use of problem solving to deal with anger. The nurse concentrates on helping the diabetic patient deal successfully with anger so that it is not directed toward self. Rage leads to feelings of guilt, and depression may be brought on by thoughts of having acquired an illness as a punishment for some real or imagined misdeed.

Aggression—Turned Inward Diabetics may become reactively depressed because of their illness. Assessment of the level of depression to determine how much of the patient's behavior is within normal limits is essential. Some depression is recognized as a normal reaction to chronic illness. Further depression can lead to suicide. Nurses must be aware of the clinical signs of depression that indicate the need for special intervention.

Observation of any depressed patient reveals that he or she looks sad, is very quiet, and may show some confusion. More severely depressed patients are apt to lack interest in their surroundings, eat little, and complain of insomnia. They may voice helplessness about their illness and become overly concerned and dependent on the nurse. Such patients appear discouraged and may show signs of grieving for their lost health. Activity is slowed and the patients offer a number of somatic complaints ranging from fatigue and generalized weakness to fear of injections. These patients may focus on the techniques of insulin administration or urine testing and may worry about minor details. Such patients may talk directly about guilt in relation to deserving their illness.

Intervention in depression centers around empathizing with what patients must feel. To accomplish this, the nurse can encourage patients to express feelings and talk about their illness in detail. Listening actively while patients talk about their worries conveys acceptance of their right to feel sad. It is useful to focus on areas outside of the illness and reinforce the *normalcy* aspect of living with diabetes.

Although depressed diabetic patients may be poor candidates for teaching, some gentle nudging for them to participate in their own care is necessary. In addition, this often allows release of some of their anger. Since depression is self-limiting, expression of the anger and guilt will speed the emotional adjustment.

Dependency Dependency is a form of regression that is seen in the acknowledgment stage. Patients with chronic illnesses learn to trust by placing themselves in the hands of competent others and offering little resistance. The nurse's task is to accept the patient in the regressed state, aware that some dependency is a necessary means of coping.

The diabetic at this time will need encouragement to participate actively in his or her own care and attend classes but should not be forced to handle equipment or test urine before showing some signs of readiness. Assuring patients that they will be able to do more for themselves increases their independence. Being alert to overdependence is an essential part of a nurse's assessment. This occurs when patients show that they are able to care for themselves but prefer to remain dependent on others. Often family members become involved and need guidelines for setting limits. Nurses should differentiate between dependency and overdependency in their assessment and gently set limits on activities that enhance dependency.

ADJUSTMENT TO DIABETES

Optimal adjustment to diabetes corresponds to the final stage of adaptation. During this stage the patient develops a keen awareness of what it means to have a chronic illness. The patient acknowledges his or her role and responsibility in maintaining a treatment regime to control diabetes and minimize its consequences.

Despite the achievement of this phase of adjustment, patients can be expected to regress at times, depending on the strength of their coping skills and the new stresses that continue to occur in the natural course of the disease. These regressive periods are considered normal behavioral reactions. One cannot say with any finality that the client has adjusted to a chronic illness and not expect to see the appearance of earlier phases of adaptation.

Factors Influencing Behavioral Reactions

It is a fact that not all illness stress produces crisis situations. Therefore, it would be unwise to suggest that all diabetics react to their illness in a similar manner. As stated earlier, patients have individual reactions to stresses, and many of these reactions have been studied. It is known that certain psychological reactions to organic disease also occur in patients reacting to diabetes. Engel's concept of psychological stress provides a comprehensive and useful framework.[5] Injury or threat of injury to the body produces psychic stress. Bellak outlines a general response to illness stress, citing (1) normal reaction, (2) avoidance reaction, (3) reactive depression, and (4) a channeling into premorbid anxiety and psychological invalidism.[6] Nurses are in a strategic position to observe patients' behavioral reactions to illness and should become astute assessors of patient needs. Utilizing a crisis theory framework is one way that nurses can assess the diabetic patient's adjustment to the illness. However, nurses must consider within the framework used the variety of factors influencing the behavioral reactions of the patient to the disease. Two major factors are the individual's basic personality and the state of the ego and its stage of maturity. Some individuals are basically anxious, withdrawn, suspicious, or aggressive. When stressed, these behaviors become dominant and the basic personality patterns come into sharper focus. For example, the person who is basically aggressive reacts aggressively when confronted with the constraints of an illness.

Nurses will need to assess the strength of the individual's coping mechanisms: which mechanisms are in operation, which ones are used chiefly, and which ones worked in the past? An even more important part of the assessment is to identify which mechanisms are no longer working or are overused. Knowing that the ego will deal with stress through symptom formation when coping mechanisms fail is an essential factor in assessing the diabetic patient's adjustment. It is not unusual, in the face of accepting a chronic illness, that lifelong coping mechanisms and problem-solving skills fail as the patient becomes overwhelmed by mounting anxiety.

Socioeconomic, cultural, and educational factors need to be considered by the nurse as indicators of the types of behavioral reactions manifested. The patient's living conditions and finances, the cultural meaning of chronic illness, and the patient's level of understanding of diabetes will guide the nurse's assessment. Patients poorly educated about their disease and its ramifications will not be able to behave in the manner necessary for them to manage their treatment regime. To many patients, "sugar" is a "bad thing," but the specifics of how diabetes will actually affect their lives and what part of the control is their responsibility is often not understood.

Teaching diabetic patients, based on the level of their education, readiness to learn, and sociocultural background, will prevent both overreactions and underreactions to the seriousness of the illness.

Age   Age, of course, is another factor influencing a patient's response to diabetes. The child will certainly react differently from the adult. The child with insulin-dependent diabetes may react both to the restrictions and to the label of being different from his or her peers. However, while the adult with insulin-resistant diabetes may seem more ready to accept the illness, or perhaps is expected to be mature enough to do so in the eyes of many professionals, she or he may not adjust that quickly. The emotional trauma faced by adult diabetics is often as threatening for them as it is for the juvenile. The emotionality of responses of those with maturity-onset diabetes is often deemphasized when compared with juvenile responses. This comparison is undoubtedly based on chronologic age. Juvenile diabetics have "their whole lives ahead" and a much longer period of time to face a variety of restrictions and fears of complications, plus they are already facing adolescent adjustment. However, many adult diabetics have high levels of anxiety about their illness and experience a variety of behavioral reactions, some requiring immediate emotional support.

Previous illness experience will also influence the behavioral reactions of diabetics to their illness. How one has coped with former illness stresses and/or is still coping with other illness experiences will determine how one is able to react to a present stress.

Support System   Another essential factor influencing a diabetic patient's adjustment is the existence or nonexistence of a support system of family and friends. Nurses should take a detailed family history. It is helpful to plot a family geneogram so that both the nurse and the patient can see who is available for support. Added support from the family decreases anxiety reactions and the need for increased support from nurses. Nurses should plan to spend time with family members since they often experience behavioral reactions similar to those of the patient. A review of the possible support system with the patient is often quite revealing. Some patients have never thought about some family members as a means of support. A diabetic man in his late seventies was forced to care for his wife who had seriously injured her leg and was immobilized in a hip cast. Ordinarily, the couple depended on neighbors and children who lived a considerable distance away. The man was not able to administer his own insulin, let alone prepare food and care for his wife, and they could not afford a housekeeper at the time. After reviewing the family geneogram and checking to see if there might be a relative who could help, the nurse and the couple came up with an 80-year-old cousin who lived in the next state. She was contacted and agreed to come, live in, and care for the two of them. Had the nurse not done this, the cousin never would have been asked. The couple had believed that because of the cousin's age and the distance, she would not be able to help. She was not only able, but the three of them enjoyed being with each other. Identifying support systems for diabetic patients can be most helpful in their adjustment.

COUNSELING THE DIABETIC PATIENT

An essential role of the nurse is to provide counseling for the diabetic patient. Because of the nature of diabetes, its chronicity, the need for ongoing education, and the need for support through the initial stages of reaction, it is imperative that the diabetic patient receive expert counseling to help maintain a therapeutic regime. Counseling enables diabetic patients to discuss their fears, anxieties, worries, and concerns about their illness, its effects, and its management. Counseling is particularly crucial for new diabetic patients who need help in accepting their diagnosis. Talking through the situation enables them to problem solve, reduce the effects of stress, and cope with their fear of the unknown. Counseling provides a base, a structure for relief of anxiety, and strengthens the diabetic patient's ability to make decisions.

The role of the health professional should be aimed primarily at helping diabetic patients achieve a life-style that can be integrated into their present role orientation. The nurse as a counselor must be well educated about diabetes and the nursing role in helping the patient manage a chronic disease without unduly increasing anxiety. As discussed earlier, many diabetics need to reduce anxiety before they can learn about and adapt to their illness.

Establishing a Therapeutic Atmosphere

Although interviewing and interpersonal skills are basic tools for any nurse-patient relationship, they become the means of achieving the purposes of counseling. The nurse is in a unique position to provide education, supervision, and support in the counselor's role.

The establishment of a milieu in which the patient feels support and concern should begin with the initial contact. A supportive environment fosters trust and allows the patient to share his or her problems without undue anxiety. If the nurse has worked with the patient prior to counseling, it is important that she or he review the records so as not to burden the patient with repetitious details. However, if the nurse has not had access to this information, she or he must collect information regarding the illness, adjustment needs, and other concerns. Assessment of the diabetic patient should be done systematically, using an assessment guide that includes the patient's mental status as well as present coping ability and adjustment to disease. Initial sessions should be devoted to establishing a data base focusing on assets as well as deficits. The following areas are essential to the diabetic patient's assessment:

1   Reason for presenting self for counseling at this time
2   Description of experience with diabetes
3   Ability to communicate
4   Level of understanding of diabetes and its outcome
5   Knowledge of treatment and management of diabetes
6   Awareness of how the patient views diabetes affecting life-style, and perceived threat
7   Review of typical day
8   Previous illnesses
9   Use of coping mechanisms
10   Readiness for learning
11   Present use of problem solving
12   Existing support systems
13   Realization of new identity and skills

Goal Setting

Goals for the patient to achieve should be decided with the patient based on the nurse's assessment of needs. Decisions about the priority of these needs should be made by the nurse in light of the resources and limitations that are operative within the particular setting of practice. For example, if the expected length of hospitalization is brief and the staff nurse is restricted from postdischarge contact with the diabetic (either by policy, time, or other constraints), referral and initiating contact with a nurse who can provide service over a longer time may be very useful.

Planning the number of counseling sessions initially indicates to the client that it is expected that he or she will receive help in a limited period of time. Six to twelve sessions are often enough to help with the initial adjustment. At the end of a planned number of sessions the nurse and patient can decide if additional counseling is necessary. Seeing the patient once a week is usually sufficient. The nurse may plan to see the patient on a more frequent basis depending on the patient's needs, availability of resources, need for referral, finances, and distance to travel. Patients may be seen for counseling in clinic settings, private offices, or in the patient's home. Telephone counseling, when deliberately planned, can also be utilized as a substitute when it is not possible for the patient and nurse to meet. Telephone counseling can be highly effective in helping patients adjust.

Mutually planned goal setting based on need assessment will determine the focus of counseling sessions. Common areas of concern for the diabetic are related to:

1 Behavioral reactions of self and family
2 Handling emergencies and complications
3 Growth and developmental needs
4 Sexuality

Emphasis on Normalcy of Behavioral Reactions

Diabetic patients may become discouraged and voice disappointment with their behavior and reactions to their illness, especially their responses to family and friends. Helping diabetic patients understand their behavioral reactions to the illness as normal responses is a priority for the nurse counselor. The counselor can do this in part by not showing undue alarm or reaction when clients report feelings of anger and depression. When the idea is conveyed to patients that these responses are normal, universal reactions, they will feel free to report behaviors that are crucial in relation to managing their physical health.

Encouraging verbalization of feelings is a technique the counselor should use initially. Patients need to describe the psychological feelings attached to the consequences of their illness. In the beginning interviews, the nurse should support patients by allowing them to talk freely without criticizing or offering advice. The nurse who can display genuineness, warmth, and empathy fosters the development of a relationship in which patients can freely disclose their fears and concerns. They may be able to explore cheating on their diet without openly seeking disapproval. Patients often expect to be criticized for not following their treatment regime. Patients should be encouraged to describe their routine concerns about buying and using equipment, giving insulin, preparing meals, and other activities of daily living.

Diabetic patients will need to develop and strengthen internal controls, modifying behavior to fit their new life-style. Too often the diabetic patient is scolded and blamed for not being in control and for not following treatment. The counselor should not add to the patient's guilt, and such criticism may be interpreted by patients to mean personal rejection. Instead, the nurse can review goals with patients and discuss the kinds of difficulties the patients have in maintaining their health regime. Explore such statements as "I forgot to take my insulin yesterday" by gathering information about the event and simultaneously assessing the emotional involvement. In response to this statement, the nurse can say simply, "Let's explore what happened. What were you thinking? What activities were you involved in? What were you feeling at the time?"

It is easy for patients to assume that they will be blamed for not following the diet. This may be true particularly for those patients who are overweight. Teaching nutrition is essential, and listening to the patient for cues and clues as to readiness is critical. Sometimes diabetic patients may be "brittle" and have difficulty convincing the health team that they have followed the prescribed diet. The perception that nurses and doctors disbelieve their reports is a direct blow to their self-concept. Often patients will experience an increase in anxiety as they try to convince the staff that they are following the prescribed routine. A young female diabetic expressed how relieved she was when the doctors and nurses discovered that her diabetes was not easy to control and that she indeed was not "sneaking" candy bars and potato chips between meals. She described the relief as a wonderful experience in contrast to all the anger she had previously felt as a result of trying to convince the staff that she was being honest and was frightened about her illness.

Scolding, cajoling, urging patients to stick to their regime "just for me," moralizing, or demanding are poor counseling techniques. Instead the nurse counselor should help patients work toward recognizing their own behavioral strengths rather than working for counselor approval or disapproval. Some patients may use the authority of the counselor as a defense and come to counseling expecting to be confronted and criticized. In this situation the nurse counselor should guide the patient, allow him or her to present facts and draw his or her own conclusions, and give the patient homework such as keeping a record of food intake or daily routine. Together patterns of eating activity can be assessed. Next, the nurse should help the patient devise his or her own behavior reinforcement for adhering to the treatment regime.

It is also necessary to help patients with feelings of "differentness" in relation to routines. This is particularly important for children who want to be like their peer group. Again, identifying family and peer support can be beneficial to the patient. Sometimes diabetics do not wish to involve family members with their problems and concerns. Yet, if they are living with their families, they need to teach family members as well as solicit their aid. For example, if patients eat meals with their families, or if another family member is responsible for cooking, then assistance is needed in order to make the diabetic diet a part of the regular routine. Diabetic patients may hesitate to join in family festivities or families may not invite them because of beliefs about food restrictions.

Often patients require supervision and help with injections and/or urine testing. Work with the total family constellation would be ideal. A responsible family member is valuable for giving support and supervision to those clients who require outside aid. Once again, a geneogram of the family, where they are located, and closeness to patient should be plotted. Such a structure enables the patient to identify sources of support that otherwise might not be obvious, as in the case involving the 80-year-old cousin. The geneogram can also be useful as a tool in helping clients work through feelings about their illness in relation to their families. Relationships with nonsupportive or unsympathetic families also should be explored.

SPECIAL CONCERNS

Handling Emergencies and Complications

Dealing with the fears of a chronic illness like diabetes is another area the patient and counselor need to explore. To tell diabetic patients that they are much better off today than they would have been a century ago is to offer them little relief. Diabetics are faced with an illness of chronic nature fraught with the possibility of many complications. It is an illness that is incurable and can only be controlled. Complications such as decrease in circulation, loss of libido, increased chances of complications with pregnancy, and loss of eyesight are frightening for such patients. Further, if the disease is not well controlled, such emergencies as insulin reaction and diabetic coma could cause the patient great alarm.

Adjusting to diabetes includes accepting the fact that complications can occur even when the patient has faithfully followed the treatment regime. Diabetic patients need to talk about their knowledge of crises and complications that can occur. Assistance with realities, perhaps through role playing, would help the patient develop strategies for critical situations prior to their occurrence. Anxiety will be decreased in both patients and their families if such planning is done ahead of time. Nurses can be very helpful if they spend time with patients and their families so that they can identify signs of complications and sources of aid in emergencies.

Growth and Development Needs

The growth and development needs of diabetics should be assessed since growth and development continue throughout life. Intervention is necessary to help increase patient autonomy in managing a lifelong illness. It is necessary for patients to quickly gain a proper perspective of how diabetes affects their total situation and those developmental tasks with which they are concerned.

The Adolescent   Growth and development needs are given particular attention in the adolescent patient. The adolescent who has diabetes needs specialized counseling with a focus on normal growth and development. Intellectual guidance to increase the patient's knowledge and ability to problem solve in acute stress situations is crucial. Adolescents with diabetes need help to see their environments in new and fresh ways and to accept their differentness without feeling apart from their peer group. Adolescent patients, who are in a precarious growth and development period, must learn to follow treatment regimes that interrupt their normal patterns of daily living. The adolescent may adapt quickly to managing treatment or may use the disease to control others.

One teenager learned to adjust her insulin dosage to keep her weight down, a dangerous practice without medical supervision. Adolescents want to be part of their peer group and desperately do not want to be out of identity with them. Therefore, they may go to extremes to deny their illness and yet be very fearful of losing control in front of the group. Going to parties with restricted eating is merely one adjustment that adolescent patients have to make. They also have fears related to having such a lifelong illness and its meaning for future life plans. Stress in parent-adolescent relationships may focus around health care practices.

The emotional problems of the diabetic adolescent need special consideration by nurses. During these years, according to Erickson, adolescents begin to think about career plans and future life.[7] This is a necessary part of their growth and development. It is also a period of increased stress, yet a time when they are supposed to begin managing their emotions in preparation for participation in the adult world. Besides being concerned with their changing body image, they are confronted with an illness that alters their life-style. Diabetic adolescents become anxious and embarrassed about the possibility of having hypoglycemic reactions in front of their peers. Diabetic adolescents have genuine concern about their future careers. Counseling is a vital part of helping such adolescents select a career or explore career development plans. It is difficult to reassure them about future careers, especially when there is evidence that job discrimination exists for diabetics. There is a need for continued public education so that diabetes may be better understood.

Besides concern about careers, concern about the effects that diabetes may have on their participation in other adult roles may be devastating. Adolescents already have concerns about sexuality. Girls may have heard about the dangers of diabetes and pregnancy and fear the loss of the mothering role; and boys may have fears of impotence and sterility.

There are also fears of blindness, amputation, and renal disease experienced by diabetic adolescents and/or their parents. Increased anxiety may depend on what they have heard about the disease. Without proper guidance and counseling, irrational behavior can sometimes occur during this period. Diabetic adolescents may use denial and enter a period of testing and risk taking; some act out their angry feelings and some become suicidal.

Counseling reveals that in spite of knowledge of their illness, some adolescents may deliberately ignore the treatment regime. Hopelessness stemming from thoughts of chronicity, loss of pleasures, and gradual deterioration has to be countered by the nurse counselor. Often the diabetic adolescent uses denial and hopes for a spontaneous cure. Because the nature of the disease fosters a "what if I do follow a routine, I'll still end up with complications" attitude, counselors are faced with a major task of helping the adolescent set goals. A factor that works against acceptance of disease restrictions is that of nonovert consequences. An adolescent may be able to cheat on the diet for some time without any obvious effects. This serves to reinforce denial.

Adolescents need good emotional support to achieve optimum diabetic management. It is extremely beneficial to counsel the diabetic adolescent in a group. Group counseling and patient education classes may be provided along with individual counseling. Peer support and learning from peers enable adolescents to feel a part of a group. The work of any counseling session should focus on patient strengths, assets, and normal living routines to develop a sense of integrity.

Sexuality Assessment of the sexual concerns of diabetic patients is a critical issue since there is now more evidence that this chronic illness may affect sexual functioning. Fears of sexual dysfunction are a special concern of diabetic patients, and impotence is often a problem in diabetic men.[8] In fact, impotence may be one of the first clinical manifestations of the disease.[9]

Men who report loss of ability to maintain an erection without subsequent loss of libido can be suspected of having diabetic neuropathy. Diabetic neuropathy interferes with the nerve supply to the sexual area. Research studies have revealed alarming data that substantiate the concerns diabetic patients have with sexual adequacy. Woods reports that 70 percent of 198 diabetic males (aged 16 to 92) with diabetes of less than a year's duration suffered from impotence. Of the men who became impotent, 30 percent did so within 1 year of the diagnosis of diabetes, and 60 percent within 5 years. This study provides supporting evidence of the magnitude of sexual problems in diabetic males.

Similarly, research has been conducted on female diabetic patients, and Kalodnz found that orgasmic dysfunction was more prevalent among diabetic women than among a control group studied.[10] Women with diabetes complain of vaginitis and a decrease in libido.

Nurses should understand current research related to diabetic sexual problems. An assessment of the patient's sexual needs should be done initially and should be a part of the routine assessment. Questions such as "How is your sex life?" or "Do you have any concerns in the sexual area?" can be asked directly. Sexual concerns are often a prime factor in the marital and family planning adjustments of diabetic patients.

It is also essential to assess the degree of anxiety surrounding the sexual problem as the patient expresses concern. Patients who complain of impotence should be referred for a complete medical work-up, since there are psychogenic, biologic, and endocrine causes of impotence. Of course, nondiabetic causes of impotence may also be present. Psychological implications are by far the most common cause of impotence in men.[11] In psychogenic impotence, the patient often reports morning erections, and morning erections are not indicative of nerve damage. Potency depends on the functioning of the autonomic nervous system, which is frequently involved in diabetic neuropathy.

In Ellenberg's study of 200 diabetic men (average age 43.2), 59 percent were impotent, and 82 percent of these had neuropathy. Of the 41 percent who were potent, 12 percent had neuropathy. His results minimize a gonadal basis, since the plasma testosterone levels were found to be normal in this sample. These findings were unrelated to the severity of the diabetes.

The nurse should differentiate among libido, potency, and sterility when counseling the diabetic patient about sexual problems. Never should an indiscriminate interchange of these terms be used. Each requires a different intervention. One can continue to have libido without loss of potency, *potency* being the ability to maintain an erection throughout coitus.

Once the cause of impotence has been determined, treatment can be instituted and the nurse can provide emotional support for the patient. If impotence results from poorly controlled diabetes and is a reflection of nutritional needs, then proper management of the metabolic aspects of the disease is necessary to restore health and vigor. Psychogenic impotence must be based on a psychological evaluation, and psychotherapy should be instituted. When drugs are the cause of impotence, they should be eliminated. Appropriate hormonal therapy should be instituted when the cause is endocrine in nature. If the cause of impotence is neurogenic, then mechanical devices have been found to be beneficial in helping some patients maintain an erection.[12]

Counseling is advocated for the diabetic who is concerned about having children. Honesty is important. Counseling is essential in helping the diabetic understand the risks that are involved as well as the present state of knowledge. It is suspected that chances of having a diabetic child are increased when parents are diabetic. Not every diabetic woman develops complications in pregnancy. With proper care, women diabetics can have safe pregnancies. Remarkable advances in the management of high-risk pregnancy have occurred in the last 5 years.[13] Nevertheless, young women with diabetes may approach pregnancy with fear. The frequency of spontaneous abortions in diabetic women is often a crucial factor underlying patient concern. Counseling helps decrease anxiety and guilt, and can assist the client in planning for parenthood or avoiding pregnancy. Once a decision is reached, the nurse should be supportive.

Support for masculinity and femininity is a special need for some diabetic patients. Male diabetics have questions regarding sterility and impotence, and it is essential for them to know all the facts involved. Over a period of time the diabetic male's chances of losing potency or developing sterility are increased. Studies show that the diabetic male is likely to become impotent within a year of the diagnosis of diabetes.[14] These facts should be shared with the patient, especially if the patient is married and wants to have children. Chances of having children are greater if the couple plans to start right away.

Woods discusses sexual dysfunction and its etiology and problems in relation to diabetes.[15] Facts listed for the diabetic include the following:

1   The incidence of sexual dysfunction among diabetics increases with duration of illness.
2   Diabetic males may become transiently impotent when their diabetes is not controlled.

3 Impotence that occurs in male diabetics who are well controlled is likely to be permanent.

4 Candidal vaginitis and lack of vaginal lubrication may contribute to sexual dysfunction in diabetic females.

5 Disturbances of fertility among diabetics may compromise their concept of self as masculine or feminine.

6 Genetic counseling for diabetic patients may help them approach the consequences of genetic transmission of diabetes in the family unit.

7 Sexual dysfunction in chronic illness may result from multiple causes.

8 Assessment of biologic, psychologic, and sociologic variables that influence sexual function provides a holistic basis for assisting the diabetic patient to experience optimum sexual function.

Sexual counseling can increase the self-concept of diabetic patients and subsequently their sexual role identity.

SUMMARY

Assisting with the personal adjustment of diabetic patients is an essential role of the nurse. Understanding the emotional reactions of patients with diabetes and teaching patients to understand the illness and its management are well within the counseling role of the nurse. Diabetics will need support in accepting the lifelong management of a chronic disease and its consequences. As a counselor the nurse works with patients to assess needs and plan goals mutually so that they may comply with a treatment regimen. In the counseling role the nurse teaches diabetics, considers growth and development needs, and focuses on their special concerns. As a counselor the nurse can give emotional support and encouragement to diabetic patients so that they may experience optimal life adjustment to their chronic illness.

REFERENCES

1 Snyder, J. C., and Wilson, M. F. Elements of a psychological assessment, *Am. J. Nurs.* 77(2):235–239, 1976.

2 Shontz, F. *The Psychological Aspects of Physical Illness and Disability* (New York: Macmillan, 1975).

3 Peplau, H. A working definition of anxiety, in S. Burd and F. Marshall (eds.), *Some Clinical Approaches to Psychiatric Nursing* (New York: Macmillan, 1963).

4 Kubler-Ross, E. *On Death and Dying* (New York: Macmillan, 1969).

5 Engel, G. L. *Psychological Development in Health and Disease* (Philadelphia: Saunders, 1972).

6 Bellak, L. *Psychology of Physical Illness* (New York: Grune & Stratton, 1952).

7 Erickson, E. H. *Childhood and Society* (New York: Norton, 1963).

8 Woods, N. F. *Human Sexuality in Health and Illness* (St. Louis: Mosby, 1975).

9 Ellenberg, M. Impotence in diabetes: the neurologic factor, *Ann. Intern. Med.*, 75:213–219, 1971.

10 Kalodnz, R. C. Sexual dysfunction in diabetic females, *Diabetes* 20:557–559, 1971.

11 Ellenberg. Loc. cit.

12 Ibid.

13 Younger, D. Management of diabetes and pregnancy, in K. E. Sussman and R. J. Metz (eds.), *Diabetes Mellitus* (New York: American Diabetes Association, 1975).

14 Woods. Loc. cit.

15 Ibid.

Physiological Alterations in Diabetes

*Violet A. Breckbill**

About 4 percent of the population of the United States has diabetes mellitus. Most of these individuals are over 40 years of age, but others experience onset of the disease in early childhood. The "brittle," juvenile, insulin-deficient patient responds effectively to insulin when treated. If untreated, the young patient gives the appearance of outright cachexia and easily goes into acidosis, becomes dehydrated, and succumbs to death. It has been said that the juvenile diabetic lives because of the effectiveness of insulin only to die of renovascular disease.

The most common form of diabetes mellitus is the maturity-onset form (after the age of 40), but there is still some mystery concerning its cause. The individual, usually overweight and female, will often have an abundance of insulin. There seems to be an intolerance of carbohydrates, a mild tendency to acidosis, and a susceptibility to premature vascular disease. Most maturity-onset diabetes can be controlled by diet, but some require insulin. The effects of insulin and oral hypoglycemics, in particular, on vascular disease remain a big controversy. From the effect it is hard to identify causative factors.

Bray has noted that as relative weight increased from country to country the prevalence of diabetes also increased.[1] However, not all obese patients

* Assisted by Karen Forbes, R.N., B.S.N., M.S.N. Candidate, Case Western Reserve University, Cleveland, Ohio.

develop diabetes. Pyke and Pease studied the relationship between diabetes and obesity in 946 patients and noted that the frequency of obesity was lowest in the diabetics under 30 and highest in the diabetics between 30 and 60.[2] There is an apparent distinction on the basis of body weight between juvenile and adult-onset diabetes. Experiments with animals would implicate obesity as a source of the "environmental stress" that can precipitate failure of the pancreas and diabetes if the pancreas is already diseased. This observation would suggest that obesity increases the demands on the pancreas to produce insulin. When the pancreas is unable to meet the demands because it is injured by chemical, viral, or genetic factors, then the demands of obesity may lead to failure of the pancreas.

Patients with diabetes mellitus of either type can develop certain microvascular complications involving kidneys, eyes, and nervous system. These complications involve small vessels in tissues that are *not* insulin sensitive. It has been suggested that all the complications involve cells that are similar histologically and have similar functions in their respective sites, such as reabsorption, secretion, etc. What meaning this suggestion has is not clear at the moment.

Lastly, Cahill and other investigators have strongly indicated a genetic basis to diabetes mellitus, both for the juvenile and the maturity-onset forms.[3] The basic lesion would appear to be some kind of cellular instability or "accelerated" senescence, probably resulting from the influence of multiple genes. Juvenile diabetes would be the result of the basic lesion plus added insult to the beta cells such as a viral or autoimmune process or a combination of both. Some viruses, such as mumps or Coxsackie B_4, have been so indicted. Maturity-onset diabetes would result from the basic lesion (studies with identical twins implicate such a lesion) plus the "fizzling out" of the beta cells of the pancreas. Enhanced need for insulin could come from obesity, as previously noted, from steroid therapy, or from other stresses.

Diabetes mellitus affects all physiological systems and functions of the organism at the levels of the cell, organ, and system. Through the interference with normal metabolism, hormonal control, nutrition, fluid and electrolyte interactions, and circulation, we end up with a big web of abnormalities in the metabolism of carbohydrates, fats, proteins, availability of insulin, and perhaps some other important life molecules as yet not identified. In this chapter, an attempt will be made to penetrate that web so that we may gain some knowledge to help diabetic patients live useful, reasonably healthy, and comfortable existences.

NORMAL PHYSIOLOGY: METABOLIC PATHWAYS RELATED TO GLUCOSE

The glucose needed for energy to support a multitude of cellular activities comes to the various areas of the body from three sources: (1) dietary intake of carbohydrates, (2) breakdown of glycogen stores within the body, and (3) conversion of other biomolecules to glucose through the process known as gluconeogenesis. In a normal individual, the level of glucose is usually maintained at 80 to 90 mg per 100 mL of blood, as measured in the fasting period before breakfast. This concentration may increase to 120 to 140 mg per 100 mL in the first hour or so following a meal, and the marvelous feedback mechanisms, through a variety of interrelated controls, return the blood glucose concentration to control level, often within 2 h after the intestinal absorption of digested carbohydrate.

Insulin

The glucose measured in the circulating blood is made available to the cells by the action of insulin, a peptide hormone. The peptide hormones appear to act through a fixed receptor mechanism at the cell membrane to activate an en-

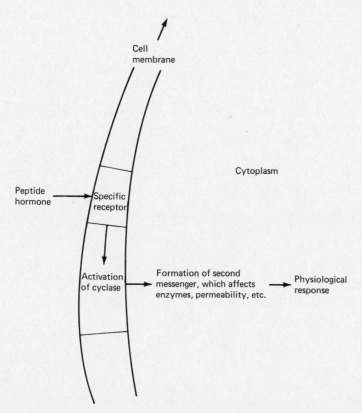

Figure 4-1 Illustration shows a peptide hormone, e.g., insulin, glucagon, growth hormone, acting at the membrane of a cell at specific receptors. A second messenger is formed which causes a whole cascade of events.

zyme within the membrane which, in turn, acts upon specific molecules within the cell to form a "second messenger" (see Fig. 4-1). Many of the peptide hormones effect their actions through the activation of adenyl cyclase, which is an enzyme found within the cell membrane. Adenyl cyclase causes the formation of a second messenger, cyclic adenosine 3,5-phosphate (cAMP), from adenosine triphosphate (ATP), which is a very important energy molecule within cells. Insulin is known to suppress the production of cAMP and would

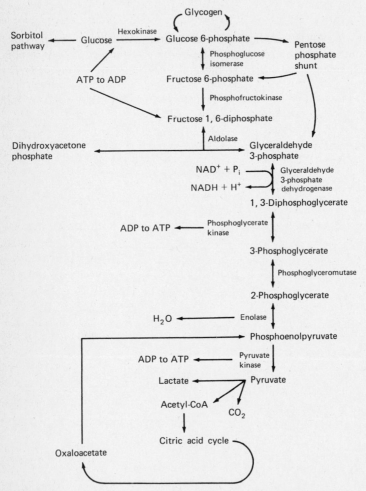

Figure 4-2 The Embden-Meyerhof pathway of glycogenesis and glycolysis is the anaerobic synthesis of glycogen or the degradation of glucose, respectively. Other pathways that glucose can enter are also shown, as well as where ATP is used and where it is recovered. The arrows indicate whether the various steps are reversible with the same enzyme. If the arrow points in only one direction or two arrows are shown, different enzymes are utilized for reversing the process, such as in gluconeogenesis.

seem to have its effects through its second messenger, cyclic guanosine 3,5-phosphate (cGMP), which is a molecule that usually has effects opposite those of cAMP within cells. Cyclic GMP is a product of enzyme activity on guanosine triphosphate, another high-energy molecule.

Insulin's second messenger, cGMP, acts on a group of enzymes in the cell and causes a series of reactions that eventually result in anaerobic glycolytic and aerobic degradation of glucose; or ultimately, if not catabolized, glucose is stored in the form of glycogen in the liver and skeletal muscle (see Fig. 4-2).

Insulin has its greatest effect on muscle and fat cells. It has its least effect on liver, brain, and red blood cells. Not only does insulin facilitate the movement of glucose into muscle and fat cells, but it also facilitates the movement of Na^+ ions and some amino acids as well. Thus insulin affects the enzymes of glycolysis and aerobic metabolism of carbohydrates. In addition, it affects the enzymes of fat metabolism in the cell, as well as the enzymes of protein metabolism. In fact, the effects of insulin on fat metabolism are at least as dramatic as its effects on carbohydrates and perhaps protein metabolism, too.

Hormones of the hypothalamus, the anterior pituitary gland, and the adrenal cortex and medulla act either synergistically or antagonistically with insulin in producing its effects. Let us now examine the pathways that normally metabolize glucose and see how various hormones influence them.

Glycogenolysis and Glycogenesis

The Embden-Meyerhof glycogenic and glycolytic phases of carbohydrate metabolism provide for storage of glucose in a limited amount within the liver and skeletal muscle and for the degradation of glucose to pyruvate, respectively. The degradation to pyruvate, a 3-carbon molecule, utilizes four molecules of ATP but produces two, so it becomes a source of energy, even though an inefficient one (see Fig. 4-2). Park et al. observed in experiments with rat tissue (in vivo and in vitro) that the insulin-sensitive step for glucose uptake by muscle involved the *transfer* rather than the *phosphorylation* of glucose, which must occur for glucose to enter the glycolytic pathway.[4]

$$\text{Glucose in medium} \xrightarrow{\text{transfer}} \begin{array}{c} \text{free glucose in} \\ \text{muscle cell} \\ \uparrow \\ \text{glucose from} \\ \text{metabolism} \end{array} \xrightarrow[\text{ATP}]{\text{hexokinase}} \text{glucose 6-phosphate, etc.}$$

Krebs Cycle

The pyruvate molecule can be reduced to lactate, another 3-carbon molecule, by adding hydrogen, or it can be decarboxylated to an acetate molecule, a

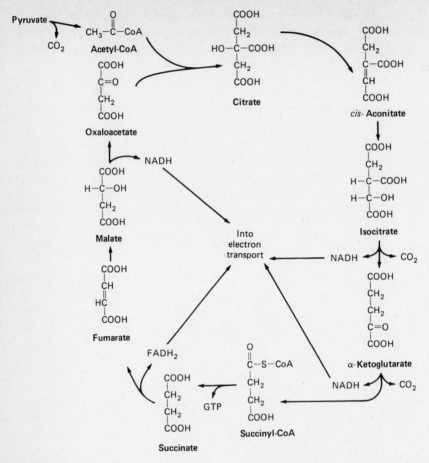

Figure 4-3 The final common pathway for oxidation of carbohydrates, fats, and amino acids is the Krebs cycle (or the citric acid cycle). Pyruvate from the glycolytic pathway is decarboxylated to acetyl-CoA. Acetyl-CoA condenses with oxaloacetate to form citrate, and the cycle begins. Oxaloacetate is recovered, and two molecules of CO_2 are given off. The released hydrogen is carried to the electron transport/oxidative phosphorylation pathways for ATP to be generated, and H_2O is formed. Fatty acids enter the cycle at acetyl-CoA; amino acids can enter at several steps. (*Adapted from L. Stryer, "Biochemistry," San Francisco, Freeman, 1975.*)

2-carbon molecule known commonly as an acetyl group, by removing a molecule of carbon dioxide (CO_2). This acetyl group combines with coenzyme A (CoA, an auxiliary molecule containing a molecule of glycine with an —SH group, pantothenic acid, and adenosine diphosphate) and is now ready to enter the aerobic pathway, the tricarboxylic or Krebs cycle, where the final products of CO_2 and water (H_2O) are derived from the initial molecule of glucose (see Fig. 4-3). CO_2 comes directly from the "spinning" of the cycle and is expired

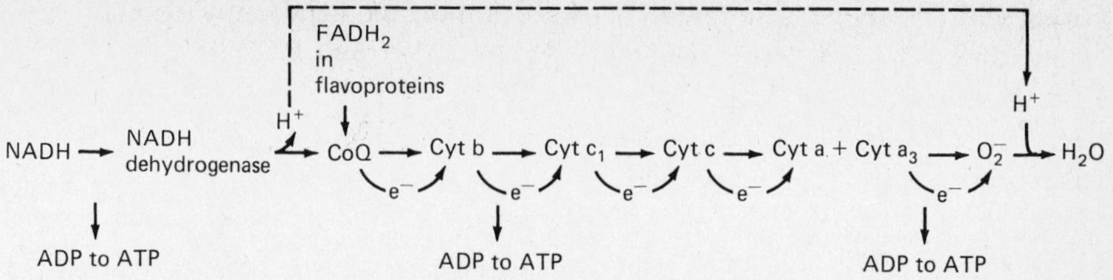

Figure 4-4 Hydrogen and then electrons are transferred from the hydrogen carriers (NADH and FADH$_2$) to oxygen to form water. Three molecules of ATP are made each time the electron transport takes place. Therefore, oxidative phosphorylation is a concomitant process. If only the electron transport takes place and no ATP is made, heat, and no energy, is the product along with the H$_2$O formed. The cytochrome molecules are iron-containing proteins that transfer the electrons along the pathway to ionize the molecular oxygen to prepare it for union with the hydrogen.

in pulmonary ventilation or becomes a part of the bicarbonate ion through the action of the enzyme carbonic anhydrase, which is found in a variety of places in the body. The water is the end product of a series of enzyme reactions through which hydrogen is passed in the mitochondria, which are the small cell organelles where the Krebs cycle, as well as fatty acid oxidation, takes place. The hydrogen is taken by carrier molecules (which are enzyme-coenzyme molecules, the coenzyme portion being various vitamin B components) to the cytochromes, a series of enzymes, and is eventually united with oxygen to form water (see Fig. 4-4). (The oxygen is transmitted to the tissues via the hemoglobin molecule in the red blood cells.) A process concomitant to the hydrogen transfer is the formation of ATP, the important energy molecule. The formation of water is called *electron transport;* the formation of ATP is *oxidative phosphorylation.* These two processes occur together, and the first is necessary for the second to take place. If hydrogen transfer occurs without the formation of ATP, only heat, but no energy, is produced. This process of oxidative phosphorylation is very efficient, and 38 molecules of ATP are produced in this way for each glucose molecule oxidized.

Pentose Shunt

The *pentose shunt* is a detour that some of the glucose can take from the first step in the glycolytic pathway, i.e., the phosphorylation of glucose to glucose 6-phosphate. From this point, another pathway is followed (see Fig. 4-5). Glucose metabolized through the pentose shunt provides molecules of the hydrogen carrier NADPH, which are necessary for fatty acid synthesis in the cytoplasm after precursors are moved from the mitochondria (see Fig. 4-6). Six-carbon fructose molecules and 3-carbon units from the shunt can reenter the Embden-Meyerhof cycle, and 4-carbon and 5-carbon tetroses and pentoses, respectively, can be generated for other important needs in the body, e.g., pentoses for the formation of nucleotides for DNA and RNA.

Glycolysis and Gluconeogenesis

Glycolysis is the aerobic breakdown of glucose through a series of decreasing energy levels influenced by various enzymes with their coenzymes and metallic cofactors. *Gluconeogenesis* is the new formation of glucose from other molecules, such as amino acids, that can be fitted into various places in the metabolic pathways utilized by glucose, or from reversing the direction of the degradation pathway of glucose. Many of the steps of the metabolic pathways are reversible, but in three specific areas there are key enzymes that control the direction of reactions so that only glycolysis may proceed and key enzymes that control the direction of the reactions so that only gluconeogenesis will occur.[5] These enzymatic differences between glycolysis and gluconeogenesis are as follows:

Glycolysis	Gluconeogenesis
Hexokinase	Glucose 6-phosphatase
Phosphofructokinase	Fructose 1,6-diphosphatase
Pyruvate kinase	Pyruvate carboxylase
	Phosphoenolpyruvate carboxykinase

The enzymes listed opposite each other either catabolize glucose in a particular step in glycolysis or anabolize glucose in gluconeogenesis.

It is absolutely necessary to take in some carbohydrates in order for the Krebs cycle to operate or for gluconeogenesis to occur. There must be a carbohydrate source for oxaloacetate, the important 4-carbon molecule in the Krebs cycle that joins with acetyl-CoA, to begin the cycle to form citric acid (see Fig. 4-3). A source of oxaloacetate must be present also for phosphoenolpyruvate to be formed to participate in gluconeogenesis. The latter molecule is made by the decarboxylation of oxaloacetate, or oxaloacetate is formed by the carboxylation of phosphoenolpyruvate, the 3-carbon molecule that precedes the pyruvate step in the glycolytic pathway (see Fig. 4-2). The molecule first formed is malate, which is an isomer of oxaloacetate and also a component in the Krebs cycle. Malate can move more easily through the mitochondrial membrane and is converted to oxaloacetate on each side of the membrane.

INSULIN AND GLUCAGON RESPONSES

The islets of Langerhans in the pancreas contain two major types of cells that have been morphologically distinguished from each other: alpha and beta cells. Beta cells secrete insulin; alpha cells secrete glucagon. Insulin is a protein

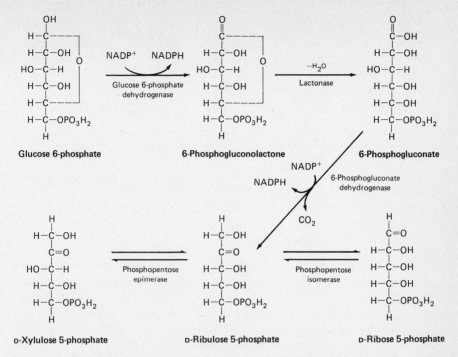

Glucose 6-phosphate

6-Phosphogluconolactone

6-Phosphogluconate

D-Xylulose 5-phosphate

D-Ribulose 5-phosphate

D-Ribose 5-phosphate

Figure 4-5 The major roles of the pentose phosphate pathway (shunt) are (1) to generate large amounts of NADPH to be used by adipose tissue in the reductive synthesis of fatty acids from acetyl-CoA and (2) to provide pentoses for the synthesis of DNA and RNA. Other molecules can be derived, e.g., glyceraldehyde 3-phosphate and fructose 6-phosphate, which can reenter the glycolytic pathway at the appropriate steps.

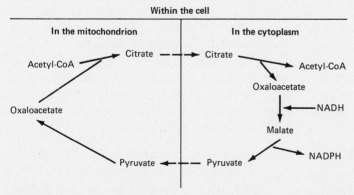

Figure 4-6 The NADPH gained in this mechanism is used for fatty acid synthesis in the cytoplasm. Oxaloacetate must be converted to another intermediate both within the mitochondrion and within the cytoplasm in order to be moved across the membrane. It is then regenerated. (*Adapted from L. Stryer, "Biochemistry," San Francisco, Freeman, 1975.*)

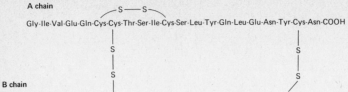

A chain

Gly-Ile-Val-Glu-Gln-Cys-Cys-Thr-Ser-Ile-Cys-Ser-Leu-Tyr-Gln-Leu-Glu-Asn-Tyr-Cys-Asn-COOH

B chain

NH_2^--Phe-Val-Asn-Gln-His-Leu-Cys-Gly-Ser-His-Leu-Val-Glu-Ala-Leu-Tyr-Leu-Val-Cys-Gly-Glu-Arg-Gly-Phe-Phe-Tyr-Thr-Pro-Lys-Thr

Figure 4-7   The insulin molecule is made up of an A chain with 21 amino acid residues and a B chain with 30 amino acid residues. Three disulfide bonds exist between the cysteine residues, as shown. This molecule began as proinsulin in the beta cells of the pancreas which contains 84 amino acids. This is the structure of human insulin; the structures of insulin obtained from various animal sources differ slightly in the position of several of the amino acids.

made up of 51 amino acids and is derived from a proinsulin molecule that contains 84 amino acids. The resulting insulin molecule is the A chain with 21 amino acids and the B chain with 30 amino acids from the original proinsulin molecule. The two chains are linked by disulfide bonds (see Fig. 4-7). Glucagon is also a protein molecule, made up of 29 amino acids. There are no disulfide bonds in its structure. Glucagon is made in the gut as well as in the islet cells. This phenomenon will be discussed later.

Insulin and Its Functions

As previously indicated, the biosynthesis of insulin takes place within the beta cells of the islets of Langerhans in the pancreas. Proinsulin, the precursor of insulin, is made on ribosomes located on the rough endoplasmic reticulum (RER). The proinsulin travels through the endoplasmic reticulum to the Golgi complex, where it is converted to insulin for storage in secretory granules, and eventually secreted (see Fig. 4-8). The proinsulin molecule is a single polypeptide chain beginning with the amino terminus of a normal B chain. Proinsulin has a connecting polypeptide (the C chain) of 33 amino acids which connects the carboxy terminus of the B chain to the amino terminus of the A chain. Proinsulin fulfills the biosynthetic need for an efficient mechanism of assembling the insulin molecule. The folding of the proinsulin aligns the molecule for the proper disulfide bonding, which occurs with the help of glutathione-insulin *trans*-hydrogenase and possibly with the help of trypsin or a trypsin-like enzyme.[6] Conversion of proinsulin to insulin takes place within the secretory granules and, once initiated, does not require energy. Studies indicate that this conversion process begins approximately 20 min after protein synthesis (the time required for transport through the endoplasmic reticulum to

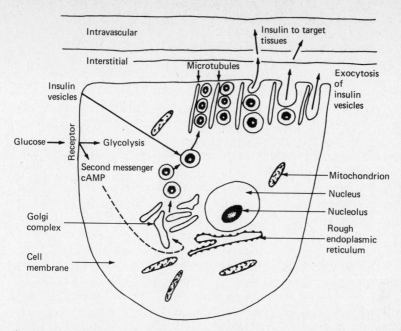

Figure 4-8 Beta cell of the pancreas. Glucose interacts with its receptor on the cell membrane which activates adenyl cyclase to produce cAMP from ATP. A cascade of events causes the insulin precursor, proinsulin, to be synthesized at the rough endoplasmic reticulum on the ribosomes and packaged in the Golgi complex. Packets or vesicles are formed and are moved with the assistance of microtubules to the luminal surface of the cell. By exocytosis, the insulin is released to the blood and transported to its target cells.

the secretory granules) and proceeds for several hours. Addition of zinc ions during the conversion process to form hexamers prevents further degradation of the insulin molecule. Proinsulin does have a small biologic activity, approximately 6 percent of that of the resultant insulin molecule, but probably acts by the same mechanism.[7]

Fifty units of insulin are secreted, on the average, each day by the normal individual. This amount represents approximately one-fifth of the insulin usually stored in the pancreas. In the process of secretion, the secretory granules, or beta granules, migrate to the plasma membrane where the granule's surface membrane fuses with the plasma membrane (see Fig. 4-8). The fused membranes then rupture and the contents of insulin and connecting peptides are released into the pericapillary space concluding the process of exocytosis. Microtubules are implicated in facilitating or directing the movement of the granules toward the cell membrane. The insulin then crosses the basement membrane of a neighboring capillary and the endothelium of the capillary to reach the blood for distribution to the target cells.

Release of Insulin

Stimulative factors and necessary cofactors for the release of insulin appear to be numerous and quite varied. Most of the hormone released is insulin, with proinsulin being secreted into the blood only after a prolonged stimulus for insulin. Insulin is secreted as a direct result of hyperglycemia, and the concentration of insulin parallels that of blood glucose. Indeed the major control of secretion appears to be a feedback mechanism of plasma glucose directly on the pancreas. As the concentration of blood glucose rises, so does the amount of insulin secreted. Similarly, if the concentration of blood glucose falls, so does the amount of insulin secreted.

Glucose is a more potent stimulator if given orally than if given by an intravenous route. The presence of glucose in the duodenum stimulates intestinal factors of gastrin, pancreozymin, secretin, and a glucagon-like polypeptide which also promotes insulin release. Intermediates of glucose metabolism, such as xylitol derived from the pentose phosphate, and readily metabolized sugars, such as mannose and fructose, stimulate insulin release. Non-metabolizable sugars, such as galactose, L-arabinose, and xylose, do not stimulate insulin release. Certain amino acids (especially arginine and leucine), fatty acids (particularly octanoate), ketones, tolbutamide, and β-keto acids also result in insulin secretion.

It appears that diet is an important factor in determining the most potent stimulator for secretion. Studies show that in high-protein diets amino acids are the most potent stimulator, while glucose is a more potent stimulator in high-carbohydrate diets.[8]

Secretion is enhanced by cAMP, glucagon, adrenocorticotrophic hormone (ACTH), and thyrotropin, or potentially any agent that increases the level of intracellular cAMP. Cyclic AMP potentiates the stimulatory effects of glucose or amino cells but is unable to stimulate secretion alone. Growth hormone and glucocorticoids also increase secretion, probably by enhancing the effects of glucose.

Zinc and calcium ions are prerequisites for release, while magnesium ions inhibit secretion. A decrease in the sodium pump or an increase in the concentration of potassium causes immediate release of insulin, while release is blocked by epinephrine and norepinephrine.[9]

The main effects of insulin action are to decrease blood glucose and free fatty acid levels. Insulin also has a stimulatory effect on protein synthesis and works synergistically with growth hormone in this effort. Insulin effects the lowering of blood glucose by promoting its transport across the cellular membrane, and the surface of the cell is felt to be the primary site of insulin action. The interaction of insulin with receptor structures on the cell surface may suffice to elicit the transport and metabolic effects of the hormone. The receptor sites must specifically recognize the insulin molecules and then transfer this information of binding to other molecules. Experiments show that there are receptor sites on lymphocytes, monocytes, fibroblasts, and adipocytes. Very few receptors are located on some cells, averaging as few as 1 per square micrometer of the membrane, leaving an average of 10,000 Å (angstrom) between receptors.[10] Cells having a large number of receptors are more sensitive to insulin than those having only a small number of receptors.

Insulin is particularly effective in skeletal muscle and adipose tissues, probably via a large number of receptors. Insulin also exerts its effects in the heart and certain smooth muscle organs such as the uterus but has no effect in the intestinal mucosa, renal tubular epithelium, or brain cells. The effects of the hormone are uncertain in the remainder of the body, but some probably exist. Liver cells are freely permeable to glucose. However, insulin does have an influence on glucose metabolism in the liver by inducing the synthesis of a specific hexokinase, *glucokinase*, after the diffusion of glucose has taken place across the hepatic cell membranes. This particular enzyme has a much higher K_m for glucose than does the nonspecific hepatic hexokinase and therefore functions primarily when the blood glucose level is elevated.*

Within the cell, insulin has been implicated in enhancing glucose transport through the mitochondrial and endoplasmic reticulum membranes.[12] If the cell membrane is treated with trypsin, the receptor sites are destroyed. Treated cells regenerate new receptor sites at a few percent per hour, which is consistent with the turnover rate of new surface membranes. The evidence supplied by the trypsin study indicates that the receptors are on the outer cell membrane but does not rule out the possibility of internal receptors as well. Studies using protein reagents and enzymes show that tyrosyl and possibly histidyl residues are important in binding interactions. Evidence indicates that sialic acid residues, as well as phospholipids, are present in the receptor molecules. Carbohydrate groups are present but are not directly involved in the insulin binding. Instead they may be involved in conveying the knowledge of binding to adjacent structures.[13]

Insulin promotes all the known pathways of glucose metabolism and storage. It stimulates the formation of glycogen in the liver and therefore influences the activity of glycogen synthetase for this process to occur (see Fig. 4-9). The net effect of insulin is to stimulate glycogen and protein syntheses and to stop glucose output by the liver. As suggested previously, the insulin molecule acts by raising the intracellular cGMP content, which acts as its second messenger, and this explains, in part, the anti-cAMP effect that insulin has in the tissues in which it has any influence.

Glucose enters the cells via a transport mechanism located in the membrane. The carrier substance in the cell membrane transports glucose to the inside of the membrane where it is released into the cytoplasm. Glucose transport is not an *active transport* mechanism; it is a process of *facilitated diffusion*. It does not occur against a concentration gradient; once the glucose

---

* K_m is the concentration of substrate at which half the active sites are filled. It is known as the *Michaelis constant*.[11]

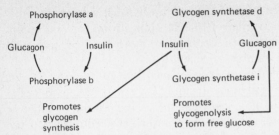

Figure 4-9 Diagram illustrates the influence of insulin and glucagon in the liver on the enzymes which promote glycogen synthesis and glycogenolysis. The two hormones have direct opposite effects on the release or storage of glucose.

concentration inside the cell reaches that of the extracellular fluid (ECF), additional glucose cannot be transported into the cell. Insulin increases the transport of glucose within seconds through its direct action on the membrane itself by means of the fixed receptor sites previously discussed. Cuatrecasas has indicated that a receptor molecule does exist for insulin, a glycoprotein with a molecular weight of 300,000 which may be the glucose carrier itself or simply the first molecule in a series of molecules that transport glucose across the membrane.[14] Once the glucose molecule is within the cell, it is phosphorylated and is ready to move through the metabolic pathways (Fig. 4-2).

In the absence of insulin (and this usually occurs in the normal individual when the blood glucose concentration becomes low), the body is provided with large amounts of glucose by the liver through glycolysis and gluconeogenesis. Phosphorylase is activated by cAMP in the *absence* of insulin and catalyzes the breakdown of glycogen (see Fig. 4-9). Glycogen synthetase, which is the enzyme for glycogen synthesis, is suppressed. Both these effects probably result from increased quantities of cAMP in the liver cells, a situation that occurs when insulin and therefore levels of cGMP are low. Very large amounts of glucose are synthesized in the liver by the process of gluconeogenesis when insulin is low. Amino acids and glycerol from fat are mobilized; these two groups of substances can enter the metabolic pathways at several places and be converted into glucose by the liver. This process can also occur in the kidney. As much as 50 to 100 g of glucose can be made in this way through the influence of glucagon, the hormone synthesized in the alpha cells. Glucagon can cause this effect for weeks at a time in starvation, and it is believed to be responsible for this regulatory mechanism for months and years in a diabetic patient. This process is discussed further in the next section.

Insulin has both a primary and a secondary effect upon fat metabolism. As indicated, insulin influences the movement of glucose into fat cells. Excess glucose in fat and liver cells promotes fat storage and thereby has the secondary effect of "sparing" the fats. Glucose enters the glycolytic pathway in adipose tissue, and large quantities of glyceraldehyde 3-phosphate are formed from the cleavage of fructose 1,6-diphosphate (see Fig. 4-2). Glyceraldehyde

3-phosphate combines with fatty acids to form triglycerides. This breakdown by-product of *carbohydrate* metabolism is necessary for fat storage to take place because once glycerol has been split from triglycerides, it cannot recombine with free fatty acids (FFA) to form *new* triglycerides. The fatty acids are either synthesized within the fat cell itself or obtained from the lipoproteins in the blood by the action of the hormone-sensitive lipase. In the absence of insulin, not only is fat not stored in fat cells, but it is released into the blood as FFA. Normally, FFA are immediately converted into triglycerides and stored again in fat cells. In the absence of insulin, glucose is less readily available, and within a short time the concentration of glyceraldehyde 3-phosphate falls so low that FFA cannot be combined into triglycerides. The FFA then cross through the cell membrane into the blood, combine with albumin to form lipoproteins, and are transported throughout the body. The FFA are used as energy in almost all the cells of the body, with the major exception of the brain cells. Brain cells do use breakdown products of fatty acids for energy in severe starvation. The excess FFA-lipoprotein molecules become a deposition problem in diabetic complications. At optimal concentrations, insulin can cause a thirtyfold increase in fatty acid synthesis and inhibit the lipolytic effects of epinephrine, adrenocorticotrophic hormone, and glucagon.[15]

Insulin has direct effects on protein metabolism, increasing total protein in the body by (1) influencing active transport of amino acids into cells, (2) accelerating the translation of the mRNA code by the ribosomes to form new proteins, and (3) increasing the transcription of DNA in the cell nuclei to form increased RNA, which in turn increases protein synthesis at the ribosomes. A secondary effect is that glucose transported into cells yields many intermediary products that play important controlling roles in cellular metabolism. Insulin works synergistically with growth hormone to affect growth. The two hormones utilize different mechanisms, but a combination of both hormones has a dramatic effect on growth through protein synthesis. The lack of insulin causes wasting of body proteins; amino acids then move into the blood and the level is elevated. These amino acids end up being used for energy or gluconeogenesis. This process becomes one of the most serious complications of diabetes mellitus. It leads to severe weight loss, along with the lipolysis previously indicated; it also leads to weakness and poor functioning of organs resulting from loss of structural and enzyme proteins.

In summary, although the effects of insulin in one part of the body are also apparent in all other parts of the body, major effects seem to be exerted in the liver, muscle, and adipose cells. The overall effects of insulin in all sensitive cells include enhanced carbohydrate metabolism, glycogen storage, fatty acid incorporation into stored fat, amino acid uptake, and protein synthesis.

Glucagon and Its Functions

When insulin was first crystallized, the preparations were found to be contaminated with a hyperglycemic factor identified as a polypeptide hormone, glucagon. This small peptide hormone (see Fig. 4-10) is secreted by the alpha$_2$ cells of the pancreatic islets of Langerhans. Glucagon has several functions completely opposing those of insulin: it raises the blood glucose and FFA concentrations; it acts directly on these processes, stimulating glycogenolysis and lipolysis through cAMP; and it also stimulates gluconeogenesis in the liver. In addition, glucagon seems to function at both ends of the spectrum of carbohydrate availability, serving a dual purpose by functioning as both a hormone of glucose need and a hormone in glucose abundance. If all its actions are mediated by cAMP, then the availability of substrate and the concentration of enzyme, rather than glucagon, may determine its net metabolic effect.

Glucagon is also secreted by alpha cells contained in the stomach and duodenum. It is called "gut glucagon," and one of its probable functions is to trigger insulin release from the pancreas.

Glucagon appears to circulate in plasma in a free state and has a half-life of 5 to 10 min. Glucagon binds avidly to hepatic and renal tissue following injection and is rapidly degraded. Intravenous administration of glucagon leads within minutes to a striking rise in glucose concentrations in the blood. This hyperglycemic response can be accounted for by the augmentation of hepatic glycogenolysis. Sutherland and his colleagues localized the biochemical site of this glycogenolytic action of glucagon at the enzyme adenyl cyclase, the activation leading to the generation of cAMP and then to the activation of the enzyme phosphorylase, which controls the rate-limiting step in hepatic glycogenolysis.

Glucagon is a potent gluconeogenic hormone. Within 45 min of its intravenous injection, amino acid levels in the blood had declined; and in about 1 h, hepatic uptake of amino acids and production of urea had peaked.[16] Glucagon activates adenyl cyclase in the hepatic cell membrane, which causes the formation of cAMP, which activates protein kinase regulator proteins, which activates protein kinases, which activates phosphorylase b kinase, which converts phosphorylase b into phosphorylase a, which promotes the degradation of glycogen into glucose 1-phosphate, which then is dephosphorylated, and glucose is released from the liver cells.

The preceding "cascade" of events is one of the most thoroughly studied of all the second messenger functions of cAMP. The cascading mechanism gives an amplifying effect. After the liver glycogen stores have been depleted, hyperglycemia continues because glucagon increases the rate of gluconeogenesis in the liver cells. This process is thought to be due to (1) the increase in transport of amino acids into the liver, (2) the increase in conversion of amino acids to glucose precursors, (3) the increase in proteolysis in extrahepatic tissues thereby supplying amino acids, and (4) the enhancement

His-Ser-Gln-Gly-Thr-Phe-Thr-Ser-Asp-Tyr-Ser-Lys-Tyr-Leu-Asp-

Ser-Arg-Arg-Ala-Gln-Asp-Phe-Val-Gln-Trp-Leu-Met-Asn-Thr

Figure 4-10 The glucagon molecule is made up of 29 amino acid residues with 15 different amino acids. It is secreted by the alpha cells of the islets of Langerhans in the pancreas as well as by the gastric and duodenal mucosa.

of lipolysis in adipose tissue, providing glyceraldehyde 3-phosphate for gluconeogenesis.

As previously indicated, glucagon directly stimulates lipolysis by fat cells by activating the hormone-sensitive lipase, possibly again via cAMP. (Remember this effect is inhibited by insulin.) Glucagon stimulates the release of both epinephrine, a lipolytic enzyme that elevates FFA in plasma, and insulin, which removes FFA from plasma. Furthermore, there is evidence that glucagon increases utilization of FFA in the liver, which should lower the concentration of FFA in plasma. The effect of "acute" administration of glucagon on ketone bodies is also variable, although chronic therapy with glucagon is consistently ketogenic.[17]

Glucagon has effects on the secretion of other hormones. It has a direct stimulatory effect on the release of insulin from the beta cells of the pancreas. This action has been convincingly demonstrated, both in vivo in humans and in vitro in the isolated perfused pancreas, to be independent of its hyperglycemic action. (This effect leads to the subject of a glucagon/insulin ratio, which will be discussed later.) In dogs the infusion of pharmacologic doses of glucagon caused a rise in the concentration of epinephrine and norepinephrine in plasma, but it is not known if this apparent releasing effect of catecholamines is of physiological importance. Glucagon has a more potent effect on liver glycogenolysis than does epinephrine or norepinephrine. However, epinephrine has a much more potent effect in causing glycogenolysis in muscle cells. Epinephrine also has a far more potent effect in causing fatty acid mobilization from adipose tissue than does glucagon, which has a similar but much weaker effect.[18]

Administration of glucagon alleviated the hypoglycemia of starving, adrenalectomized rats; but in the absence of cortisol, the gluconeogenic effect of glucagon was substantially reduced, in part, perhaps, as a consequence of diminished availability of amino acids. Thus cortisol and glucagon presumably function in concert as gluconeogenic hormones, whereas insulin and growth hormone serve as protein anabolic hormones.

The pharmacologic doses of glucagon also cause a rise in K^+ and a fall in serum PO_4^{3-}. They increase urinary excretion of Na^+, Cl^-, uric acid, HCO_3^-, and water, presumably by increasing glomerular filtration. Large doses of glucagon diminish gastrointestinal motility and gastric secretion and induce anorexia and nausea.

A decrease in blood sugar increases glucagon secretion. When blood glucose falls as low as 70 mg per 100 mL of blood, the pancreas secretes very large quantities of glucagon and this secretion rapidly mobilizes glucose from liver; glucagon protects against hypoglycemia. The normal fasting level of glucagon in human blood ranges from 0.3 to 2.0 mg/mL. At the end of 3 days of complete starvation in normal human volunteers, a rise in levels of glucagon in plasma was observed.[19] Glucagon participates in adjustment to glucose deprivation, particularly during the first 5 days of starvation when cerebral energy needs require that increased gluconeogenesis replace exogenous sources of glucose.

Recent evidence that the infusion of arginine stimulated glucagon secretion is also in keeping with this gluconeogenic role.[20] Glucagon also plays a role in releasing insulin after an oral load of glucose. Glucose in the gastrointestinal tract causes the release of a local intestinal glucagon-like immunoreactive substance rather than the release of glucagon from the alpha cells of the pancreas.

In summary, glucagon increases the blood glucose concentration by breaking down glycogen stores and accelerating the formation of new glucose through gluconeogenesis, the process of utilizing amino acids, glycerol, and other precursor molecules such as pyruvate and lactate to make glucose.

THEORY OF DISEASE

Regulation of Blood Glucose Concentration

Five hormones are involved in the control of blood glucose levels: insulin, glucagon, growth hormone, epinephrine, and the glucocorticoids (collectively called cortisol). Insulin and glucagon are secreted by the islets of Langerhans of the pancreas. Growth hormone is secreted by the anterior pituitary gland, with the ultimate control of its secretion through two peptide hormones of the hypothalamus: a somatotrophic stimulating hormone and a somatotrophic inhibitory secretion, *somatostatin.* Epinephrine is from the adrenal medulla, and cortisol is from the cortex of the adrenal gland. Of these five hormones, insulin is the only one that lowers blood glucose; the other four hormones elevate the blood glucose level. Somatostatin does not directly affect the blood glucose level but has its controlling effects on the secretion of insulin and glucagon. Its interesting effects will be discussed later.

Insulin   Diabetes mellitus includes many biochemical abnormalities, but the essential sign of diabetes is sustained hyperglycemia, i.e., an elevated blood glucose level. These abnormalities are often attributed to an *inadequate* secretion of insulin or to a partial or total lack of *functioning* insulin. The change in the plasma levels of insulin is abnormal in response to carbohydrate loads in both the obese and diabetic patients. Thus the insulin defect could be due to a failure in its synthesis, release, or action; an altered insulin molecule has also been implied from several research endeavors.[21,22] Exciting advances have been made in this area, and it now appears that a specific receptor may be present on the membrane surface of the beta cell which recognizes and interacts with glucose. The interaction of glucose and the specific receptor initiates the formation of chemical messengers that convey this information to certain organelles with the resultant release of the appropriate number of packets of stored insulin molecules into the blood. Calcium appears to be one of the intracellular messengers; it then reacts with a contractile protein in the beta cells causing the protein to contract and move packets of insulin to the surface where they are ejected into the fluid surrounding the beta cell. These contractile proteins are probably the microtubules and microfilaments that have been mentioned before (see Fig. 4-8). It has been shown experimentally in the spiny mouse, which has a hereditary form of diabetes, that the beta cells are deficient in the contractile protein responsible for the movement of the packets of insulin to the cell surface.

When plasma levels of insulin are monitored in relation to blood glucose concentrations it is found that the *overt* diabetic patient has a slower, reduced secretion of insulin in response to glucose intake. The obese person has a nearly normal glucose tolerance, but it is achieved with a very high insulin level. The obese, mildly diabetic individual shows a slower but still higher rise in plasma insulin, which is associated with hyperglycemia and a slow recovery. It would appear that the concentration of circulating insulin, measured by radioimmunoassay, is not always indicative of physiologically active hormone.

In spite of hyperglycemia, cells are deficient in glucose and are living essentially in a low-carbohydrate, high-fat energy supply, resulting in ketosis. Diabetes mellitus is an intracellular starvation resulting from insufficient insulin. In muscle, glucose utilization diminishes with a decrease in the activity of the glycolytic pathway. The metabolic needs of muscle are then met by increased utilization of FFA and/or ketone bodies. Similar amounts of amino acids are taken up, but increased amounts are released into the blood. In adipose tissue, glucose uptake and utilization also decrease as the activity of the Embden-Meyerhof pathway decreases and formation of glyceraldehyde 3-phosphate and the pentose shunt are curtailed. Triglycerides are released in increasing amounts into the blood as FFA.

In diabetes, metabolism of glucose in the liver becomes almost completely production of glucose. The increased level of amino acids and FFA in the blood, coupled with a decrease in the breakdown of glucose, enhances gluconeogenesis. As a result of the influx of FFA, the formation and release of ketone bodies increase. The increased FFA and ketone body production (see Fig. 4-11) seem to inhibit the enzyme citrate synthetase, with the resulting diminished conversion of oxaloacetate with acetyl-CoA to citrate in the Krebs cycle (see Fig. 4-3). Acetyl-CoA cannot be utilized through the aerobic glycolytic pathway, so it piles up and is diverted into ketone bodies. Note the close interplay between gluconeogenesis and ketogenesis. Is the hormone glucagon the culprit in this pathophysiological collaboration?

Glucagon The hyperglycemia of diabetes mellitus results partly from increased hepatic glucose output and partly from underutilization. All the substrates supplied to the liver from the periphery, i.e., the increased amino acids and FFA released from muscle and adipose tissue, certainly play an important role in regulating glucose production. The regulatory effects of hormones, especially insulin and glucagon, on hepatic glucose production and release are most important. The role of glucagon in particular has become interesting. Unger suggests that insulin deficiency alone does not account for the hyperglycemia in diabetes.[23] An excess of glucagon is thought to be at least partially responsible for the high glucose levels seen in diabetics. As mentioned before, high levels of glucagon stimulate the release of glucose from the glyco-

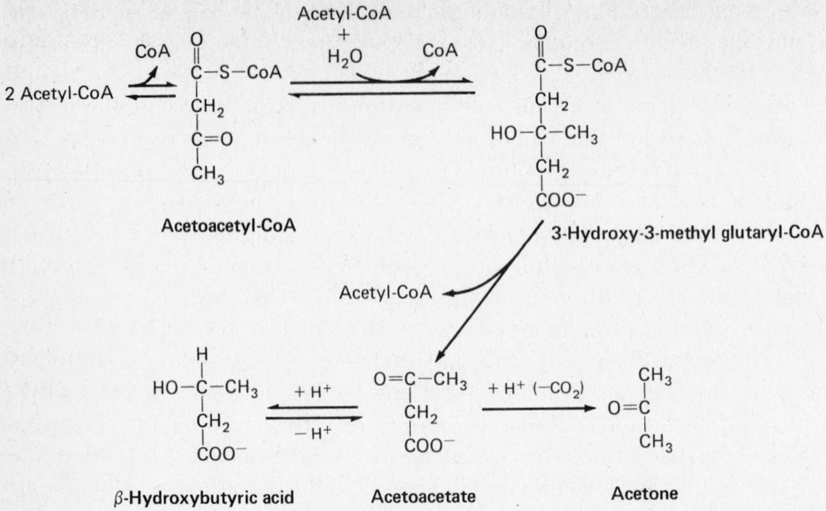

Figure 4-11 Ketone bodies are formed from excess acetyl-CoA. After the combining of three and then the deletion of one molecule of acetyl-CoA, acetoacetate is formed. When acetoacetate is reduced (that is, hydrogen is added), β-hydroxybutyrate is formed; when acetoacetate is decarboxylated (that is, a carbon dioxide group is removed), the end product is acetone. (*Adapted from L. Stryer, "Biochemistry," San Francisco, Freeman, 1975.*)

gen stores and cause the production of new glucose from the supply of FFA and amino acids made available because of the lack of insulin.

An increase in serum amino acids stimulates pancreatic glucagon. Arginine was shown to stimulate glucagon release in rat pancreas.[24] The primary metabolic effect of glucagon is hyperglycemia as a result of increased glycogenolysis and gluconeogenesis, as previously indicated. When glucose needs are not being met, glucagon first increases hepatic production by glycogenolysis and then later promotes the synthesis of new glucose from nonglucose precursors. These effects come about through the activation of adenyl cyclase and an increase in the amount of cAMP in the hepatocytes.[25] Glucagon appears to exert its effects in glycogenolysis on the enzymatic steps between glucose 1-phosphate and glycogen to decrease the glycogen content in liver. Cyclic AMP conveys the message delivered by glucagon at the membrane to the effector enzymes in the cytoplasm, which results in the stimulation of phosphorylase activity and depression of glycogen synthetase activity[26] (see Fig. 4-9). This action promotes the phosphorylytic breakdown to glycogen to glucose 1-phosphate, to glucose 6-phosphate, and, finally, to glucose, with the catalysis by phosphoglucomutase and glucose 6-phosphatase, respectively. Glucagon has no effect on the glycogen stores in skeletal muscle.[27]

Glucagon stimulates lipolysis in adipocytes;[28] this mechanism is also mediated through cAMP. As glycogen stores are depleted, lipids are hydrolyzed to glycerol and fatty acids; the glycerol can take part in gluconeogenesis along with amino acid precursors pyruvate and lactate.

The significance of an insulin/glucagon ratio is emphasized by Unger.[29] He believes that the ability of the body to change from a low insulin/glucagon ratio when fuel is unavailable to a very high ratio when fuel is abundant is a sign of good health. The inability to respond to fuel availability is seen in uncontrolled diabetes mellitus, acute injury, and severe infections. In these catabolic diseases, the insulin/glucagon ratio remains low, with the consequence of inappropriate production of glucose from endogenous sources even though exogenous glucose is in sufficient supply. Amino acids are not converted to new proteins, and the person is in negative nitrogen balance and exhibits weight loss.

Somatostatin A major breakthrough came several years ago when a recently isolated hormone, somatostatin, was found to suppress both insulin and glucagon. It was then possible to vary the concentrations of insulin and glucagon independently and investigate the effects. It quickly became apparent that glucagon plays a crucial role in the pathology of diabetes. The somatostatin-induced suppression of glucagon release in diabetic humans and animals restores blood sugar concentrations to normal and alleviates certain other symptoms of diabetes.[30] Glucagon and insulin appear to coexist in a delicate balance (ratio); high concentrations of insulin suppress glucagon release and low concentrations stimulate glucagon release. It has been shown that hyperglucagonemia occurs in conjunction with diabetic insulin deficiency in humans and in dogs and rats with chemically induced diabetes. Hyperglucagonemia has also been observed in association with stress hyperglycemia caused by severe injuries, burns, heart attacks, and hemorrhagic shock. An increased concentration of glucagon accompanying hyperglycemia might be an effect rather than a cause, but there was no way to examine this role until the discovery of somatostatin.

Somatostatin is a 14-amino-acid peptide with a disulfide bond between the third and last amino acid (see Fig. 4-12). It was first isolated from sheep brain, and the first effect observed was the inhibition of the release of somatotropin (the growth hormone from the anterior pituitary gland). It is also produced in cells of the pancreas near the alpha and beta cells that secrete glucagon and insulin. Another observation made was that the concentration of glucose in baboon blood fell during the administration of somatostatin. It was then noticed that with appropriate doses of somatostatin the secretion of both insulin and glucagon could be completely and quickly inhibited. The site of action of somatostatin is the pancreas. The important aspect of the suppression of insulin release is that hyperglycemia was not produced if glucagon release was suppressed also. There is a rapid appearance of hyperglycemia if somatostatin

H-Ala-Gly-Cys-Lys-Asn-Phe-Phe-Trp-Lys-Thr-Phe-Thr-Ser-Cys-OH

Figure 4-12 The 14 amino acids making up somatostatin, the somatotrophic inhibitory releasing hormone, are shown here. A disulfide bond exists between the two cysteine residues. Somatostatin influences the blood glucose level indirectly by its action on the secretion of insulin and glucagon.

and glucagon are given simultaneously, and it cannot be alleviated by a simultaneous infusion of insulin. It was also shown that when glucagon was infused into laboratory animals a hyperglycemia was observed that could not be abolished by insulin. These findings suggest that glucagon may be even more important than insulin in the maintenance of normal levels of glucose in the blood.

In healthy individuals it has been demonstrated that somatostatin reduces the concentrations of glucagon, insulin, and glucose in the blood. All these results suggest that reduction of glucagon concentrations in the blood with somatostatin should alleviate the symptoms of diabetes, and this, in fact, has been shown by Gerich.[31]

All the preceding findings strongly indicate that the presence of a relative or absolute excess of glucagon is an essential factor in the development of diabetes. The most reasonable conclusion might be that the major role of insulin is the regulation of the transfer of glucose from the blood to storage in insulin-responsive tissues such as liver, fat, and muscle. The role of glucagon, however, is the regulation of the liver-mediated mobilization of stored glucose so that the glucose can be used by vital tissues, such as the brain, in times of stress, including starvation. The principal consequence of insufficient insulin in the blood would then be a reduced rate of removal of glucose from the blood, which would be manifested as hyperglycemia after meals. The consequence of a high concentration of glucagon in the blood would be the liver-mediated release of an inappropriately high concentration of glucose in the blood, producing a persistent hyperglycemia.

Glucagon also appears to regulate the oxidation of fatty acids in the liver and is probably involved in ketoacidosis, with the increased production of ketone bodies. Release of ketone bodies lowers the pH of the blood, inducing coma and possibly death. There was a definite correlation shown between the concentrations of glucagon and ketone bodies in a group of patients with ketoacidosis in experiments conducted by a group of investigators in England. It has also been reported that when insulin is withdrawn from insulin-dependent diabetics, there are increases in the concentrations of many compounds associated with ketoacidosis, e.g., β-hydroxybutyric acid, free fatty acids (FFA), and glycerol, that can be correlated with the increase of glucagon in the blood.

Conventional therapy for ketoacidosis is administration of insulin. The primary effect of insulin is probably suppression of the release of glucagon, but insulin can only mediate a limited reduction of glucagon. It would seem that a more effective therapy might be the administration of somatostatin. One laboratory has recently demonstrated that infusion of somatostatin prevents development of ketoacidosis in insulin-dependent diabetics deprived of insulin. Some drawbacks to giving this peptide are (1) it has a very short half-life of 4 min; (2) it can be given only by infusion; (3) it is difficult to give to young diabetics because it is antagonistic to growth hormone; and (4) it has caused some hemorrhages in experimental animals by interfering with the aggregation of platelets for clotting. The last drawback has been disputed by Gerich and his associates.

Epinephrine   Epinephrine opposes the action of insulin by causing glycogen breakdown in the liver and muscle and plasma glucose increases. Epinephrine inhibits the release of insulin from the pancreas, and it stimulates the breakdown of triglycerides in fat tissue by increasing the activity of the hormone-sensitive lipase. This hormone is reflexly released by the preganglionic sympathetic nerves to the adrenal medulla in response to exercise, pain, hypotension, and stress. Studies indicate that the autonomic nervous system has a modulating effect on insulin secretion and may play a role in the causation or enhancement of the severity of diabetes. A low plasma glucose level stimulates epinephrine release, and this response is probably mediated through a glucose receptor in the brain (hypothalamus).

Growth Hormone   When there is an overproduction of growth hormone, the individual will not only exhibit excessive growth but also diabetes. Growth hormone increases adipose tissue breakdown of triglycerides, releasing fatty acids into the blood, and inhibits the uptake and oxidation of glucose by many body tissues. The only effect that growth hormone and insulin have in common is the transfer of amino acids into the cells. Growth hormone acts like glucagon and epinephrine and is considered a hyperglycemic stimulant.

Cortisol   Like growth hormone, cortisol is a potent inhibitor of glucose uptake by many tissues; it therefore elevates blood glucose levels. It is required for normal gluconeogenesis in the liver, and it facilitates the conversion of amino acids into glucose by the liver, as well as the breakdown of muscle protein. Glucose levels do not determine the secretion of cortisol, but stress would be a very important factor in its release via ACTH from the anterior pituitary gland.

From the preceding considerations of the interactions of the various hormones it would appear that a very delicate balance is maintained in regulating blood glucose concentrations in the healthy individual. LaVia and Hill believe that some of the inherited disorders of metabolism may actually represent a variety of different biochemical lesions that give rise to a common clinical picture.[32] Diabetes mellitus may prove to consist of a group of genetically, etiologically, and pathogenically distinct metabolic disorders involving all the regulators discussed.

CHANGES AT THE CELLULAR LEVEL

As implied previously, changes can occur in the normal secretion of the various regulators of blood glucose concentrations, particularly insulin, which is needed to transport glucose into about 65 percent of the cells that make up the body weight. Various causal theories as to what would make a change in secretion will be discussed later. A thickening of the basement membrane in the capillaries becomes very evident in diabetes mellitus and has been described as a duplicated basement membrane, i.e., the cell appears to lay down two such membranes. As to which comes first, the laying down of the thickened membrane and the inability of glucose to be transported through it or a change in the cellular metabolism due to an overabundance of glucose that diverted derivatives of glucose metabolism into a duplication of the existing membrane, who is to say?

With the lack of insulin, storage of fat does not occur in the adipose tissue, so FFA are available to be broken down by the liver and rebuilt into cholesterol, new triglycerides (not stored), and ketone bodies. All these end products of abnormal excessive precursors for fatty deposits are poured into the blood and do great harm in a variety of tissues. Along with the production of faulty fat products, a second process known as gluconeogenesis is occurring. Normal gluconeogenesis is a protective mechanism to make glucose for the brain in periods of normal fast; excessive gluconeogenesis, with the depletion of necessary structural and enzymatic proteins, is a pathological complication of diabetes mellitus.

With insulin either deficient or defective in its activities, many intermediate products pile up from the inability of the metabolic pathways to operate because of missing or deficient enzymes. This so-called metabolic debris is not easily removed from the cells and ends up as unwanted deposits in or near the cell membranes. Let us look at some of these cellular changes in more detail.

Basement Membrane

Utilizing a light microscope, the normal basement membrane appears as a homogeneous unit situated between the epithelial and endothelial capillary cells. This membrane appears to be 1 to 2 μm in diameter. With the advent of the electron microscope, a meshwork of fine filaments was found to be embedded in the homogeneous substance. Utilizing the highest power of resolution, the basement membrane was found to be a few hundred angstroms thick in blood vessels and between 200 and 400 Å in the renal glomeruli.[33]

The basement membrane is composed of two types of carbohydrate units, both of which are bound to a peptide chain. The first is a heteropolysaccharide unit composed of sialic acid, fucose, galactose, mannose, and/or hexosamines. The usual makeup is three molecules of galactose, three of mannose, five of N-acetylglucosamine, three of sialic acid, and one of fucose, resulting in a molecular weight of 3200. This heteropolysaccharide is a branched structure with a sequence of sialic acid or fucose, galactose, and N-acetylglucosamine linked to an inner core of mannose and N-acetylglucosamine. The first carbon in the inner glucosamine is linked to an asparagine in the peptide chain. The second basic unit is a disaccharide unit. A glucose molecule via a glycosidic bond is linked to the second carbon in a galactose molecule. The galactose molecule is, in turn, linked by a glycosidic bond to a hydroxyl group of a hydroxylysine residue in the peptide chain (see Ref. 33). The basement membrane does not usually contain any lipids or mucopolysaccharides. Approximately one-fifth of the amino acid residues in the peptide chain are glycine; there are also substantial amounts of hydroxyproline and hydroxylysine. Vascular basement membrane is produced by the endothelial and smooth muscle cells in larger blood vessels and by pericytes in smaller vessels. The glomerular basement membrane is produced within the cisternae of the endoplasmic reticulum of the epithelial cells. The basement membrane is insoluble at physiologic pH, but it may be digested by mild alkali and digestive enzymes. This membrane acts both as a supportive structure and as a selective filter; it must be traversed by diffusing molecules into the cells.[34]

Structure of the Diabetic Basement Membrane Biosynthesis of glycoproteins in general, and specifically of those in the basement membrane, is related to carbohydrate metabolism. The exact relationship between the altered carbohydrate metabolism in the diabetic and the unusually thick basement membrane is not established fact. In skin the thickened basement membrane is manifested in two ways. The first, and more common, type shows a stratified pattern with several concentric layers resembling the original "normal" membrane. These layers alternate with less electron-dense layers in which single filaments, intermingled with collagen fibrils, are only occasionally seen. The second type shows a more uniform composition of a loose, but sometimes compact, granular texture. These changes are unevenly distributed, often being more evident on one side of a capillary. Although it is hard to distinguish, the thickening seems to extend from the capillary into both arterioles and venules. In severe cases the thickening may be 10 times greater than normal. In interstitial capillaries of skeletal muscle, the widened basement membrane is characterized by redundant bands of amorphous basement membrane material between muscle fibers, and strands of endothelial cytoplasm project intraluminally. Enlarged vesicles, and in some cases small, oval subsarcolemmal nuclei with masses of electron-dense vacuolated material, are seen in the cytoplasm. Myofibrils may be replaced by irregular areas of granular sarcoplasm. Many of the capillary basement membranes are laminated and contain strands of collagen and unidentified oval structures with granular contents. In other areas, fragments of endothelial and pericapillary cell cytoplasm were found within the layers of the basement membrane. No differences could be seen in the mitochondrial membranes.[35]

The changed material found in diabetic vessels stains solidly periodic acid Schiff (PAS)-positive, while nondiabetic vessels show only a PAS coating. This finding suggests the presence of increased amounts of carbohydrates within the membrane. These membranes fail to react with colloidal iron stain, again suggesting the composition to be that of a neutral polysaccharide or mucoprotein.[36]

Proposed Theories of Basement Membrane Thickening Within the body there are three types of cells in regard to insulin and glucose utilization. In cells such as muscle, insulin is needed for glucose to penetrate the cell membrane but has no effect on the phosphorylation of the glucose once it is within the cell. Other cells such as hepatocytes are freely permeable to glucose, but they do require insulin for induction of the synthesis of a specific hexokinase glucokinase. This kinase is then responsible for the utilization of glucose and storage of glycogen in the liver. Finally there are cells (brain, kidney, lens, and blood vessels) that are freely permeable to glucose and are able to utilize glucose without the aid of insulin. They would also be subjected to very high levels of glucose when the blood glucose level is elevated with no control of concentration resulting from gradient or active transport mechanisms. In the diabetic state the third pattern is favored, resulting in increased glycoprotein synthesis, including those within the basement membrane. However, the rate of basement membrane degradation is very slow, and has been shown to be even slower in the diabetic rat as compared with the normal rat. The net result of increased production and decreased removal is the accumulation and widening of this membrane.[37]

In contrast, Vracko holds that the basal lamina provide a microskeleton for cellular regeneration. The thickening is due to an accumulation of an abnormally large number of normal basal lamina, each layer being deposited by a new cell generation. This theory depends on an accelerated rate of cell turnover, which to date is unsupported and requires further evaluation and documentation.[38]

Those who accept the genetic theory believe that microangiopathy is not a complication but rather a concomitant of the diabetic state. A single gene or, more likely, multiple genes determine both the vascular changes and the alterations in carbohydrate metabolism. The evidence usually cited to support this hypothesis is the occurrence of the lesions in those individuals with a family history (and therefore a genetic predisposition) but without any signs of metabolic alterations or clinical diabetes. Arguments against this proposal include the fact that characteristic diabetic lesions occur in diabetes resulting from trauma or pancreatectomy and hence lack any genetic predisposition to the disease.[39]

One of the more recently proposed and fascinating theories is that of the *sorbitol* pathway, which is thought to be responsible for the metabolism of excess glucose in non-insulin-dependent tissues. Being insulin-independent, this pathway is not rate limited by glucose transport and may be accelerated in the presence of *excess* glucose. The pathway is a two-step procedure (see Fig. 4-14). Aldose reductase is a nonspecific enzyme that may react with many aldoses. It normally has a low affinity for glucose and galactose. In the diabetic state the activity of large pools of free intracellular aldoses (excess glucose) results in a shift in the first reaction to the right, forming large quantities of sugar alcohols, specifically sorbitol and possibly galactitol. Sugar alcohols penetrate cell membranes poorly and hence must go through the second reaction, which is slow in most tissues, and slowly leak out of the cell or accumulate within the cell. The accumulation results in hypertonicity within the cell and osmotic swelling.

Another theory, put forth by Spiro and others, deals directly with the biosynthesis of the capillary basement membrane. Although the biosynthesis is not fully understood, many steps appear to be open to or controlled by environmental influences. Besswenger and Spiro believe that the overall rate of synthesis is determined by the availability of sugar moieties for attachment to the peptide chain.[40] Since glucose is thought to be shunted into insulin-independent glycoprotein formation in the diabetic state, this rate-limiting step will be accelerated. It has been determined that in the diabetic membrane there are increased quantities of hydroxylysine residues in the peptide chain, the site of the disaccharide unit linkage. In the normal membrane there are 11.3 disaccharide units for each heteropolysaccharide unit. In the diabetic this ratio is increased to 14.6:1.

Two specific glycosyl transferases are responsible for the assembly of the disaccharide unit. The activity of the first, UDP-glucose:galactosyl hydroxylysine–basement membrane glycosyl transferase, has been shown to increase in diabetic rats. This increased activity further increases with age and/or duration of diabetes. Insulin therapy is effective in returning this enzyme to normal levels of normal weight and blood glucose levels are maintained. Insulin therapy is less effective if it is delayed by a period of no treatment. Studies also indicate that the second enzyme, galactosyl transferase, which attaches the galactose to hydroxylysine, is also elevated in the diabetic patient. Unfortunately, the normal level of this enzyme is so low, and further decreases with age, that it has not been possible to accurately measure it to date. UDP-galactose:N-acetylglucosamine glycoprotein galactosyl transferase, an enzyme responsible for the synthesis of asparagine-linked carbohydrate units, does not show increased amounts of activity. All these proposals and findings are consistent with the clinical observations of an increased number of hydroxylysine-linked disaccharide units but no increase in the asparagine-linked heteropolysaccharide units.[41]

Vascular Lesions

Warren et al. believe that the complications demonstrated as vascular lesions are a direct result of the altered carbohydrate metabolism.[42] They have found that α_2-globulin levels of serum, the *seromucoid* fraction of serum, and the urinary excretion of polysaccharides were elevated. They have also found that the level of protein-bound hexoses was elevated and was in direct relationship to the severity of vascular changes. A mechanism to account for these elevations has yet to be proposed.

Proposed Theories of Vascular Changes   Immunologists also have an explanation for vascular changes. This group of scientists believes that the lesions represent an accumulation of insulin-insulin antibody complexes, specifically of the IgG and IgM varieties. Studies have shown that the vascular lesions specifically bind fluorescent-conjugated insulin, fluorescent-conjugated antihuman globulin, and complement. Support for this view can be found in the fact that if a rabbit is immunized with an insulin-adjuvant mixture for a 30-month period and then challenged with small doses of insulin every other day for 6 weeks, proliferative vascular lesions identical to those of the diabetic are produced. Support is also given by the fact that similar lesions are also found in chronic glomerulonephritis, systemic lupus erythematosus, rheumatoid arthritis, and malignant lymphoma, all of which have a strong autoimmune component. Those who argue against this theory point to the fact that insulin naturally sticks to anything. Because of this property, it is argued that the proposed antibody-insulin binding is not a specific immunologic binding.[43]

Many investigators think that the small vessel disease is a continuation of the large vessel arteriosclerosis. Diabetes, in disrupting the carbohydrate metabolism, also affects lipid metabolism, as discussed before. Insulin normally inhibits lipase in adipose tissue, and in the relative absence of insulin, the plasma levels of FFA are usually more than doubled. The FFA levels often parallel the blood glucose levels. In addition, there are increased cholesterol synthesis, increased levels of nonesterified and esterified fatty acids, and elevated triglycerides. It appears that early, severe atherosclerosis of large vessels develops because of the altered carbohydrate and lipid metabolism; it also seems almost conclusive that the microvascular disease is not an extension of the same mechanism. The characteristic lesion of the microvascular disease is a thickened basement membrane, not plaque formation.

Effects of the Peripheral Vascular Lesions   Although the basement membrane is thickened in the diabetic state, it is also leaky and functions imperfectly as a filter, giving further evidence of a structural defect. Within the glomerulus, the vascular lesions result in increased rates of albumin excretion, β_2-microglobulin excretion, and glomerular filtration, with an increased albumin/β_2-microglobulin ratio. In dermal capillaries there are increased capillary filtration coefficients and transcapillary escape ratios of albumin. The increased urinary protein excretion is interpreted as evidence of a functional abnormality of the glomerular membrane causing increased permeability. The increased β_2-microglobulin excretion rate indicates a decreased renal tubular reabsorption for protein. The increased transcapillary escape rate of albumin represents an increased extravasation of albumin.[44]

Banson and Lacy, while studying the capillaries of toes, speculated that the thickened basement membrane might interfere with the normal exchange of substances and predispose to the development of infections and gangrene.[45] The widening of the capillary basement membrane could physiologically embarrass oxygen diffusion and excretion of metabolic wastes. Diffusion constants of the basement membrane are unknown at the present time, so it is impossible to measure the magnitude of the proposed disruptions. It has also been shown that diabetic capillaries fail to respond to vasodilating agents, probably because of the thickened basement membrane. In the peripheral vessels of the lower extremities of people with long-standing diabetes mellitus, when sodium and iodide tracer substances are injected into the anterior tibial muscle, an increase in permeability to inorganic ions occurs, and yet, a decrease in permeability to water molecules is seen. It is probable that in the diabetic state there is a new distribution of pores, with more small pores and fewer large ones. These changes result in a decreased permeability to proteins.[46]

In conclusion, large vascular disease appears to be due to plaque formation, as in atherosclerosis, but at an unusually early age. It seems reasonable to assume that this plaque formation is due to the altered lipid metabolism. Many attribute the peripheral neuropathy to a compromised blood supply to the peripheral nerves. Within recent years, others attribute the neuropathy to cellular swelling resulting from the sorbitol pathway. Perhaps the most perplexing problem is that of microvascular disease. Our knowledge of normal basement membrane formation, structure, and metabolism is incomplete. The altered enzyme levels and activity appear to be most consistent with histologic and chemical changes.

Cellular Changes Due to Metabolic, Hormonal, and Nutritional Influences Leading to "-opathies"

The changes in secretion from the beta and alpha cells in diabetes mellitus would appear to be a relative lack of functioning insulin and an increased level of circulating glucagon. All of the effects from these changes have been discussed in previous sections. Some of the basic cell changes have been elaborated, and now those changes will be discussed more explicitly in relation to pathologic alterations in the cells that appear to be insulin-independent in respect to glucose utilization.

Microcirculatory Alterations Leading to Diabetic "Triopathy" When the specific complications of diabetes in humans are discussed, the term *triopathy* is given to the pathologic involvements of the eyes (*retinopathy*), the kidneys (*nephropathy*), and the nervous system (*neuropathy*). These complications will be discussed further in Chapter 10.

Neuropathy Almost 100 percent of diabetic patients have one or more alterations in their peripheral nerves. The common pattern is "mixed distal polyneuropathy." A number of different nerves are involved which supply the peripheral tissues, mainly the lower limbs, and affect mainly sensation first, motor responses later, and leading, as the lesion progresses, to total anesthesia. The autonomic nervous system is involved; and since this "vegetative" nervous system involves many basic functions, such as movement of food through the gastrointestinal tract, contraction of the urinary bladder, opening of urethral valves for urination, and, in the male, erection and ejaculation, the sequelae of autonomic neuropathy are manifold.

The basic physiological interrelationships between Schwann cells, the axons of the nerve cells, and the nerve cell viability and function are not known; nor is it known whether the primary lesion in the diabetic patient is in the axon or in the Schwann cell or, possibly, in the myelin, which is supposedly produced by the Schwann cell. Spritz focused on the level of myelin in diabetic nerve and found that it decreased in humans and experimental diabetic animals, as it also does in aged humans. More recent studies in animals have shown a number of metabolic deficiencies, such as the rate of protein synthesis. The parallel of age and diabetes may explain the higher susceptibility of middle-

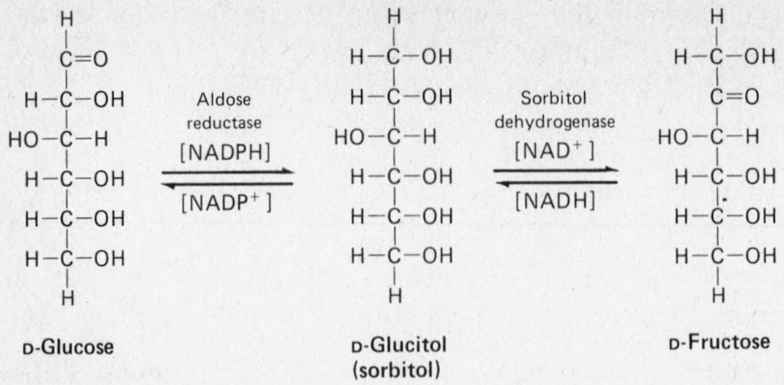

Figure 4-13 This polyol pathway, the interconversion of D-glucose and D-fructose by way of D-glucitol (sorbitol), may be the source of D-fructose in cerebrospinal and seminal fluids. The pathway exists in many tissues, including those of the peripheral nerves, and it may be important in diabetic patients in whom episodes of hyperglycemia are common.

aged and older diabetic patients to distal polyneuropathy than of children with more severe degrees of insulin deficiency. Gabbay has studied the accumulation of sorbitol, an abnormal by-product of glucose metabolism (see Fig. 4-13), and has correlated its accumulation with delayed nerve conduction velocity in experimental diabetic animals. He also has been successful in using chemical agents to block the enzyme system responsible for sorbitol synthesis (administration of 3,3-tetramethylene glutaric acid inhibits aldose reductase). Winegrad studied another material, myoinositol, which is similar to sorbitol but, in contrast, is deficient in diabetic nerve. When the animal is supplemented with myoinositol, the delayed nerve conduction velocity is corrected. Finally, Matschinsky has demonstrated that the rate of flow of nutrients and other materials from the cell body in the spinal cord along the axon is delayed in diabetic nerve and has suggested that the delayed axonal flow may play a role in the etiology of diabetic neuropathy.[47]

Neuropathy, in general, is associated with poorly controlled diabetes, and there is evidence that those who are under careful control have a lower incidence of this complication. The brain, along with the rest of the body, develops widespread microangiopathy. Such microcirculatory lesions may lead to generalized neuronal degeneration. There is a predisposition to cerebral vascular infarcts and brain hemorrhages, perhaps related to the hypertension seen so often in diabetes. In addition, hypoglycemia and ketoacidosis may both damage brain cells. Degenerative changes also have been observed in the spinal cord. None of these neurologic disorders, though, are specific for diabetes mellitus.[48]

Neuropathy has subsided with improvement in blood glucose level control, although unfortunately it has also occurred and become very serious in individuals who have been thought to be under good control. Some physicians have used vitamin B-complex, and, specifically, injections of vitamin B_{12} have been helpful in some patients. Some investigators have suggested the use of another alcohol, myoinositol (related to one of the components of vitamin B-complex), which seems to aid the transmission and velocity of a nerve impulse.

Pancreatic Changes

The pancreas may show no anatomic changes, as in mild maturity-onset diabetes, or there may be slight atrophy of the islets of Langerhans, as seen in aged nondiabetic individuals. However, in the great majority of patients, one or more characteristic alterations are usually evident: (1) reduction in the size and number of islets; (2) increase in the size and number of islets (this is seen in nondiabetic newborn of diabetic mothers; the hyperplasia is in response to the mother's hyperglycemia); (3) beta-cell degranulation resulting in depletion of stored insulin; (4) glycogen accumulation within the beta cells reflecting poor control with long periods of hyperglycemia; (5) amyloid replacement of the islets—virtual islet obliteration with a fill-in of pink amorphous material; and (6) leukocytic infiltration of the islets resulting from insulitis seen in growth-onset diabetes due to a possible autoimmune reaction.

Depressed Glucose Metabolism

In diabetes mellitus with a relative lack of insulin, the major abnormalities are an uncontrolled and accelerated rate of lipid catabolism and an increase in the rate of ketone body formation. The excess free fatty acids in the blood cause an inherent depression of cellular glucose utilization along with the severe depression of glucose metabolism resulting from the direct effect of insulin lack.

On entering the cells, the excess fatty acids are immediately catabolized in the mitochondria to acetyl-CoA. This molecule enters the Krebs cycle and provides energy required by the cell (see Fig. 4-3). Second, two of the important products of this energy process are citrate and ATP, both of which have a strong inhibitory effect on phosphofructokinase, the enzyme required to initiate glycolysis in the cell. Therefore, the use of glucose for energy almost ceases, and consequently, glucose uptake and utilization by the cells are further depressed.[49] The preceding process is referred to as the *glucose–fatty acid cycle*. It approximately doubles the depressive effect of insulin lack on cellular uptake and utilization of glucose.

KETOACIDOSIS
Anabolic Insulin Effects

In adipose tissue, fatty acids under the influence of insulin are synthesized from acetyl-CoA and malonyl-CoA in the cytoplasm of the cells. A high concentration of glyceraldehyde 3-phosphate is formed from glycolysis (see Fig. 4-2). This 3-carbon phosphorylated molecule combines with the fatty acids, and the triglycerides thus formed are stored rather than released from the adipocytes. Insulin inhibits the breakdown of fatty acids and their release because of its inhibitory effect upon the hormone-sensitive lipase of adipose tissue. It also prevents free fatty acids from accumulating in the blood and liver (which is the secondary place for new triglyceride synthesis to take place). Normal triglyceride levels in the blood are maintained by removal of fatty substances due to the activity of lipoprotein lipase, which is activated by insulin.

Insulin has three major effects on fat metabolism: (1) it stimulates the production of glyceraldehyde 3-phosphate, which is then utilized in triglyceride synthesis; (2) it inhibits the action of the hormone-sensitive lipase of adipose tissue preventing an excess of FFA in the blood and liver; and (3) it activates lipoprotein lipase to maintain optimum levels of lipoprotein substances in the circulation.

Ketosis

Many of the fatty acids that enter the liver are oxidized to form acetyl-CoA; and this, in turn, is converted to acetoacetyl-CoA. Acetoacetyl-CoA is converted in turn into acetoacetic acid. Normally, most of the acetoacetic acid is released into the circulating blood and passes into the peripheral cells where it is converted again to acetyl-CoA and used for energy in the usual manner. However, in insulin lack the acetoacetic acid concentration rises (as FFA are mobilized from the adipose tissue) in far greater quantity than can be used for energy elsewhere in the body. A small increase occurs in acetoacetic acid almost immediately after the onset of insulin lack and is followed by a much greater increase after several days of insulin deficiency, as often occurs in severe diabetes mellitus. Some of the acetoacetic acid is then reduced to β-hydroxybutyric acid or decarboxylated to acetone (see Fig. 4-11). These three molecules, acetoacetic acid, β-hydroxybutyric acid, and acetone, are called *ketone bodies,* and their presence in large quantities in the circulating fluids is called *ketosis*. Acetoacetic and β-hydroxybutyric acids can cause severe acidosis and coma in diabetic patients.[50]

Metabolic Acidosis

The acid-base imbalance derives from excessive ketone body production, hyperventilation, and impaired kidney function. The pH of the blood has been lowered, which results in the stimulation of the medullary respiratory centers causing "air hunger" or *Kussmaul's breathing,* which is intermittent periods of rapid, deep respiratory movements coupled with a severe dyspnea. The compensatory rapid respiratory movements are an attempt to increase the $[HCO_3^-]/[CO_2]$ ratio. This eventually reduces the total CO_2, creating more problems. The urine becomes quite acidic, and electrolyte imbalances occur when the renal capacity for exchanging plasma cations, such as Na^+ and K^+, with H^+ and NH_4^+ ions is exceeded. Sodium and potassium are then lost in the urine. The great loss of electrolytes, with a concomitant water loss, during metabolic acidosis of diabetes leads to dehydration, hypovolemia, and hypotension. Very low blood pressure reduces glomerular filtration. These changes will affect the nervous system, and consciousness is lost. Furthermore, an increase in the blood lactic acid may also complicate the ketoacidosis of diabetes.

Acidosis results from a shift from carbohydrate to fat metabolism for energy. When this occurs, the level of acetoacetic acid and other keto acids may rise from 1 meq/dL to as high as 30 meq/dL of blood. A second effect, as previously mentioned, is a decrease in the plasma cations caused by the following: keto acids have a low threshold for excretion by the kidneys; therefore, when the keto acid level rises in diabetes, as much as 100 to 200 g of keto acids can be excreted in the urine each day. Because these are strong acids having a pK of about 4.0 (pK is the measure of dissociation of ions making up a molecule of acid), very little can be excreted in the acidic form, but instead a large portion excreted is combined with sodium derived from the extracellular fluid (ECF). As a result, the Na^+ ion concentration in the ECF decreases, and loss of this basic ion adds to the acidosis that is already caused by excessive keto acids in the ECF. In addition to the acidosis, the dehydration is believed to exacerbate the coma.

Hyperosmolality and Osmotic Diuresis

Diabetic coma may also be due to *hyperosmolality* of the blood that is caused primarily by hyperglycemia (hyperosmolar coma) as well as by metabolic acidosis. Another factor, *osmotic diuresis,* must also be mentioned. As was noted, hyperglycemia results in glycosuria, and so much glucose finally "spills" over into the urine. It cannot be reabsorbed through the tubule cells because the threshold has been exceeded. As a result, there is an increased urinary loss of water and, along with the water, a profound loss of electrolytes, causing delection of extra- and intracellular fluids, resulting in dehydration, weakness, and weight loss. These several complications acting together—ketoacidosis and/or hyperosmolality, and osmotic diuresis—upset the normal balance and end in systemic metabolic acidosis and possible death.

CURRENT CAUSAL THEORIES

Three major forms of diabetes mellitus have been recognized: (1) hereditary diabetes, by far the most common type; (2) diabetes associated with other endocrine disorders; and (3) diabetes associated with destructive pancreatic disease.[51]

Although a familial disease, the precise mode of inheritance is not known. Familial clustering of diabetes was described in the ancient Hindu literature, and genetic factors have been reported repetitively ever since.[52] Diabetes is inherited neither as a simple dominant trait nor as a recessive one; there appears to be a common inherited predisposition to both juvenile and maturity-onset diabetes. The possibility cannot be ruled out that diabetes represents a heterogeneous group of disorders having in common hyperglycemia as a nonspecific manifestation. The disorders of insulin kinetics and impaired carbohydrate metabolism are accompanied by alterations in lipid and protein metabolism. It is probable that a tendency to develop diabetes is inherited and that the onset of the disease is *precipitated* by other factors, e.g., pregnancy, infection, or obesity.

Diabetes is encountered in Cushing's syndrome, acromegaly, and pheochromocytoma, and following glucocorticoid therapy. Under these circumstances, the disease appears as a result of the overabundance of hormones that are antagonistic to insulin. We have discussed the antagonistic effects of growth hormone, the catecholamines such as epinephrine, and cortisol. The specific effects of glucagon that add profoundly to the hyperglycemia of diabetes have demonstrated that this hormone may be just as responsible for the disease as a relative lack of insulin. The synthesis of analogs of somatostatin should be able to carefully delineate the individual effects of insulin and glucagon in the disease; some of the analogs inhibit glucagon secretion specifically and others inhibit only the secretion of insulin.[53] More is involved than merely a lack of insulin. A delayed secretory response (in the obese, maturity-onset diabetic), resistance to insulin function in the peripheral tissues, and inappropriate glucagon secretion probably all contribute to the disordered metabolism of carbohydrates, fats, and proteins.

While the alpha- and beta-cell dysfunctions are certainly in part inherited, environmental influences such as stress, infection, nutrition, and obesity play a significant role in the expression of the diabetic state.

Currently, attempts are being made to isolate virus from patients with newly diagnosed diabetes mellitus. For years, reports of the appearance of juvenile diabetes after measles, mumps, and even after the common cold have been made. A study in England correlated juvenile diabetes with Coxsackie B virus infection, and other investigators have implicated the encephalomyocarditis virus also. The leukocyte invasion of the islets of Langerhans in recent-onset juvenile diabetes in relation to a viral infection was taken as a possible indication of an autoimmune reponse. Since most of these viruses affect such a large part of the population, why do most children escape diabetes? Do those who succumb have the added complication of a destructive pancreatic disease such as a chronic pancreatitis and/or fibrocystic disease?

SUMMARY

Insulin, a relatively small hormone, has a variety of effects, as is discussed throughout the chapter. Most of the current knowledge of the structure, function, and importance of this hormone has been gained over a period of almost 65 years from the beginning experiments of Banting and Best. Unfortunately, much of this knowledge is no more than theory and gives rise to many research questions concerning exact mechanisms of action. The implications that other hormones may be involved are relatively new contributions. Glucagon, for example, was first considered simply a nuisance factor or contaminant of insulin that caused a hyperglycemic effect.

It is clear that diabetic patients suffer from premature large and small vascular disease at unusually high frequencies. This appears to have become a problem following the widespread use of insulin and oral hypoglycemic drugs which allow people to live for longer periods of time. Unfortunately, the mechanisms that are responsible for these abnormalities are not clearly defined.

Large vascular disease appears to be due to plaque formation, as in atherosclerosis, but at an unusually early age. It seems reasonable to assume that plaque formation results, at least in part, from the altered lipid metabolism.

Microvascular disease, as previously indicated, appears to depend on the changes in the basement membrane. Knowledge of normal basement membrane formation, structure, and metabolism is incomplete. The altered enzyme levels and activity appear to be the most consistent with histologic and clinical changes; yet, at the same time, this syndrome is the most resistant to potential treatment.

Many investigators attribute peripheral neuropathy to a compromised blood supply to the peripheral nerves. Others, especially in recent years, suggest that the neuropathy is due to cellular swelling resulting from the sorbitol pathway.

The one treatment followed by most clinicians is an attempt to keep blood glucose near normal physiological levels at all times, a difficult goal to achieve with the current level of knowledge and modes of therapy. Hope lies in the future with research directed at the basic pathology of diabetes, not at specific complications.

Areas of Research

Beta-Cell Implants Although blood glucose is fairly well controlled and ketosis prevented, injected insulin fails to restore either blood glucose or blood insulin levels to the body's normal patterns of fluctuation based on metabolic needs. The injected insulin enters arterial circulation without going to the liver first, as it would normally in natural secretion from the pancreas. Some investigators have suggested that the resultant peripheral hyperinsulinemia may be an important factor in causing the complications of diabetes.

Surgical transplantation of a pancreas has been tried at several medical centers, but rejection of the foreign tissue by response of the patients' immune systems has completely destroyed the transplants. The beta cells, the insulin-producing cells, have survived longer than the rest of the gland in most of the transplants.

A number of experiments are currently being conducted in animals—rats, monkeys, and baboons—to see if beta cells grown in tissue cultures in vitro (in the laboratory) can be implanted and reverse the effects of chemically induced diabetes. Some improvements have been shown, particularly when the beta cells were implanted into the liver or at a site near the liver so that the insulin produced went into the portal system, its natural flow before it goes throughout the peripheral circulation. The cells continued to produce insulin in response to blood glucose elevation after being implanted into the diabetic animals.

In animals that had been kept diabetic for a long time and had developed vascular complications, the beta-cell implants appeared to impede the progress of the complications, and even slight reversals were observed.

With all the advances in making artificial membrane "sacs," a "beta-cell pouch" or "sandwich" has been attempted at Joslin Research Laboratory which permits insulin to flow out from the beta cells into the blood and glucose to pass into the beta cells from the blood. Nutrients pass into and maintain the beta cells, but antibodies that would come from the host do not pass into the pouch, and antigens from the beta cells do not pass into the blood.

Other researchers at Joslin have been trying to develop an artificial pancreas. It would be a mechanical device containing a sensor that would release insulin into the blood when glucose levels increased and decrease the response when the glucose level fell. The insulin pump would be a unit that could be supplied by an injection from an external catheter. Where the artificial pancreas would be implanted—leg, arm, abdomen, or within the portal circulation—has not been decided.

If any concrete results come from the research efforts involving the causal effects of viral infections in the onset of diabetes mellitus, then the possibilities of vaccines being developed to immunize people to prevent infection by the specifically identified organisms are possibilities for the future prevention of the disease in some of the population.

Molecular Structures and Manipulation of Mechanisms   Investigators in the United States and Japan have been able to synthesize the insulin molecules. There is now an opportunity to determine whether there is a structural difference between the insulin molecule produced by the islet cells of diabetics and that of nondiabetics. That there is a difference has been implied but not proven for a number of years.

We have also noted previously that an enzyme does exist that can be used to block the synthesis of sorbitol from glucose. Similar enzyme therapy may be discovered and found to be helpful in inhibiting other defective metabolic pathways or shunts.

The use of analogs of somatostatin, i.e., molecules of the hypothalamic peptide hormone that have had some substitution in their peptide structures, are now being used to influence specifically either the activities of insulin or glucagon, which many people feel exist in a very delicately balanced ratio in health or are in imbalance in diabetes mellitus.

Biofeedback and Recombinant DNA   Two exciting and provocative areas of research to help diabetic patients are in biofeedback and recombinant DNA experiments. Biofeedback is essentially a conditioning process. Some patients have learned to dilate their own blood vessels, which seems to improve general circulation and reduce the insulin dosage needed for control. Moreover, it is now science fact, not fiction, that researchers using recombinant DNA have been able to engineer laboratory-bred bacteria to make the genes for insulin. Use of bacteria to produce insulin could provide an almost limitless supply of the hormone, which is becoming limited in supply from animal sources such as pigs and cattle.

Genes from rat cells that carry genetic instruction for making insulin have been transplanted, or "spliced," into the DNA of bacteria. After the transplantation, succeeding generations of the bacteria continue to make numerous copies of the insulin genes. The next step in the research is to induce the transplanted genes to make the bacteria produce insulin. If the experiments are successful in rats, the same experiments will be tried with splicing of the bacterial genes into human DNA to make human insulin (if permitted!). A natural, ready source of this vital hormone would be available internally to treat diabetes and hopefully prevent or decrease its devastating complications in humans.

REFERENCES

1 Bray, G. New developments in diabetes: obesity and insulin resistance, *Calif. Med.,* **119:**22, 1973.
2 Pyke, D., and Pease, J. Diabetic ketosis and coma, *J. Clin. Pathol.,* **22:**57, 1969.
3 Cahill, G., and Lacy, P. *Report of the Committee on the Etiology and Pathology of Diabetes to the National Commission on Diabetes,* DHEW Publication NIH-76-1023, Washington, D.C., 1975, vol. 3, part 3.
4 Park, C. R., et al. Effect of insulin on free glucose content of rat diaphragm in vitro, *Am. J. Physiol.,* **12:**12, 1955.
5 Stryer, L. *Biochemistry* (San Francisco: Freeman, 1975).
6 Lehninger, A. *Biochemistry,* 2d ed. (New York: Worth, 1975).
7 Narahara, H. *Biological activity of proinsulin,* in I. Fritz (ed.), *Insulin Action* (New York: Academic, 1972).
8 Farina, J., et al. Aspects of intermediary metabolism and insulin level in the penguin (*Pygocellis papua*), *Gen. Comp. Endocrinol.* **27:**209, 1975.
9 Harper, H. *Review of Physiological Chemistry,* 15th ed. (Los Altos, Calif.: Lange, 1975).
10 Stryer. Loc. cit.
11 Ibid.
12 Guyton, A. *Textbook of Medical Physiology,* 5th ed. (Philadelphia: Saunders, 1976).
13 Cuatrecasas, P. Membrane receptors, *Annu. Rev. Biochem.,* **43:**169, 1974.
14 Ibid.
15 Halperin, M., and Robinson, B. Sites of insulin action on lipogenesis, in I. Fritz (ed.), *Insulin Action* (New York: Academic, 1972).
16 Unger, R. H. Glucagon, in E. Astwood (ed.), *Clinical Endocrinology* (New York: Crane & Stratton, 1968), vol. 2.
17 Ibid.
18 Guyton, A. *Basic Human Physiology: Normal Function and Mechanisms of Disease,* 2d ed. (Philadelphia: Saunders, 1977).
19 Unger, R. H. The essential role of glucagon in the pathogenesis of diabetes mellitus, *Lancet,* **1:**14, 1975.
20 Ibid.
21 Ullrich, A., et al. Rat insulin genes: construction of plasmids containing the coding sequences, *Science,* **196:**1313, 1977.
22 Heald, F., and Hung, W. (eds.). *Adolescent Endocrinology* (New York: Appleton-Century-Crofts, 1970).

23 Unger, Glucagon.
24 Gerich, J., et al. Characterization of the glucagon response to hypoglycemia in man, *J. Clin. Endocrinol. Metab.*, **38**:77, 1974.
25 Unger, Essential role of glucagon.
26 Lehninger. Loc. cit.
27 Ibid.
28 Dikstein, S. *Fundamentals of Cell Pharmacology* (Springfield, Ill.: Thomas, 1973).
29 Unger, Essential role of glucagon.
30 Maugh, T. H., II. Diabetes therapy: can new techniques halt complications? *Science*, **190**:1281, 1975.
31 Gerich. Loc. cit.
32 LaVia, M., and Hill, R., Jr. *Principles of Pathobiology*, 2d ed. (New York: Oxford Univ. Press, 1975).
33 Ellenberg, M., and Rifkin, J. *Diabetes Mellitus: Theory and Practice* (New York: McGraw-Hill, 1970).
34 Ibid.
35 Zacks, S., et al. Interstitial muscle capillaries in patients with diabetes mellitus: a light and electron microscope study, *Metabolism*, **11**:381, 1962.
36 McMillan, D., et al. Forearm skin capillaries of diabetic, potential diabetic and nondiabetic subjects, *Diabetes*, **15**:251, 1966.
37 Lazarow, A., and Speidel, E. The chemical composition of the glomerular basement membrane and its relationship to the production of diabetic complications, in Siperstein, M. D., et al. (eds.), *Small Blood Vessel Involvement in Diabetes Mellitus* (Washington, D.C.: American Institute of Biological Science, 1964).
38 Williams, R. *Textbook of Endocrinology*, 5th ed. (Philadelphia: Saunders, 1974).
39 Warren, S., et al. *The Pathology of Diabetes Mellitus*, 4th ed. (Philadelphia: Lea & Febiger, 1966).
40 Besswenger, P. J., and Spiro, R. Human glomerular basement membrane: chemical alterations in diabetes mellitus, *Science*, **168**:396, 1970.
41 Spiro, R., and Spiro, M. Effects of diabetes on the biosynthesis of the renal glomerular basement membrane, *Diabetes*, **20**:641, 1971.
42 Warren. Loc. cit.
43 Blumenthal, H., Goldenberg, S., and Berns, A. Pathology and pathogenesis of the disseminated angiopathy of diabetes mellitus, in B. S. Leibel and G. A. Wrenshall (eds.), *On the Nature and Treatment of Diabetes* (New York: Excerpta Medica Foundation, 1965).
44 Parving, J., et al. The effect of metabolic regulation on *micro*vascular permeability to small and large molecules in short-term juvenile diabetes, *Diabetologia*, **12**:161, 1976.
45 Banson, B., and Lacy, P. Diabetic micro angiopathy in human toes with emphasis on ultrastructural change in dermal capillaries, *Am. J. Pathol.*, **45**:41, 1964.
46 Ussing, J. The role of the basement membrane in epithelial and endothelial permeability, in J. Ostman and R. Milner (eds.), *Diabetes Proceedings of the Sixth Congress of the International Diabetes Foundation.* (New York: Excerpta Medica Foundation, 1969).
47 Cahill and Lacy. Loc. cit.
48 Robbins, S., and Angell, M. *Basic Pathology*, 2d ed. (Philadelphia: Saunders, 1976).
49 Guyton, *Textbook of Medical Physiology*, p. 1047.

50 Montgomery, R., et al. *Biochemistry: A Case-Oriented Approach*, 2d ed. (St. Louis: Mosby, 1977).
51 Walter, J. *An Introduction to the Principles of Disease* (Philadelphia: Saunders, 1977).
52 Cahill and Lacy. Loc. cit.
53 Brown, M., et al. Somatostatin: analogs with selected biological activities, *Science*, **196**:1467, 1977.

Diagnosis of Diabetes Mellitus

Anas A. El Attar

Glucose in the blood arises from two sources: diet and liver glycogen. In diabetes, the liver increases its formation of glucose from amino acids, lactic acid, and glycerol, and thus greatly augments its output of glucose. Liver glycogen is depleted and blood sugar is elevated. If the extrahepatic tissues were able to utilize glucose sufficiently well to equalize the increased hepatic glucose output, hyperglycemia would not be possible.

It is pertinent to note that reduction in the death rate among diabetic patients is the result of a combination of factors, the most prominent of which are early diagnosis, availability of insulin, improved care, antibiotics, and preventive measures such as weight reduction and preventive personal hygiene. Well-cared-for diabetics have lower morbidity and mortality rates, and those who receive treatment shortly after the onset of their disease live longer than diabetic patients in general.

Improved methods of diagnosis will lead to earlier treatment and longer life expectancy for diabetics. The diagnosis of diabetes mellitus depends on adequate history, examination, and proper use and interpretation of laboratory procedures. The following summaries of the functions and pathogeneses of the pancreas, liver, adipose tissues, and muscles are presented to provide basic understanding of the biochemical and pathologic changes that take place in diabetic patients.

REVIEW OF PHYSIOLOGY

Pancreas

The pancreas is composed of two major types of tissues: the aceni and the islets of Langerhans. The aceni secretes a digestive juice that contains enzymes for digesting all three major types of food: protein, carbohydrate, and fat. The pancreatic digestive juice also contains large quantities of bicarbonate ions, which play an important role in neutralizing the acid chyme emptied by the stomach into the duodenum.

The islets of Langerhans do not have any means of emptying their secretions externally; they secrete insulin and glucagon directly into the blood. The islets of Langerhans of the human body contain two major types of cells: alpha cells, which secrete glucagon, and beta cells, which secrete insulin.

Insulin affects carbohydrate, fat, and protein metabolism. Insulin has three basic effects on carbohydrate metabolism: (1) it enhances the rate of glucose metabolism; (2) it decreases blood glucose concentration; and (3) it increases glucogen stores in the tissues.

The response of the beta cells (insulin-secreting cells) to changes in blood glucose concentration provides an extremely important feedback mechanism for regulating blood glucose concentration. The rise in blood glucose increases insulin secretion, and the insulin in turn causes transport of glucose into the cells, thereby reducing the blood glucose concentration back toward the normal value. At the normal fasting level of blood glucose (80 to 90 mg per 100 mL), the rate of insulin secretion is minimal (10 ng/min per kilogram of body weight). If blood glucose concentration is suddenly increased to a level 2 to 3 times normal and is kept at this high level thereafter, insulin secretion increases markedly in three separate stages:[1]

1   Insulin secretion increases up to tenfold about 5 min after an acute elevation of the blood glucose, and it decreases about halfway back to normal in another 5 to 10 min.

2   After 15 min insulin secretion rises a second time, reaching a new plateau in 2 to 3 h. This rate of secretion is even greater than that in the initial phase.

3   Over a period of a week or so, the rate of insulin secretion increases still more, often doubling the rate at the end of the first few hours.

Glucagon, a hormone secreted by alpha cells of the islets of Langerhans, has several functions that are opposed to those of insulin. The most important of these is an increase in blood glucose concentration by (1) breakdown of glycogen (glycogenolysis), (2) increased reservoirs (gluconeogenesis), and (3) increase in the conversion of amino acids and glycerol to glucose (gluconeogenesis).

Diseases of the pancreas, e.g., acute or chronic pancreatitis as well as cholylithiasis of the ampulla of Vater, may result in a disturbance of the function of the secreting cells of the islets of Langerhans (alpha and beta cells). In these conditions, disturbance of carbohydrate metabolism occurs and is diagnosed and treated primarily by proper assessment and treatment of the underlying cause.

Liver

The liver has many physiological functions, e.g., metabolic pool; storage of protein, fat, and carbohydrates; secretion of bile, enzymes, etc.; detoxification; breakdown of hemoglobin; and formation of gamma globulin.

The liver plays many special roles in the metabolism of glucose. The most important of these are

1   In the presence of excess insulin, excess glucose, or both, the liver stores large quantities of glucose from the blood.
2   In the absence of insulin, or when the blood glucose concentration falls very low, the liver gives glucose back to the blood.

Thus the liver acts as an important blood glucose buffer mechanism, helping to keep the blood glucose concentration from rising too high or falling too low. Consequently, liver diseases such as cirrhosis could trigger or aggravate an underlying metabolic ailment. Hence, assessment of liver function is in order for proper assessment of and appropriate management planning for the diabetic patient.

Body Tissues and Metabolic Function

In human adipose tissue, an apparently larger proportion of the glucose uptake is utilized for formation of the glycolytic intermediate alpha glycerophosphate, which is rapidly esterified to free fatty acids that form triglycerides, the primary storage form of fat within the adipose cell. Insulin, by virtue of its action on glucose metabolism, thus has an effect on enhancing fat accumulation in the adipose tissues. Insulin also promotes accumulation of fat in the adipose tissues by a direct action on lipid metabolism.

In human muscle tissues, insulin increases transport of glucose across the cell membrane. In contrast to the fat cell, the glucose taken up by the muscle tissues is either metabolized to lactate or carbon dioxide or is converted to glycogen. Insulin has an important primary action on muscle protein metabolism, whereby it stimulates the uptake of amino acids and their incorporation in protein. The feedback rate of amino acids and protein-stimulating insulin secretion thus provide the proper hormonal milieu to ensure uptake of ingested amino acids in muscle and adequate repletion of body protein.

TYPES OF DIABETES MELLITUS

Diabetes is a genetically determined disorder of metabolism which, in its fully developed clinical expression, is characterized clinically by fasting hyperglycemia, arteriosclerotic and microangiopathic vascular disease, and neuropathy. Diabetes mellitus with fasting hyperglycemia is the most common recognizable form of the disease; however, diabetes mellitus may be recognized without this condition. The typical vascular and neuropathic manifestations of diabetes may occur in a patient with a genetic predisposition to diabetes who has relatively mild carbohydrate intolerance and normal fasting blood glucose levels. It must be realized that there is no sharp dividing line between normal and abnormal carbohydrate metabolism in the first-degree relatives of the diabetic patient.[2]

There is a common agreement that diabetes is a disease in which inherited susceptibility plays an important role. This implies that the disease may have its origin at conception and may exist for prolonged periods before there is any recognizable abnormality of carbohydrate metabolism.[3] Genetic diabetes mellitus may be classified according to the natural history of diabetes as divided into four stages: prediabetes and subclinical, latent, and overt diabetes.[4]

The Earliest Stage: Prediabetes

The prediabetic state exists prior to the onset of identifiable diabetes mellitus, whether it be overt, latent, or subclinical. This stage denotes the interval of time from conception until there is demonstration of impaired glucose tolerance in an individual predisposed to diabetes on genetic grounds. During the prediabetic period, glucose tolerance and cortisone-glucose tolerance tests are normal. A delayed or decreased elevation in plasma insulin level in response to such stimuli as glucose or amino acids has been demonstrated in groups of genetic prediabetic individuals and in other nondiabetic relatives of diabetic patients. Vascular changes, as evidenced by thickening of the capillary basement membrane of muscle obtained by biopsy, has been reported by Siperstein et al.[5]

Subclinical Diabetes

Subclinical diabetes may be suspected because of evidence of insufficient functional reserve of the islet cells. The fasting blood sugar level and the glucose tolerance test are normal under normal circumstances. The patient may have a normal standard glucose tolerance test but an abnormal cortisone-glucose tolerance test. An individual of normal physiological condition may have a normal glucose tolerance test, but in a state of physiological stress, e.g., pregnancy, an abnormal glucose tolerance test may be detected.

Latent Diabetes

In the latent stage the patient has no symptoms of the disease, but a definite diagnosis of diabetes mellitus can be established by laboratory procedures, namely, by a modestly elevated fasting level of glucose and/or a definitely abnormal glucose tolerance test.

Overt (or Frank) Diabetes

Overt diabetes is the most advanced of the stages. Classical symptoms may be present. There is fasting hyperglycemia and glycosuria; a glucose tolerance test is not necessary for diagnosis. This stage may be subdivided into the ketosis-prone and ketosis-resistant types of diabetes. Clinically, diabetes mellitus may be classified as (1) insulinopenic and (2) insulinoplethoric.

Insulinopenic (Type 1) Diabetes   This is a state of hyperglycemia caused by absent or diminished insulin secretion of the pancreatic beta cells in response to glucose. There are two types of insulinopenic diabetes: 1A severe and 1B mild.

1A Severe   This type usually occurs in juveniles or nonobese adults, and the postglucose serum insulin response is absent. This type of diabetes is treated by insulin and diet.

1B Mild   This type occurs in nonobese adults, and the postglucose plasma or serum insulin is greater than 50 ng at 1 h. This type is treated by (1) eucaloric diet alone, (2) diet plus insulin, or (3) diet plus oral hypoglycemic agents. The need for insulin is established by the presence of ketosis and/or the failure of dietary oral drugs.

Insulinoplethoric (Type 2) Diabetes   This is a state of hyperglycemia resulting from the end-organ resistance to insulin action; it occurs usually in obese adults. The postglucose plasma or serum insulin is less than 100 ng at 2 h. This type is treated usually by hypocaloric diet and weight reduction. Insulin or hypoglycemic agents are used for symptomatic control only.

CRITERIA FOR DIAGNOSIS OF DIABETES MELLITUS
History

A standard medical history should be taken very carefully in every case seen in medical practice. The diabetic patient may present for the first time with a current complaint which, on the surface, appears to be a well-defined and unrelated ailment such as cellulitis, abscess formation, peripheral neuritis, or complicated pregnancy. In proper medical history, diabetes could be suspected by a history of diabetes among the family, overweight, polyuria, and/or gradual impairment of vision. For proper evaluation of signs and symptoms of diabetes mellitus, special emphasis should be devoted to the hereditary aspect, past medical history, social and occupational history, and current medical ailment and treatment.

Once diabetes mellitus is detected in the history, a detailed diabetic history is in order. This detailed diabetic history has to include the following information:

1 Duration
2 Previous or current medical treatment including diet and/or medication
3 Results of previous laboratory tests
4 Changes in weight and appetite
5 History of any complications
6 Pregnancy history

7 Dietary habits
8 Socioeconomic factors
9 Review of previous medical records

This information is very helpful in current assessment of and future management planning for the diabetic patient.

Clinical Findings

The classical symptoms of polyuria, polyphagia, thirst, recurrent blurred vision, parasthesias, and fatigue are manifestations of diabetes mellitus. Frank nocturnal enuresis or change in nocturnal habit may signal the onset of diabetes mellitus. Paleness of the patient, polyuria, and light-colored urine may direct attention to a possible underlying diabetic ailment. Pruritis vulvae and vaginitis are frequent initial complaints of an adult female. Weight loss despite normal or increased appetite is primarily a feature of the insulinopenic variety, whereas weight loss is unusual in diabetics who have a normal or increased level of circulating insulin. Diabetes should be suspected in obese patients, in those with peripheral neuritis, in patients with recurrent inflammatory ailments, gangrenous processes, bed sores, or early vascular changes, and in women who have delivered large babies or had polyhydraminos, preeclampsia, or unexpected fetal losses.

In chronic diabetes, the patient may present with ocular, cardiovascular, neurologic, and/or skin and mucous membrane signs.

The mild diabetic is most commonly obese and, except for vaginitis in females, may have no characteristic physical abnormalities related to diabetes. However, evidence of neuropathy may be apparent early in the disease. In acute diabetic syndrome, the patient may show apparent weight loss from a combination of dehydration, loss of subcutaneous fat, and muscle wasting. In diabetic coma, in addition to change in the level of consciousness, the patient may present with signs of fluid and electrolytic imbalance, e.g., diabetic ketoacidosis. In chronic diabetic syndrome, the patient may present with any one or a combination of the following signs.

Neurologic Signs　Bilateral atrophy of the first interosseous muscles of the hand is characteristic of diabetes mellitus. The ankle jerk may be absent but the knee jerk may be retained. Sensory neuropathy may be noted in dullness of perception of vibration, pain, and temperature, particularly in the lower extremities. Autonomic neuropathy includes evidence of postural hypotension, alternating bouts of diarrhea and constipation, and inability to empty the urinary bladder.

Eye Signs　Diabetic blepharitis, premature cataracts, and refractive changes occur in the lens. Diabetic retinopathy may be of the "background" variety consisting of microaneurysms, intraretinal hemorrhages, and hard exudates. Proliferative diabetic retinopathy may be seen in the formation of new capillaries and duplication of small veins. Complicated diabetic retinopathy may present in the form of retinal detachment, preretinal or vitreous hemorrhage, and fibrosis.

Cardiovascular Signs   Gangrene of the feet has a high incidence after age 40 and can be manifested by changes in temperatures of the feet in the early stage. Hypertension develops with progressive renal involvement, and coronary and cerebral arteriascleroses with all their sequelae seem to be accelerated in people with diabetes.

Dermatologic Signs   Chronic pyogenic dermatitis may occur, especially in poorly controlled diabetic patients. Necrosis of subcutaneous adipose tissues may occur in females and is usually located over the anterior surface of the legs or dorsa of the ankles. Brownish, rounded, painless atrophic lesions of the skin may be noted on the pretibial area. Candidal infection and vulvovaginitis are common among chronically diabetic females.

Laboratory Procedures

Urine Analysis   Urine testing as a preliminary screening procedure for diabetes is the cheapest method available; however, it is not very productive. Although the finding of glycosuria suggests diabetes mellitus, it should always be corroborated by blood glucose measurements. When glycosuria is detected, several possibilities should be considered.

1   True glycosuria. This could be secondary to hyperglycemia associated with diabetes or due to renal glycosuria in the presence of normal fasting blood sugar.
2   False glycosuria. This could be due to the presence in urine of sugars other than glucose (e.g., maltose, lactose, fructose, galactose, mannose, xylose, and arabinose) or nonsugar substances, (e.g., uric acid, ascorbic acid, salicylates, methyldopa, levodopa, phenylpyruvic acid, PAS, streptomycin, and penicillin).

The Clinitest modification of Benedict's test using 5 drops of urine with 10 drops of water provides a rapid, easy, and semiquantitative estimate of the degree of glycosuria. The low concentration of 0.25 percent glucose in urine is required to show a trace reaction (green). The color progresses from yellow through orange until a brick-red color indicates a glucose concentration of 2 percent or more. A more specific and convenient method is the paper strip impregnated with glucose oxidase and a chromogen system (Clinistix, Tes-Tape, etc.) which is sensitive to as little as 0.1 percent glucose in urine. The disadvantage of the paper-strip method is that it fails to estimate the quantity of glycosuria.

Qualitative detection of ketone bodies can be accomplished by a nitroprusside test (Acetest or Ketostix).

Blood Testing   For glucose determination, serum or plasma fractions rather than whole blood are preferable because of their stability, the absence of striking effects from hematocrit differences, and the ease of handling in automated equipment. However, whole blood is still widely used and can be valuable when the appropriate precautions are observed. In the past, a "fudge factor" of 20 mg per 100 mL has been used to differentiate between venous and capillary glucose levels. This is somewhat arbitrary and inaccurate. Whenever possible, venous blood should be used. The sample is preserved by freezing (serum) or the addition of an anticoagulant (ethylenediaminetetraacetic acid). If serum is used, samples should be refrigerated and separated from corpuscles within 1 h of collection. Glucose oxidase and orthotolidine methods are most reliable, with normal plasma values ranging from 70 to 150 mg per 100 mL.

Screening Blood Tests   Tests on plasma rather than urine are preferable for detection of the unidentified diabetic. Although fasting plasma glucose tests are not recommended for screening because of their insensitivity, they are of great significance if elevations are above 120 mg per 100 mL. The following are considered indications for screening with 1- or 2-h postprandial glucose determinations:

1   Predisposition to infection
2   Overweight
3   Obstetrical complications
4   Accelerated vascular disease
5   Suggestive signs and symptoms of diabetes
6   Family history of diabetes
7   Peripheral neuritis
8   Other metabolic and/or endocrinic disorders
9   Cholecystitis
10   Pancreatitis
11   Accelerated degenerative disease processes

The screening test is most dependable when it embodies a standard early-morning glucose load of 50 to 55 g. The glucose level following a meal containing carbohydrate, fat, and protein is highly variable, although still useful. A 1-h glucose value of 160 mg per 100 mL or more or 2-h postprandial levels of 120 mg per 100 mL or more (in the presence of a normal fasting blood level) indicate the need for an oral glucose tolerance test.

If the fasting plasma glucose is over 120 mg per 100 mL, further evaluation of the patient with a glucose challenge is seldom necessary. If the screening level of plasma glucose after a glucose load is greater than 140 mg per 100 mL without fasting hyperglycemia, a standard oral glucose tolerance test may be done.

Oral Glucose Tolerance Test   This procedure consists of the administration of 1.75 g of glucose per kilogram of ideal body weight in 300 mL of water after an overnight fast to subjects who have been receiving at least 150 to 200 g of

Table 5-1 Glucose Tolerance with Aging
(Plasma Glucose in mg per 100 mL)

Age	Normal			Probable diabetes, 2 h	Diabetes, 2 h
	Fasting	1 h	2 h		
0–30	110	185	165	166–185	> 185
30–40	112	191	175	176–195	> 195
40–50	114	197	185	186–205	> 205
50–60	116	203	195	196–215	> 215
60–70	118	209	205	200–235	> 235
70–80	120	215	215	216–245	> 245

Source: R. Andres; adapted from T. E. Prout, *Diabetes Mellitus,* 4th ed. (New York: American Diabetes Association, 1975).

carbohydrate daily for 3 days before the test. For proper evaluation of the test, the subjects should be normally active and free of acute illness. Medications which may impair glucose tolerance include diuretics, contraceptive drugs, glucocorticoids, nicotinic acid, and phenytoin.

Since tolerance to a glucose challenge is apparently age-dependent, age-adjusted standards are required for proper interpretation of glucose responses. One method adapted from Andres is shown in Table 5-1.

Insulin levels may be obtained during the glucose tolerance test. Normal insulin levels range from less than 10 to 25 mU/mL in the fasting state to 50 to 130 mU/mL 2 h postprandial. Values below 50 mU/mL at 1 h and below 100 mU/mL at 2 h in the presence of sustained hyperglycemia implicate a lack of sensitivity of the pancreatic beta cells to glucose. However, an insulin value above 100 mU/mL at 1 or 2 h postprandial suggests unresponsiveness to the action of the insulin.

Capillary Morphometry Under aseptic standard surgical procedures, usually using a local anesthetic, a biopsy specimen of the quadriceps muscle is removed and sent to the pathology laboratory. Basement membrane of capillaries is abnormally thickened in all cases of overt spontaneous diabetes mellitus in adults with fasting hyperglycemia of 140 mg per 100 mL or more. A normal basement membrane of the capillaries is usually noted in acquired states of carbohydrate intolerance due to pancreatitis, Cushing's syndrome, or pheochromocytoma.

COMPLICATIONS OF DIABETES MELLITUS

In addition to the pathological changes described above (neurologic, eye, cardiovascular, and dermatologic), special attention is directed to the following complications.

Diabetic Ketoacidosis

Biochemical and Physiological Changes Diabetic acidosis may be described as a complex of disturbed pathophysiological processes consisting of biochemical alterations, fluid and electrolytic defects, and systemic manifestations which result from an absolute or relative deficiency of insulin. In general, diabetic acidosis is most commonly referred to as *diabetic ketoacidosis*. Diabetic ketoacidosis does not always lead to diabetic coma, nor is coma in diabetics always due to diabetic ketoacidosis. Equally pertinent is the point that diabetic acidosis is not always ketotic.

It has been estimated that 15 to 20 percent of all diabetic ketoacidosis occurs in cases not previously diagnosed as diabetes mellitus. The early recognition of the presence of ketoacidosis is of paramount importance, since this leads to early treatment and a decreased morbidity and mortality. The essentials of the treatment of diabetic acidosis have not changed greatly in the last 15 years, but an improved understanding of the disturbed physiological-biochemical state has led to the development of modifications that have been greatly instrumental in improving the recovery rate in diabetic acidosis.

Small but significant concentrations of insulin are normally present in the plasma in the fasting state. Diabetic ketoacidosis is most frequently observed in patients with juvenile diabetes. The levels of insulin found in the plasma of patients with untreated juvenile diabetes after an overnight fast are extremely low or unmeasurable; moreover, they do not rise significantly in response to the usual physiological stimuli (e.g., the ingestion of carbohydrate or protein). It is not surprising, therefore, that in juvenile diabetes the omission of insulin or the development of conditions that reduce the apparent effectiveness of insulin, such as infection or acute emotional disturbance, can result in the rapid development of hyperglycemia and hyperketonemia that can lead to ketoacidosis. In contrast, unless they are subjected to unusual stress, patients with maturity-onset diabetes rarely develop ketoacidosis, since they are able to maintain appreciable levels of plasma insulin at all times.

Insulin deficiency greatly increases the rate of free fatty acid release from adipose tissue and results in the markedly elevated levels of free fatty acids that are found in the plasma of patients in diabetic ketoacidosis. The rate at which free fatty acids are taken up by the liver is largely a function of their concentration in plasma.[6] They do not accumulate in gross quantities within the liver but are rapidly activated to their CoA derivatives. These compounds may be utilized for either the synthesis of triglycerides and phospholipids, which may ultimately appear in circulation as lipoproteins, or they may be transported into the mitochondria by a carnitine-dependent mechanism.

A major point in understanding how insulin deficiency leads to hyperketonemia is that insulin plays a role in determining the rate at which free fatty acids are released from adipose tissue.[7] Although the concentration of plasma free fatty acids (FFA) is usually quite low (less than 0.6 meq/L), this lipid fraction turns over very rapidly, and the oxidation of fatty acids transported from the adipose tissue in this fashion accounts for a major fraction of the basal metabolic rate during fasting. The rate of release of free fatty acids from adipose tissue appears to be controlled by a "hormone-sensitive lipase" that catalyzes the hydrolysis of adipose tissue triglycerides to glycerol and fatty acids. The activity of this enzyme system is increased by a number of agents, including epinephrine, and is decreased by insulin.[8]

The proper diagnosis and treatment of diabetic acidosis depends on a full understanding of the disturbed physiology and biochemistry of this clinical disorder. The basic defect is an inability to metabolize glucose normally because of lack of insulin. As a consequence, fat breakdown in the tissues is accentuated, and nonesterified fatty acids (NEFA) are released into the circulation. These are transported in association with serum albumin to the liver where they are converted to acetoacetic acid and β-hydroxybutyric acid. These highly acidic substances deprive the body of a valuable fixed plasma base, which culminates in acidosis. Concomitantly, the elevation of blood sugar accompanied by glucosuria produces a marked fluid and electrolyte loss, which causes dehydration and a reduction of ionic reserves. Schematically,

Insulin lack →
      increased NEFA release by adipose tissue into serum →
           increased NEFA to liver →
        increased rate of fatty acid oxidation →
      increased rate of formation of 4-carbon keto acids →
                release of the keto acids into the circulation

The development of hyperglycemia, ketosis, acidosis, and dehydration is responsible for the clinical picture of dry skin, Kussmaul's breathing, torpor, and "fruit odor" breath. The treatment of this diabetic acidosis must be all-inclusive if it is to deal adequately with the consequences of the cellular starvation and ketotic state.

Symptoms and Signs of Diabetic Ketoacidosis   Anorexia, nausea, vomiting, and abdominal pain are symptoms that frequently bring the patient to the physician. In a known diabetic, these symptoms, particularly if preceded by a period of polydipsia, polyuria, and weight loss, or a history of decreased insulin intake or infection, obviously suggest the possibility of ketoacidosis. The major problems in diagnosis arise in patients not previously known to be diabetic or in maturity-onset diabetics who have not previously required insulin. Delays in diagnosis commonly result from attributing the symptoms of young patients to "gastroenteritis." Similarly, ketoacidosis in elderly patients suffering from severe infections or cardiac problems may be missed until chance laboratory determinations suggest its presence.

Diabetic ketoacidosis must be considered in the differential diagnosis of coma and stupor even when an obvious cause such as alcohol intoxication appears to be responsible. Abdominal pain may be sufficiently severe to suggest an acute surgical abdomen, particularly in children. Since tenderness, guarding, and decreased bowel sounds may be present in association with leukocytosis in patients with ketoacidosis without significant intra-abdominal disease, continued reevaluation of the cause of the abdominal pain must be made during the course of therapy. It should be noted that there is an increased incidence of acute pancreatitis in adults presenting in diabetic ketoacidosis, and this possibility should be considered. There is usually no difficulty in distinguishing diabetic ketoacidosis from hypoglycemic coma on clinical or laboratory grounds.

The patient in diabetic ketoacidosis may not appear to be seriously ill or may be comatose and moribund. The physical findings of immediate concern are those suggesting severe dehydration and circulatory insufficiency (hypotension and tachycardia), marked impairment of cerebral function (stupor or coma), decreased respiratory response to the acidosis, and the presence of a precipitating infection or an acute abdominal or cardiac catastrophe.

Laboratory Findings   If diabetic ketoacidosis is suspected, the diagnosis can be rapidly confirmed by demonstrating hyperglycemia and hyperketonemia. This requires only a matter of minutes with commercially available test reagents (Dextrostix, Ketostix, or Acetest tablets). These methods are only semiquantitative, and the blood sugar should subsequently be determined by standard laboratory procedures.

The vast majority of patients in diabetic ketosis will have a blood sugar level greater than 400 mg per 100 mL, and many will have levels in the neighborhood of 1000 mg per 100 mL or more.

At the onset, further laboratory studies of value include a complete blood count and urinalysis, and determinations of blood glucose, urea nitrogen, and serum electrolytes, as well as arterial pH and P_{CO_2}. The plasma bicarbonate and arterial P_{CO_2} are usually significantly reduced. The serum potassium deserves specific attention. It is characteristically normal or elevated despite significant total body potassium depletion. The finding of low serum potassium should alert the physician to the necessity for vigorous replacement therapy. The blood urea nitrogen and hematocrit are commonly elevated from dehydration and impaired renal function.

Significantly elevated arterial lactate concentrations are rarely observed initially in diabetic ketoacidosis.[9,10] However, lactate levels may be slightly elevated and have been reported to rise following the initiation of therapy.[11] The presence of a degree of acidosis which cannot be accounted for by ketoacidosis should raise the possibility of lactic acidosis, particularly in the elderly, hypotensive patient.[12] Increased serum glutamic-oxaloacetic transaminase levels recently reported in patients with ketoacidosis may be an artifact of automated analytic techniques.[13,14] Leukocytosis is common, even in the absence of significant infection.[13,14]

Dehydration   Dehydration is characteristic of diabetic ketosis. It results from a complexity of metabolic alterations starting with intense glycosuria and polyuria not infrequently accompanied by vomiting or diarrhea. Dehydration is aggravated by coexisting fever and infection plus increased losses of fluid during the deep, rapid, Kussmaul's respiration. Clinically, dry skin, soft eyeballs, dry mouth, hypotension, and reduced urine output all signal dehydration and the need for corrective measures.

The extracellular location of large amounts of glucose increases effective extracellular osmolality and promotes the movement of water from cells, thereby causing intracellular dehydration.

Acidosis   The characteristic pH disturbance is acidosis. Since acidosis may lead to coma, peripheral circulatory failure, insulin failure, and insulin resistance, it is an extremely important consideration. Acidosis results from the accumulation of hydrogen ions donated by the 4-carbon ketone acids which are the products of increased fat catabolism. β-Hydroxybutyric acid and acetoacetic acid displace bicarbonate, and the concentration of carbonic acid increases. In order to compensate for this, respiratory activity becomes rapid and deep, and the excess of carbonic acid is eliminated as carbon dioxide. Typical Kussmaul's respirations are not generally observed until the serum pH values are 7.2 or less. Since this respiratory excretory mechanism is inadequate to handle the H^+ excess, the pH of the serum continues to fall and may reach extremely low values of 7.0 or less. In seriously ill patients, the respiratory compensatory activity may be impaired as a result of supervening muscular fatigue and respiratory center narcosis.

The renal mechanisms for protection against acidosis are also working maximally. Even with normal kidneys, these mechanisms are insufficient to deal with the overwhelming load of hydrogen ions. The fact that renal impairment is frequently present in diabetics suggests an even greater reduction in the ability of the kidney to compensate for the pH changes.

The seriousness of the acidosis and the depth of coma are usually well correlated, and morbidity and mortality figures in diabetic ketoacidosis correlate statistically with the degree and duration of acidosis.

Electrolyte Disturbances   Two cations, sodium and potassium, and two anions, bicarbonate and chloride, must be given major consideration in diabetic ketoacidosis. In general, acidosis causes a loss of intracellular electrolytes (K^+, Mg^{2+}, phosphate). The magnesium and phosphate alterations are rarely marked in degree and as such do not pose a formidable problem.

Hyponatremia is much more common than hypernatremia in diabetic acidosis. Patients with diabetic acidosis often have considerable vomiting and diarrhea, which are known to deplete sodium stores. In the developing stage of diabetic ketoacidosis, the excessive urinary output also contributes to the loss of sodium.

Alterations in potassium levels are of particular interest in diabetic ketoacidosis since failure to appreciate low as well as high levels of potassium may be life-threatening. The diuresis in diabetic ketoacidosis is not solely water, but includes many electrolytes such as Na^+ and K^+. In diabetic ketoacidosis, the gastric contents are quite high in K^+, which is lost with vomiting and/or diarrhea. Therefore, the general picture is one of the total body

K^+ depletion. Although serum K^+ may be normal or elevated as a result of protein catabolism, the shift of K^+ from the cells, and reduced renal excretion, serum levels indicating low K^+ may be found if there is dilution by the hyperosmolar effect of hyperglycemia. In addition, during insulin therapy, the reduction in blood sugar is accompanied by a transfer of K^+ from the extracellular spaces into the intracellular compartments, which, after 4 to 6 h, may lead to severe hypokalemia.

The serum HCO_3^- is usually below 15 meq/L in moderately severe acidosis and below 10 meq/L in severe acidosis. It should be noted that plasma bicarbonate may be an unreliable index of hydrogen ion concentration in diabetic acidosis; serum pH determinations are recommended.

In the diabetic who has been out of control for an extensive period of time and then develops ketoacidosis, there may be a depletion of phosphate. This ion is essential to the restitution of normal carbohydrate metabolism, which depends on the formation of phosphorylated intermediates.

The concentration of calcium and magnesium ions may be decreased, but this rarely poses a significant problem.

Nonketotic Comas

Diabetic patients may develop a nonketotic coma as a result of inherent pathological and biochemical changes in the course of the disease, disturbances in diet and/or treatment, the presence of associated complications, or a problem unrelated to diabetes mellitus. Nonketotic coma may be one, or a combination of more than one, of the following five types:

1 Coma unrelated to diabetes mellitus
2 Hypoglycemic comas
3 Lactic acidosis
4 Hyperosmolar (hyperglycemic-hypernatremic) coma
5 Cerebral edema and coma

Comas Unrelated to Diabetes Mellitus This group of nonketotic comas could occur among nondiabetic individuals as a result of stroke, circulatory shock, drug poisoning, uremia, hepatic insufficiency, and so forth. In some instances, of course, the diabetes contributes indirectly to the coma, e.g., through arteriosclerosis or glomerulosclerosis.

Hypoglycemic Comas Excesses of administered insulin are far more common causes of hypoglycemia. Such excesses may result from unnecessarily increased dosages of insulin, decreased food intake, or diminished insulin requirements as a result of improvement in glucose tolerance during exercise or following recovery from illness or an emotional problem.

Hypoglycemia in undiagnosed or untreated diabetes may produce stupor or coma which may be misdiagnosed as other conditions, e.g., neurologic or cardiac. Proper systematic management of the comatose or confused patient is recommended. The reader is advised to review the causes of stupor and coma.

Sulfonylurea-induced hypoglycemic coma is more apt to develop in patients with mild diabetes, renal failure, hepatic disease, or congestive heart failure. Starvation or malnutrition increase the frequency of hypoglycemia by decreasing the binding of the sulfonylurea to plasma proteins, lowering its urinary excretion, or decreasing glucose production or release. Sulfonamide, ethionamide, or phenformin treatment has evoked hypoglycemia.

Though recovery from hypoglycemic coma is usually prompt, its occurrence is not to be taken lightly, since hemiplegia, epilepsy, emotional disturbances, intellectual deterioration, and death can occur.

Lactic Acidosis   Stupor or coma and metabolic acidosis with or without Kussmaul's breathing can result from an accumulation of lactic acid in excess of the usual concentrations present in the basal resting state in health, that is, in excess of 7 mmol/L or 12 mg per 100 mL with disturbance of the normal lactate/pyruvate ratio.

Lactic acidosis must be differentiated from excesses of lactate produced by physiological manipulations such as hyperventilaton, exercise, or infusion of pyruvate, alkali, or sodium chloride solution. Such physiological excesses of lactate are attended by proportionate increases in lactate and pyruvate, with maintenance of a normal lactate/pyruvate ratio. However, true lactic acidosis usually follows pathophysiological variables such as hypoxia, hemorrhage, impending or actual circulatory collapse, infection with gram-negative bacilli, injection of epinephrine or norepinephrine, or the administration of cyanide. These pathophysiological disturbances produce increases in the lactate and lesser rises in pyruvate, with a consequent increase in the lactate/pyruvate ratio. Lactic acidosis may also develop without apparent cause.[15]

Since lactic acidosis may develop in any diabetic patient with general or regional hypoxia,[16] this possibility should always be raised whenever the serum bicarbonate is substantially reduced without a demonstrated elevation in urine or plasma ketones. Ordinary diabetic ketoacidosis is not generally accompanied by an increase in lactic acid levels.

Hyperosmolar (Hyperglycemic-Hypernatremic) Coma   The fourth type of nonketotic coma results from hyperosmolarity of extracellular fluids as a consequence of excess blood glucose (600 mg per 100 mL or higher) and/or sodium (150 meq/L or higher). However, in patients with hyperglycemia, serum sodium may be normal or low. Ketone bodies are, of course, absent or minimal, and serum bicarbonate is normal or only slightly reduced. In the initial reports, most patients in this type of nonketotic coma were in the older age group, the diabetes was generally of recent onset or diagnosis, and inadequate regulation of diabetes, dehydration, and acute illness frequently preceded the coma. This type of coma results from extracellular hyperosmolarity with resultant dehydration of cells. Hyperosmolar coma has followed the use of adrenocorticosteroids,[17] immunosuppressive agents,[18] diuretics,[19] intravenous Dilantin,[20] peritoneal dialysis,[21] high-carbohydrate diets and mafenide burn ointment,[22] and heat stroke.[23]

The hyperosmolarity usually arises from a combination of dehydration and excess glucose. Hyperosmolar coma can also result from sugars other than glucose, such as sorbitol.[24] The dehydration follows continued osmotic diuresis and inadequate perception of or response to thirst. Fluid loss through the skin contributes to water deficits in burn patients treated with mafenide ointment, which increases insensible water loss.[25]

Cerebral Edema and Coma   Coma and death have occurred following apparently successful treatment of diabetic ketoacidosis.[26] Papilledema and diabetes insipidus were observed in some of these patients, and cerebral edema and brain damage have been noted at necropsy. These developments could be related to therapy with alkali or to an accumulation of fructose, sorbitol, or other osmotically active components within brain cells during therapy of ketoacidosis.

Alternatively, it may be that during insulin therapy the decrease in the glucose level of brain tissue is less rapid than the fall in extracellular glucose, and water therefore moves into the brain as a result of the osmotic disequilibrium this produces. Thus a patient may develop coma while receiving insulin treatment, a condition which has to be detected as early as possible.

Kidney Disease

The edematous diabetic with proteinuria, pallor, retinopathy, hypertension, and a steadily rising blood urea level is a familiar sight on medical wards and in medical practices. Now comparatively protected from death from diabetic coma and overwhelming sepsis, the diabetic lives longer today but often is the victim of insidious and progressive destruction of renal tissue.

Physicians caring for patients with diabetes mellitus, particularly those with onset of disease at a relatively early age, are frequently frustrated by the fact that despite a relatively sophisticated ability to recognize and treat hyperglycemia and ketosis and their attendant disorders, they are almost ineffective bystanders in dealing with the vascular and renal deterioration associated with this disorder.

Every diabetic should be assumed to have renal disease. If the physician finds this assumption untenable, he or she will at least agree that the potential for developing renal disease is exaggerated in the diabetic patient. The problem then centers around the early detection and examination of the renal lesion with respect to both severity and type. The recognition that these patients may have acute and chronic pyelonephritis, arteriolar nephrosclerosis, intercapillary glomerulosclerosis, or any combination of these not only gives the physician a basic understanding of the nature of the problem but also provides a stimulating diagnostic and therapeutic challenge.

It is recommended that employment of generally available clinical laboratory studies will allow a reliable and clinically useful characterization of the

renal lesion. Laboratory studies pertinent to the evaluation of diabetic nephropathy include routine urinalysis, blood urea and creatinine levels, quantitative estimation of bacteriuria, urine culture, 24-h urinary protein excretion,
creatinine clearance, serum albumin level, and intravenous pyelogram.
Moreover, in some cases, renal biopsy may be advised. Proper evaluation and
treatment of any underlying urinary ailment is recommended.

Pregnancy

Normal pregnancy applies substantial stresses to carbohydrate metabolism. In
the prediabetic woman, these stresses may unmask overt diabetes; in the established diabetic, they may decrease insulin sensitivity and bring about unusual
instability of control with a strong tendency to ketosis. A rise in insulin requirements commonly begins during the second trimester and continues, often
at an increased pace, during the third, right up to delivery.

As the mother's insulin requirements increase, she is apt to become less
stable and show an unusual tendency to hypoglycemia on the one hand and
ketosis on the other. Since ketosis is itself an important cause of fetal death, the
physician must provide careful instruction for any pregnant diabetic, especially
the patient with previously stable diabetes of recent onset who may, for the first
time, be faced with the necessity for meticulous management in the place of the
relatively relaxed approach she has so far found appropriate.

Meanwhile, the diabetic is spared none of the usual hazards of pregnancy;
among these, hyperemesis, urinary tract infections, and toxemia present special
problems.

In contrast to the good prognosis offered by modern treatment to the
diabetic mother herself, there remains a very high risk of fetal mortality. Most
of the fetal deaths occur after the 28th week of pregnancy, as well as in the
presence of extensive vascular complications of long-standing diabetes.

Among the factors contributing to this excess fetal mortality are (1) diabetic ketosis, (2) toxemia, (3) hydramnios (increased in incidence in diabetes),
and (4) increased size of fetus in diabetic mothers. Ketoacidosis sharply increases fetal mortality to levels which approach 65 percent in frank coma. The
incidence of toxemia is probably increased only in long-standing diabetes with
vascular complications, but it is the consensus that toxemia, when it does occur
in diabetic mothers, carries an unusually high risk to the fetus.

Diabetes may be discovered for the first time during pregnancy, and even if
the defect of carbohydrate metabolism is mild and asymptomatic, it raises
special problems of management.

A patient with a normal or nearly normal fasting blood sugar level, a
diabetic glucose tolerance curve, and occasional glycosuria may have an underlying metabolic ailment. Although some of these patients will recover normal
carbohydrate tolerance after delivery, the abnormality cannot be dismissed, for
many of these patients are latent diabetics who will go on to develop florid
diabetes and who, even now, may show an increased incidence of large babies.
In this group of patients, the advantages of possibly ensuring normal fetus size

at term by controlling the blood sugar with insulin during pregnancy must be balanced against the inconvenience to the patient and the risk that hypoglycemia in the mother may cause abnormal fetal development.

DIFFERENTIAL DIAGNOSIS

Subjective complaints (symptoms), objective findings (signs), and laboratory findings of diabetes mellitus could be similar to the observations noted among other diseases. Symptoms of polyuria could be noticed in diabetes mellitus as well as in diabetes insipidus. Proper assessment and interpretation of the appropriate laboratory tests will help in establishing the underlying diabetic problem (mellitus or insipidus).

Nondiabetic glycosuria could be seen in a case of renal glycosuria. A proper evaluation has to be done to differentiate between glycosuria and lactosuria.

Attention has to be directed to hyperglycemia that occurs in nondiabetic patients, e.g., resulting from obesity, muscle disorders, acromegaly, Cushing's syndrome, liver disease, lipoatrophy, hemochromocytosis, thyrotoxicosis, pheochromocytoma, chronic pancreatitis and chronic cholecystitis, and cholelithiasis.

PRINCIPLES OF ASSESSMENT

The reader is referred to Chapters 6 and 7 for discussion of management by nutrition and by pharmacological agents. The following are essentials for proper assessment that result in ideal management planning for diabetic patients. See "History," under "Criteria for Diagnosis" above. In addition, proper history should include the dietary habits, caloric value, presence of any underlying disease, and any use of prescribed or nonprescribed medications.

History should also include

1 How long the diabetic condition has been known to the patient
2 How the diabetic condition is being controlled, by diet and/or by medication
3 Whether the patient has changed the kind of diet and/or medication, and if so, what the changes were, when and how frequently they occurred, and what the response of the patient was to these changes
4 What kind of monitoring (individual and/or laboratory) procedures the patient follows
5 What the patient's socioeconomic status is
6 What degree of knowledge the patient has pertaining to diabetes

Periodic Checkup and Laboratory Monitoring

The patient must be advised to have periodic checkups and laboratory testing at any facility the patient desires, e.g., diabetic clinic, outpatient clinic, or physician's office. Proper record keeping has to be maintained, and patients must be reminded whenever they miss an appointment for a periodic checkup.

Monitoring Complications

Patients also must be informed of the possibility of complications that may occur or be aggravated by the underlying diabetic condition. Special information sessions have to be devoted to (1) control of the diabetic condition (by proper follow-up of diet and/or medication, periodic checkups, and laboratory monitoring), (2) preventive actions directed toward personal hygiene of teeth, feet, and skin ulcerations, and (3) immediate medical consultations for development of any signs of complications, e.g., peripheral neuropathy, visual changes, infectious process, ketoacidosis, or nonketotic coma.

REFERENCES

1 Guyton, A. C. *Textbook of Medical Physiology*, 5th ed. (Philadelphia: Saunders, 1976).
2 Fajans, S. S., and Conn, J. W. Prediabetes, subclinical diabetes, and latent clinical diabetes: interpretation, diagnosis and treatment, in B. S. Leibel and G. S. Wrenshall (eds.), *On Nature and Treatment of Diabetes* (New York: Excerpta Medical Foundation, International Congress Series 84, 1965), chap. 46, pp. 641–656.
3 Conn, J. W., and Fajans, S. C. The prediabetic state: a concept of dynamic resistance to a genetic diabetogenic influence, *J.A.M.A.*, **31**:839–850, 1961.
4 Fajans and Conn. Loc. cit.
5 Siperstein, M. D., et al. Studies of muscle capillary basement membranes in normal subjects, diabetic and prediabetic patients, *J. Clin. Invest.*, **47**:1973, 1968.
6 Greville, G. D., and Tubbs, P. K. The catabolism of long-chain fatty acids in mammalian tissues, *Essays Biochem.*, **4**:155, 1968.
7 Jeanrenaud, B. Adipose tissue dynamics and regulations revisited, *Rev. Physiol. Biochem. Exper. Pharmacol.*, **60**:57, 1968.
8 Ibid.
9 Marliss, E. B., et al. Altered redox state obscuring ketoacidosis in diabetes with lactic acidosis, *N. Engl. J. Med.*, **283**:978, 1970.
10 Oliva, P. G. Lactic acidosis, *J.A.M.A.*, **48**:209, 1970.
11 Watkins, P. J., et al. Lactic acidosis in diabetes, *Br. Med. J.*, **1**:744, 1969.
12 Marliss. Loc. cit.
13 Chen, J. C., et al. Diabetic ketosis: interpretation of elevated serum glutamic-oxaloacetic transaminase (SGOT) by multi-channel chemical analysis, *Diabetes*, **19**:730, 1970.
14 Cryer, P. E., and Daughaday, W. H. Diabetic ketosis: elevated serum glutamic oxyloacetic transaminase (SGOT) and other findings determined by multi-channel chemical analysis, *Diabetes*, **18**:781, 1969.
15 Danowski, T. S., and Nabarro, J. D. N. Hyperosmolar and other types of non-ketoacidotic coma in diabetes, *Diabetes*, **14**:162, 1964.
16 Tranquada, R. E., et al. Lactic acidosis, *Arch. Intern. Med.*, **117**:192, 1966.
17 Spenney, J. G., et al. Hyperglycemic hyperosmolar non-ketoacidotic diabetes, *Diabetes*, **18**:107, 1969.
18 Ibid.

19 Boyer, M. H., Hyperosmolar anacidotic coma in association with glucocorticoid therapy, *J.A.M.A.*, **202:**1007, 1967.
20 Goldberg, E. M., and Sanbar, S. S. Hyperglycemic, nonketotic coma following administration of Dilantin (diphenylhydantoin), *Diabetes*, **18:**101, 1969.
21 Fernandez, J. P., et al. Cerebral edema from blood-brain glucose differences complicating peritoneal dialysis: second membrane syndrome, *N.Y. State J. Med.*, **68:**677–680, 1968.
22 Oakes, D. D., et al. Hyperglycemic non-ketotic coma in the patient with burns: factors in pathogenesis, *Metabolism*, **18:**103, 1969.
23 Monteleone, J. A., and Keefe, D. M. Transient hyperglycemia and aketotic hyperosmolar acidosis with heat stroke, *Pediatrics*, **44:**737, 1969.
24 Raja, R. M., et al. Hyperosmotic coma complicating peritoneal dialysis with sorbitol dialysate, *Ann. Intern. Med.*, **73:**993, 1970.
25 Oakes. Loc. cit.
26 Taubin, H., and Matz, R. Cerebral edema, diabetes insipidus and sudden death during treatment of diabetic ketoacidosis, *Diabetes*, **17:**108, 1968.

Chapter 6

Management by Nutrition

Janice N. Neville

What are the nutritional needs of people with diabetes mellitus? Basically they are the same as the nutritional needs of anyone: (1) sufficient energy (calories) to grow normally and to work without developing excess body fat, (2) protein, fat, carbohydrate, vitamins, minerals, and water for body structure and metabolism, and (3) management of dietary practices to minimize risk of chronic degenerative conditions and to limit detrimental metabolic arrangements.[1] West has identified four therapeutic goals:

  1 Reversal of the diabetic state toward or to normal with improvement in glucose tolerance and β-cell reserve and amelioration of resistance to insulin

  2 Mitigation and regulation of glycemia, including the control of symptoms of diabetes and prevention and therapy of hypoglycemia

  3 Prevention or reduction in progression of certain complications of diabetes, e.g., vascular disease, neuropathy, cataract, and ketosis

  4 Management of certain complications of diabetes, e.g., pregnancy, renal failure, and hypertension[2]

The most important goal of therapy is to obtain, maintain, and prolong a satisfying, productive, and healthy life. In the final analysis, the patient's adherence to any aspect of the treatment regimen, including dietary management, will be based in large part on personal perceptions of satisfaction in life. Levine stated it simply:

> Since the disease has a duration of thirty years or more,* treatment ought to be so designed that the patient, most of the time, should not feel himself an invalid. A sensible diet with a normal food distribution; a modicum of exercise of the type suitable to the patient; oral agents if effective; insulin if it is required and livable demands for rigidity of treatment.[4]

Nurses, physicians, and dietitians or nutritionists working with patients might well do some soul-searching. A review of the dimensions and persistence of failure in dietary control suggests that such failure may result in large part from regimens that are not "livable" and inadequate communication and education[5,6] rather than lack of patient interest or cooperation.

Dietary management has been part of the treatment of diabetes for centuries. A recent review traces some of the concepts and suggests that high-carbohydrate, low-calorie therapy may have been initiated by Will in 1675 to replace the sugar loss in urine.[7] Avoidance of dietary carbohydrate was urged by Rollo in 1797, and the proposed diet was rancid meat and fat. The high-fat, low-carbohydrate calorically restricted diet was championed by many up to the insulin era and beyond. Some liberalizing of the diet occurred in the 1930s and 1940s. Concepts of dietary control ranged from very strict regimens to moderate-to-free ones. Review of the literature of that era (and of today) reveals sharp disagreement as to the constraints to be imposed on the patient. Despite the almost universal admonition to observe individual differences in severity of the condition; individual, social, and cultural needs; and practical constraints of understanding, home, and work, standard regimens with timing of hypoglycemic medication and meal patterns are handed to the patient with the expectation that the patient will adjust. If the patient does not adjust, he or she may be characterized as uncooperative, a cheat, a failure, or, at the mildest, uninterested in his or her own health and well-being.

Recently the voices of moderation have been heard. It has been suggested that insulin (when needed) can be so prescribed that the medication regimen is adapted to the patient's life pattern. The priorities in dietary management are different depending on the type of diabetes, e.g., insulin-dependent and obese or normal weight. Recent research has confirmed the importance of dietary management in mitigating diabetes but has raised questions about long-held beliefs in limitations of dietary carbohydrate for all and inflexible dietary management programs.[8,9]

---

* Remember that age of diagnosis varies: 8 percent at 24 years or before; 22 percent from 25 through 44; 50 percent from 45 through 64; and 20 percent at 65 or over.[3] The average duration of 30 years or more should not be interpreted as life expectancy after diagnosis. Unfortunately, it has been used this way, introducing another element of fear.

NUTRITIONAL NEEDS

Everyone needs the same nutrients, and the amounts needed are based on certain predictable patterns of growth and physical activity. The National Academy of Sciences' *Recommended Dietary Allowances* (*RDA*) (Table 6-1) provides a guide for the kinds and amounts of nutrients. These guidelines were first published in 1940 and are reviewed and revised periodically as more knowledge of nutritional needs is obtained through research. The table does not list all the vitamins and minerals known to be required. The energy levels in Table 6-1 are based on average needs for Americans of normal weight for height who lead relatively sedentary lives; they are not meant to be used as dietary prescriptions. The text of the *RDA* does discuss all nutrients, amounts, and rationale, as well as methods for evaluating energy requirements.[10]

The child or adult with diabetes mellitus needs protein to provide amino acids for replacement of body structure and growth, fat to provide essential fatty acids, energy, and to enhance absorption of fat-soluble vitamins, and carbohydrate to provide energy and fiber. Calcium, phosphorus, magnesium,

Table 6-1 Food and Nutrition Board, National Academy of Sciences–National
Designed for the maintenance of good nutrition of practically all healthy people in

	Age, years	Weight kg	Weight lb	Height cm	Height in	Energy, kcal[b]	Protein, g	Vitamin A activity, RE[c]	IU	Vitamin D, IU	Vitamin E activity,[d] IU
Infants	0.0–0.5	6	14	60	24	kg × 117	kg × 2.2	420[g]	1400	400	4
	0.5–1.0	9	20	71	28	kg × 108	kg × 2.0	400	2000	400	5
Children	1–3	13	28	86	34	1300	23	400	2000	400	7
	4–6	20	44	110	44	1800	30	500	2500	400	9
	7–10	30	66	135	54	2400	36	700	3300	400	10
Males	11–14	44	97	158	63	2800	44	1000	5000	400	12
	15–18	61	134	172	69	3000	54	1000	5000	400	15
	19–22	67	147	172	69	3000	54	1000	5000	400	15
	23–50	70	154	172	69	2700	56	1000	5000		15
	51+	70	154	172	69	2400	56	1000	5000		15
Females	11–14	44	97	155	62	2400	44	800	4000	400	12
	15–18	54	119	162	65	2100	48	800	4000	400	12
	19–22	58	128	162	65	2100	46	800	4000	400	12
	23–50	58	128	162	65	2000	46	800	4000		12
	51+	58	128	162	65	1800	46	800	4000		12
Pregnant						+300	+30	1000	5000	400	15
Lactating						+500	+20	1200	6000	400	15

[a] The allowances are intended to provide for individual variations among most normal people as they live in the United States under usual environmental stresses. Diets should be based on a variety of common foods in order to provide other nutrients for which human requirements have been less well defined. See text for more detailed discussion of allowances and of nutrients not tabulated.

[b] Kilojoules (kJ) = 4.2 × kcal.

[c] Retinol equivalents.

[d] Total vitamin E activity, estimated to be 80 percent α-tocopherol and 20 percent other tocopherols.

[e] The folacin allowances refer to dietary sources as determined by *Lactobacillus casei* assay. Pure forms of folacin may be effective in doses less than one-fourth of the recommended dietary allowance.

and vitamin D are needed, as are iron, B-complex vitamins, and so on. The same factors that determine dietary nutritional adequacy for any child or adult determine dietary nutritional adequacy for the person with diabetes mellitus. Weight control and normal growth are important aspects of dietary management for everyone, including the patient with diabetes. It has been said that the patient with diabetes has to do what everyone ought to do. This is based on concern for mitigation of the risks of degenerative disease for the diabetic person as well as control of blood glucose levels.

Perhaps the general public and people with diabetes would be better served if there were less emphasis on diet management for the control of diabetes and more emphasis on diet management for health in general. Those who have worked with families know that frequently the child with diabetes is singled out for special restrictions in food, play, rest, and social activities. The rational diet for the child with diabetes is the rational diet for his or her siblings and friends. Regularity in meals, consistency in food patterns, and control of the intake of rich desserts and candies are all desirable dietary goals for the entire family.

Research Council Recommended Daily Dietary Allowances (Revised 1974)[a]
the United States

| | Water-soluble vitamins | | | | | | Minerals | | | | | |
Ascorbic acid, mg	Folacin,[e] μg	Niacin,[f] mg	Riboflavin, mg	Thiamine, mg	Vitamin B₆, mg	Vitamin B₁₂, μg	Calcium, mg	Phosphorus, mg	Iodine, μg	Iron, mg	Magnesium, mg	Zinc, mg
35	50	5	0.4	0.3	0.3	0.3	360	240	35	10	60	3
35	50	8	0.6	0.5	0.4	0.3	540	400	45	15	70	5
40	100	9	0.8	0.7	0.6	1.0	800	800	60	15	150	10
40	200	12	1.1	0.9	0.9	1.5	800	800	80	10	200	10
40	300	16	1.2	1.2	1.2	2.0	800	800	110	10	250	10
45	400	18	1.5	1.4	1.6	3.0	1200	1200	130	18	350	15
45	400	20	1.8	1.5	2.0	3.0	1200	1200	150	18	400	15
45	400	20	1.8	1.5	2.0	3.0	800	800	140	10	350	15
45	400	18	1.6	1.4	2.0	3.0	800	800	130	10	350	15
45	400	16	1.5	1.2	2.0	3.0	800	800	110	10	350	15
45	400	16	1.3	1.2	1.6	3.0	1200	1200	115	18	300	15
45	400	14	1.4	1.1	2.0	3.0	1200	1200	115	18	300	15
45	400	14	1.4	1.1	2.0	3.0	800	800	100	18	300	15
45	400	13	1.2	1.0	2.0	3.0	800	800	100	18	300	15
45	400	12	1.1	1.0	2.0	3.0	800	800	80	10	300	15
60	800	+2	+0.3	+0.3	2.5	4.0	200	1200	125	18+[h]	450	20
80	600	+4	+0.5	+0.3	2.5	4.0	1200	1200	150	18	450	25

[f] Although allowances are expressed as niacin, it is recognized that on the average 1 mg of niacin is derived from each 60 mg of dietary tryptophan.

[g] Assumed to be all as retinol in milk during the first 6 months of life. All subsequent intakes are assumed to be half as retinol and half as β-carotene when calculated from international units. As retinol equivalents, three-fourths are as retinol and one-fourth as β-carotene.

[h] This increased requirement cannot be met by ordinary diets; therefore, the use of supplemental iron is recommended.

Source: Adapted from *Recommended Dietary Allowances,* 8th ed., National Academy of Sciences, Washington, D.C., with permission.

The majority of patients with diabetes in developed nations are overweight and obese adults. It is generally accepted that weight control with return to normal weight for height is the single most important aspect of dietary management, yielding returns in control of blood glucose and lipid levels. Control of body weight, and return to normal weight, is a goal for all adults, with or without diabetes.

Perhaps there would be fewer problems in patient acceptance of dietary management if that management were presented as the positive force for everyone's health that it truly is. More often it is presented to the patient, and family, as a necessary and unpleasant evil. The diet is given as a guide to deprivation and a loss of freedom in food choice. Dietary control *is* an integral part of management for the diabetic, but dietary control is an integral part of management for *anyone*.

Dietary Goals

In defining dietary goals it is necessary to differentiate the type of diabetes mellitus. In affluent societies such as the United States, the majority of patients have adult-onset diabetes and are fat. Relatively few are lean. A recent report estimates that 10 million people in the United States have diabetes known (1.6 percent of the population), unknown (0.6 percent), or are destined to develop it (2.8 percent).[11] The prevalence in children is about 1 in 1000. It is rare in preschool children and present at an approximate rate of 0.1 percent in school children. In adults, however, the situation is quite different, with some estimates of more than one-third of elderly Americans having impaired glucose tolerance.[12] Dietary goals for the insulin-dependent lean diabetic are different from those of the obese diabetic. They differ for people with growth-onset diabetes as opposed to maturity-onset diabetes. The general dietary goals are outlined in Table 6-2.

West estimates that about one-fourth of the known diabetics in the United States are being treated with insulin, about half with oral agents, and the remainder with no antidiabetic medication.[13] Many of the obese adult-onset diabetics could be managed without insulin or oral agents if dietary management were successfully handled.[14] It is important to differentiate between obesity and leanness, as well as insulin dependence. For the obese adult, weight reduction is the most important aspect of management—the essential dietary goal. For the normal or underweight patient, priorities differ.

Priorities

Diet for the child with diabetes is the same as for the nondiabetic child. The symptoms of diabetes mellitus in children are similar to those in adults, although the child is more likely to be underweight. Diagnosis may follow examination because of growth failure despite excellent eating or failure to recuperate with expected ease after an ordinary childhood infection. It may follow a

Table 6-2 Dietary Goals

Dietary component	Classification of diabetes mellitus		
	Growth onset		Maturity onset
	Child	Adult	
Total calories (most important)	Sufficient for growth, activity	Maintain weight, activity	Maintain desirable weight; weight reduction usually needed
Protein (RDA + 0.5)	1.5–2.5 g/kg	0.8–1.5 g/kg	0.8–1.5 g/kg
Fat	Varies to meet caloric need, 20 to 45 percent of calories; low saturated fat (10 percent calories) with polyunsaturated fat (10 percent) often prescribed for those with hyperlipoproteinemia.		
Carbohydrate: Amount	Varies to meet caloric need and management philosophy, 45 percent of calories appears acceptable.		
Type	Complex carbohydrates and simple carbohydrates that are normal components of food; concentrated doses of simple carbohydrates such as sucrose, syrups, honey, etc., should be avoided in low-calorie diets, limited in high-calorie diets.		
Distribution	Adjust to available insulin (relate to medication).		
Vitamins	Normal	Normal	Normal
Minerals	Normal	Normal	Normal
Meal size (most important)	Adjust to available insulin; consistency	Adjust to available insulin; consistency	Adjust to insulin/lifestyle; consistency
Meal frequency (most important)	Adjust to life-style and medication; consistency	Adjust to life-style and medication; consistency	Adjust to life-style; consistency

visit to a hospital emergency room. The child and the family may find it difficult to handle the emotional turmoil engendered by the diagnosis and the volume of information given on hygiene, foot care, medication, diet, and prevention of ketoacidosis. It is no surprise that many families find the stress very difficult to handle.

At first the child's requirements for energy and other nutrients may be higher than those of the usual child, since nutritional stores may be depleted until insulin therapy is instituted. After the initial period of regulation, energy intake is gradually adjusted to the appetite and weight response of the child. Priority should be given to increased frequency and number of feedings, with special attention to the day-to-day consistency in calories, carbohydrate, protein, and fat and the timing of meals. Food is used to prevent or treat hypoglycemia, and extra food is provided for unusual exercise. Prevention of starvation ketosis is important. Consistency in the ratios of carbohydrate, fat, and protein for each feeding on a day-to-day basis is desirable, since insulin requirement immediately after a high-carbohydrate meal is higher than after a low-carbohydrate meal.[15] The dietary prescription should be reviewed periodically to ensure adequate food to meet changes in body size and activity.

The same priorities exist for the lean insulin-dependent adult as for the child. For the obese adult, the major priority is weight reduction.[16] Benefits occur even if desirable body weight is not obtained. Protection or improvement of the beta-cell function is defined as a very urgent priority. If insulin or hypoglycemic agents are being used in the treatment of the obese patient, the timing of meals and consistency in meal size and content are important. Generally the obese adult is resistant to ketosis.

Calorie Requirement

How many calories should be provided? A standard used for children under 12 years as a starting point is 1000 cal plus 100 cal for each year of age. This should be adjusted as the child's response in weight and growth are observed. For adults, calories can be planned initially on the basis of general guidelines which consider the desirable body weight and general activity level: 20 kcal/kg for weight reduction, 25 kcal/kg for patients in bed, 30 kcal/kg for light activity (including ambulatory hospitalized patients), 35 kcal/kg for moderate activity, and 40 to 50 kcal/kg for people with habitually heavy work. Older people usually require somewhat fewer calories in relation to body size than young adults. A carefully taken quantitative dietary history can serve as a guide to previous intake when obtained by a dietitian skilled in the interviewing techniques required.[17,18] This, in conjunction with the weight history and estimation of activity, provides useful data on energy needs. Estimation of activity can be obtained by questioning the person about typical daily patterns of sleep and rest, sitting and standing, light, moderate, and heavy activity. Light activity includes walking at a moderate pace (2.5 to 3 mi/h), household activities such as washing clothes, garage work, carpentry, electrical and carpentry trades, and sports such as golf, volleyball, sailing, and table tennis. Moderate activity includes walking at 3.5 to 4 mi/h, weeding and hoeing, scrubbing floors, loading and stacking, and sports such as cycling, skiing, dancing, and tennis. Heavy work includes walking uphill with a load, using a pick and a shovel, felling trees, and sports such as climbing, swimming, basketball, and football.[19]

There is a tendency to restrict calories for all people with diabetes. It is essential to ensure sufficient energy for children and lean adult patients for growth, productivity, and general well-being. A common problem for these patients is that the diet that seemed adequate in the hospital is not sufficient after discharge. Activity at home can be quite different than activity in hospital, even for the ambulatory patient. This should be taken into account when determining the discharge diet prescription.

In general, pregnant women should have a moderate increase of 300 to 800 kcal per day in the last half of pregnancy, but total weight gain should not exceed 25 lb. An insufficient energy supply for the nonobese diabetic can compromise protein status.

Protein

The levels of protein recommended per kilogram of body weight are illustrated in Fig. 6-1. Traditionally, diets for people with diabetes have been generous in protein, since carbohydrate restriction has been a priority. In Table 6-2, the dietary goal for protein is listed as the recommended levels from the *RDA* plus 0.5 g/kg. Protein should provide not less than 10 percent of the energy needed to maintain desirable weight. Most Americans choose diets higher in protein, some up to 25 percent of calories. For children and pregnant women, protein should be provided at levels exceeding 1.5 g/kg daily. This provides a wide limit for adjusting the protein content of the diet to meet patient preferences. It is not necessary to require patients to adjust to high-protein diets and increased use of costly meat and dairy products. However, if a patient prefers a protein-rich diet, the prescription can be adjusted. Typical diet prescriptions provide about 20 percent of the total calories as protein. As mentioned, this can be adjusted to higher or lower amounts. Protein status also depends on the energy supply of the diet. A child or lean adult adhering to a diet with insufficient energy to meet needs is a potential candidate for protein malnutrition. Protein is needed for essential body functions but may be used for energy when calorie intake is too low to meet needs and there are no body fat reserves available.

Carbohydrate

The question of carbohydrate in the diet is controversial. Management and philosophy vary. Historically, diets for diabetics have been limited in carbohydrate, but recent research has demonstrated improved glucose tolerance

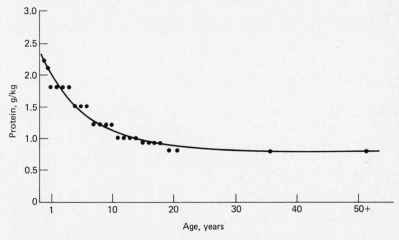

Figure 6-1 Recommended allowances for protein. Additional amounts are recommended for pregnant women. (*"Recommended Dietary Allowances,"* 8th ed., National Academy of Sciences.)

in patients with increased CHO intake.[20] The standard diets developed in 1950 by the American Diabetes Association, the American Dietetic Association, and the U.S. Public Health Service are low in carbohydrate and high in fat.[21] These groups have endorsed change,[22] but the old diets are still in wide use. There is also a problem in convincing physicians, nurses, and dietitians that the traditional pattern of carbohydrate restriction can be changed. When the energy content of the diet is controlled at appropriate levels, diets high in carbohydrate are well tolerated. A usual and acceptable level for most Americans is 45 percent of calories. Concern with risk of coronary artery disease has led groups such as the American Heart Association to recommend a reduction in fat intake to moderate levels (about 35 percent of calories), as well as a change in the kind of fat. Adherence to these guidelines will increase the proportion of carbohydrate.

A second question relating to carbohydrate concerns the type—sugars or starch. Most authorities recommend that the increase in carbohydrate intake be achieved with starch rather than sugars. Concentrated sources of simple sugars (sucrose, honey, syrups, jellies, fructose, etc.) may be used with discretion for patients requiring very high calorie levels. Sugars tend to produce sharp elevations of blood glucose. This may be a problem in the insulin-dependent patient. There may be deleterious hyperglycemic effects on small and large vessels, and in certain circumstances, sucrose and other sugars including fructose may raise serum triglyceride levels. Most Western diets include generous intakes of sugars and sweets. Most children and adults would benefit from obtaining more of their carbohydrate intake from vegetables, grains, and fruits. These foods provide starch, sugars, and fiber, together with protein, vitamins, and minerals. Nutrient contributions are high in relation to calorie value. Concentrated sweets contribute relatively little in nutritional value in proportion to calories. Many believe that small amounts of sugar ordinarily used in cooking can be allowed and that concentrated sweets should be permitted on special occasions. This is no different from the guidelines for good dietary practice for anyone of any age, with or without diabetes. There are others who recommend that no simple sugars or sweets be permitted at all.

Fat

The proportion of fat has been high in most diabetic diets and in American diets in general. The usual American diet has provided approximately 45 percent of the calories as fat, much of it saturated fat. The high prevalence of heart disease in the general public has led to recommendations for change in usual dietary patterns to reduce fat intake to about 35 percent, to decrease intake of saturated fat to 10 percent or less, and to increase intake of polyunsaturated fat to 10 percent or more of total calories.[23,24] This is endorsed for people with diabetes.[25] Limitation in dietary cholesterol is often advised. The change in type of dietary fat tends to limit dietary cholesterol, since most is found in the saturated fats.

One effect of the limitation of concentrated sweets and fat in the diet is to increase the volume of food on the plate. This should be an advantage for the obese patient, although it may be a challenge for those needing higher caloric intakes. This can be handled by careful planning of meal frequency and size with the patient.

A "modernized" diet for a patient in a Western society has been described as

1   Calories adequate to reach or maintain optimum weight
2   Protein level not critical, ranging from 12 to 24 percent of calories
3   Carbohydrate providing 10 to 15 percent of calories from the sugars naturally present in milk, fruit, and vegetables and the 30 to 40 percent remainder from starches, i.e., vegetables and grains, with sharp limitation on refined sugars
4   Fats limited to 25 to 35 percent of calories, with saturated fat making up 10 to 15 percent of calories and mono- and polyunsaturated fats providing the rest[26]

Since hypertriglyceridemia is frequent in people with diabetes, there has been concern about the increased proportion of carbohydrate calories. Incidence of hyperlipidemia is higher in uncontrolled diabetics (judged by fasting blood glucose levels) but persists in some controlled diabetics.[27] A recent study of adult patients reported that the controlled patients with hypertriglyceridemia had significantly higher values for intake of total calories, sucrose, and alcohol. Body weight was also a factor. The authors suggest weight reduction, stricter regulation of fasting blood glucose, and emphasis on principles of diet treatment including restrictions of total calories, sugar, and alcohol as the important targets for management of hypertriglyceridemia in outpatient adults.[28] Reasonable control of the blood glucose but not at the price of hypoglycemic attacks in patients with juvenile diabetes is advocated.[29]

Meal Pattern

The size and number of meals and snacks are also defined in establishing dietary goals. Consistency in the timing of meals is very important for insulin-dependent patients and must be related to insulin action (see Chapter 7). Consistency in carbohydrate content of meals is also important (i.e., lunch today, lunch tomorrow), since insulin requirements immediately after a meal vary with carbohydrate content even if total calories are kept the same by adjusting protein and fat content. Total insulin requirement for the day is apparently not affected with isocaloric exchanges.[30] For the patient not requiring insulin, consistency is not as crucial, though there are advantages for all people in establishing regular patterns of food intake.

Typical diet prescriptions provide for three meals a day and one or more snacks. Frequently these prescriptions are written without considering the patient's habits, desires, and actual needs. Patient preference and life-style should be taken into account. Insulin types and dosage can be adjusted within certain limits. Timing and distribution of meals for the insulin-dependent patient are of high priority. A number of alternatives exist in the time-action characteristics of various insulins, and certainly many alternatives in meal planning can be used to create a therapeutic program the patient can accept and manage. For the obese patient who does not require insulin, the priority is development of regular patterns of eating, with diets lower in total caloric value. There is little need to impose arbitrary patterns of meals and snacks. The obese patient does not need food to treat hypoglycemia nor extra food when undertaking unusual exercise. However, the insulin-dependent lean patient does.

The diet for the patient with diabetes mellitus is the normal diet with attention given to growth and development needs in the young and weight control at all ages.

DIETARY MANAGEMENT

Management will vary with the philosophies and goals of supervising physicians or units. Goals range from very strict to liberal to "free" diets. When the goal is to keep blood glucose within normal limits and urine sugar minimal or absent, management is usually quite rigid and may include the weighing of all foods, restricted menus and food choices, and carefully regulated insulin dosage. In contrast, the goal may be limited to prevention of ketosis (disregarding hyperglycemia and glycosuria) and control of body weight. This is often called the "free" diet regimen. Unfortunately many interpret the free diet as "no diet at all," thus mistaking freedom for license and forgetting that nutritional principles are still to be observed. Most patients on so-called free dietary regimens actually have modifications of one sort or another, e.g., restricted intake of concentrated carbohydrate foods, particularly of sweets; limitations on the number of feedings per day, with appetite at the meal providing some restraint; and regular meal schedules. When people advocating the free diet are questioned, the definition of *free* is generally found to be the normal diet, with all the principles of careful food choice and moderation that normal nutrition implies. In pediatric units with a liberal approach to dietary management, the basic goals of diet are there as part of the total regimen, even though the child in the hospital may choose his or her food from a regular house menu rather than receive a special, weighed "diabetic diet."

Most frequently, dietary management falls between the strict and the liberal. The aim is to keep blood glucose at almost normal levels for most of the day, using insulin as needed and avoiding hypoglycemia. Urine is sugar free or has only traces of sugar most of the day. Diet is adequate nutritionally and normal weight is maintained.

Perhaps the most important philosophy for all to observe is that treatment is directed to the person not the disease. There is need to adjust continuously to the demands of life—growth, exercise, illness, and work. The patient must know what the goals of therapy are, and must participate in planning the dietary regimen to meet those goals. The patient needs sufficient information to manage the diet at home, at school, at work, and socially. No matter what the philosophy of the physician, nurse, or dietitian, the treatment will depend on the patient's acceptance and ability to implement it.

The dietary prescription should include total calories for the day and distribution of protein, fat, and carbohydrate. Distribution and size of meals should be consistent for any patient, and matched to insulin activity for the insulin-dependent patient. In the past there were many elaborate schemes for dividing total carbohydrate into thirds, fifths, sevenths, and even eighteenths for meals and snacks. Available glucose from protein and fat, as well as from carbohydrate, was calculated. This practice has been changed, and patient preferences in meal frequency and size are taken into consideration. For the insulin-dependent patient, a combination of insulins with different periods of onset and peaks of activity can be used so that meals and snacks fit the patient's circumstances and patterns. For most lean insulin-dependent patients, smaller main meals and two or three snacks permit more effective treatment.

West suggests a checklist to aid in the formulation and implementation of diet prescriptions for specific patients.[31] The concept is useful. To assess patient needs, the following questions are provided as a guide for physician, nurse, and dietitian. The answers form the basis for the diet prescription and appropriate counseling. Whether the patient is newly diagnosed or not, the information gathered from these questions helps identify the degree of precision needed for dietary management and serves as the foundation for initial and continuing patient education.

1   What are the main purposes of the diet prescription? Control of body weight? Blood sugar? Urine sugar? Prevention of ketosis? Are there any other conditions such as cardiac or renal failure, hyperlipidemia, etc., requiring diet modification? What is most important? Are there other priorities?

2   Does the patient require insulin? What kind, when, and how much? Has an oral hypoglycemic agent been prescribed?

3   What caloric level is appropriate? For how long? (Consider growth, pregnancy, weight loss or gain, changes in activity.)

4   How are the calories to be provided? Are there any special requirements for levels of protein, fat, carbohydrate? Are there special requirements for the type of fat or carbohydrate? Can concentrated carbohydrates and sweets be used? Under what circumstances can alcohol or sugar substitutes be used?

5   To what degree is day-to-day consistency important in caloric intake, meal size, and frequency of feedings? Can meals be modified, postponed, or skipped?

6   Is the distribution of food during the day important? Are there specific requirements for timing or size of feedings because of insulin action, patient preferences, or schedule?

7   What adjustments, if any, are to be made for exercise or glycosuria? Should food be used to prevent or treat hypoglycemia?

8   Is the diet prescription feasible? Practical? Livable? Is the volume of food acceptable? Have economic and social factors been considered? Does the patient have any constraints on food choice such as religious observances, vegetarian practices, likes, dislikes, or allergies to consider? Are meals and snacks timed to fit comfortably into the patient's schedule?

9   Does the patient understand the dietary principles? Does the patient have the facts? How much information does the patient have? Can the patient use the information? What additional information does the patient need? How much responsibility has the patient assumed for dietary management?

10   What technique is the patient using for control of diet? Is food unmeasured, estimated, measured, or weighed? What sort of diet plan is used, e.g., counting calories or carbohydrate, a menu guide, food groupings, or an exchange system?

11   Do current dietary practices provide a nutritionally adequate intake of energy, protein, fat, carbohydrate, vitamins, and minerals? Do the dietary practices meet the main purposes and priorities as defined for question 1? What changes, if any, are needed?

12   Has the patient made the dietary plan with the help of the professional or is the plan imposed on the patient? What changes, if any, does the patient want?

The Dietary Priority

For many patients the dietary priority is to control calories. Weight reduction and protection of beta-cell function are the goals of therapy for obese patients, and a reduced energy intake is the first priority. Insulin is not usually needed. Although consistency in dietary patterns is desirable, it is not crucial. Extra food for unusual exercise or for hypoglycemia is not needed, and these patients are resistant to starvation ketosis. Foods containing refined sugars (sucrose, glucose, fructose, honey, or syrups) are usually restricted because of caloric value and in order to avoid sharp elevations of blood glucose.

In some instances, the patient may be told simply to control carbohydrate intake. This can be misinterpreted as meaning that the purpose is to eat as little carbohydrate as possible. In some cases, only carbohydrate limitation is prescribed, with the assumption that such restriction will reduce caloric intake, which is not always true. For patients requiring insulin, control of calories and carbohydrate may be prescribed, with the recommendation that each feeding include protein.

Control of carbohydrate, protein, and fat, as well as calories, is more generally recommended and is effective for the patient requiring insulin. Timing of meals, size of feedings, and consistency in ratios of protein, fat, and carbohydrate are important for insulin-dependent patients. Food can be distributed to meet patient preferences, with insulin dosage then determined.

Portion Control

Should food be weighed or measured? The amount of food eaten is important whether calories alone, carbohydrate alone, calories and carbohydrate, or calories, protein, fat, and carbohydrate are to be controlled. Some people are very good at estimating portion sizes. Others need some help in visualizing how much food is the right amount. The *weighed diet* is prescribed by some physicians. It consists of a meal plan with gram weights of the foods to be eaten. Foods are weighed to ensure proper portion sizes. Although this may be used as the continuing basis of diet therapy, often this quantitation is used during hospitalization and for some time at home as a mechanism for acquainting patients with portion sizes, after which, less rigorous measures are expected.[33] The *measured diet* uses household measures of ounces and cups. Effective control of intake of calories or carbohydrate does require portion control. It is useful for patients to weigh or measure food portions when first learning the diet. After they have become familiar with the amounts of food, estimates can be made. Weighing or measuring food at every meal can become tedious for most people and is not usually necessary once the patient develops some skill in judging portions. The scales, measuring cups, and spoons can then be used periodically to check portion sizes. If trouble develops, such as episodes of hyper- or hypoglycemia or inappropriate weight change, portion sizes should be checked by weighing or measuring. If the difficulties persist, the diet prescription or insulin dosage (if insulin is taken) should be reviewed by the physician. The *unmeasured diet* is often prescribed for the young juvenile-onset diabetic. The number of feedings is specified, and the patient is told to eat sufficient food to satisfy the appetite at the meal or snack times specified. Close attention is paid to timing, and drastic swings in blood sugar are avoided. The value of this regimen lies in its flexibility, permitting caloric intake to meet energy demands, and beneficial psychological aspects. Sweets such as cake might be a part of the meal. The unmeasured diet may be considered "no diet at all" by some professionals or by patients trained to use weighed or measured diets who are shocked to see a young patient eat cookies or similar sweets. The unmeasured diet is a diet regimen, however. It relies on appetite as a guide for consumption of adequate amounts of food to meet caloric needs, chosen from meals with desserts in moderation and wholesome foods for regularly scheduled snacks. There is controversy about inclusion of sweets in the diet, with some physicians allowing them on a once-a-week basis, others allowing them with meals if appetite persists after consumption of an adequate variety of foods, and still others not permitting them at all. If trouble develops, food intake and medication patterns are checked, with changes made as needed. This might require use of a measured diet.

TOOLS FOR DIETARY MANAGEMENT

Once the goals have been established and the diet prescription written, there are a variety of tools that can be used to help the patient determine a schedule for the number of feedings and the kinds and amounts of food to be eaten.

Exchange Lists

Since 1950 meal planning with exchange lists has been used as a practical measure.[34] Common foods are divided into groups with approximately the same amount of carbohydrate and fat. Specific foods within the lists differ slightly from the nutritive value given as average for the group, but these differences tend to cancel out because of the different foods eaten from day to day. The diet is worked out using the exchange system to meet the dietary prescriptions for energy, carbohydrate, protein, and fat. After the total number of exchanges is determined (keeping in mind the vitamin and mineral needs as well), they are then distributed into a meal/snack pattern. The meal pattern should take into account insulin activity and the patient's usual patterns. The patient can select foods from the exchange list after the menu is planned. In this way the menu provides a guide for controlling calories, carbohydrate, meal size, and frequency as necessary but allows the patient some freedom of choice in the specific foods to be eaten. In 1976 the exchange lists were revised so they could be used more easily for fat modifications.[35] A guide is available for the professional, with detailed information on developing the nutritional care plan and calculating specific diets.[36] Changing fat intake to decrease saturated fat and increase polyunsaturated fat intake is recommended to reduce the incidence of hyperlipoproteinemia in patients with diabetes.[37,38] The exchange system can be used for any patient, young or adult, lean or obese, requiring insulin or not.

The values for calculating the diet using the exchange systems are listed in Table 6-3. Procedures for calculating the diet will now be presented in detail.

Table 6-3 Food Exchange Lists
Caloric Values, Carbohydrate, Protein, and Fat

		Macronutrients			
Food list	Amount	Carbo-hydrate, g	Pro-tein, g	Fat, g	Calories
From *Meal Planning with Exchange Lists* (1950)					
Milk (regular and other)	1 cup	12	8	10	170
Vegetables A	as desired	N	N	N	170
Vegetables B	½ cup	7	2		35
Fruit (raw or unsweetened)	varies	10			40
Bread (and starchy vegetables)	varies	15	2		70
Meat	1 oz		7	5	75
Fat	1 tsp		7	5	45
From *Exchange Lists for Meal Planning* (1976)					
Milk (nonfat and other)	1 cup	12	8	T	80
Vegetables (nonstarchy)	½ cup	5	2		25
Fruit (raw or unsweetened)	½ cup	10			40
Bread (and starchy vegetables)	varies	15	2		70
Meat (lean):	1 oz		7	3	55
Medium fat (lean + ½ fat)	1 oz		7	5.5	80
High fat (lean + 1 fat)	1 oz		7	8	100
Fat	1 tsp			5	45

Source: Adapted from American Diabetes Association, Inc., American Dietetic Association, and Chronic Disease Program, U.S. Public Health Service, *Meal Planning with Exchange Lists* (Chicago: American Dietetic Association, 1950); and American Diabetes Association, Inc., American Dietetic Association, and National Institutes of Health, U.S. Public Health Service, *Exchange Lists for Meal Planning* (Chicago: American Dietetic Association, 1976).
Note: N = negligible; T = trace.

First, the amount of milk, vegetable, and fruit exchanges are determined, taking into account the patient's preferences. Second, total the remaining carbohydrate and divide by 15 to determine the number of bread exchanges. Total carbohydrate should be within 3 or 4 g of the prescription. Third, protein is totaled, subtracted from the prescription, and then divided by 7 to determine the number of meat exchanges. Fourth, the fat from all foods is totaled, subtracted from the prescription, and divided by 5 to determine the number of fat exchanges. Then the diet is checked for accuracy, and the daily food allowance is divided into a meal pattern. If there are particular foods the patient wants, these can be fitted into the appropriate exchange list or worked into the dietary pattern for daily use. The guidelines for professional use suggest that meals provide 20 to 40 percent of the calories and carbohydrate and snacks provide 10 percent. Three meals per day are usual for the non-insulin-dependent person, three meals and a bedtime snack for the insulin-dependent person. This will vary depending on the patient and on the blood glucose levels. The lists of foods for the 1950 and 1976 exchange systems are presented at the end of this chapter.

The basis for food grouping is illustrated in Figs. 6-2 to 6-4. In Fig. 6-2, the contributions of protein, fat, and carbohydrate to the total energy value of food items is illustrated. Milk and its products, such as yogurt, supply protein, fat, and carbohydrate. Cheese is grouped with meat because its protein, fat, and carbohydrate values are more similar to meat than to milk. Peanut butter is also grouped with meat for the same reason, with a reduction in fat exchanges on the day peanut butter is used to keep calories close to the prescribed level. Most vegetables are listed in vegetable exchanges, but certain vegetables, such as potatoes, corn, dried peas and beans, and winter squash, are in the bread exchange list because in servings ordinarily consumed they provide an amount of carbohydrate equivalent to bread. The concentration of calories in moderate portions of food can be seen in Fig. 6-3. Many patients find the volume of food greater than expected because of limitations on the intake of concentrated sweets and the absence from the list of foods concentrated in fats and sweets. In appropriate circumstances, items such as a doughnut, soft drinks, or even sugar may be included in the diet plan.

The exchange lists are often criticized for not including mixed dishes. Since they do include the common staple food items, they are relatively easy to convert for mixed dishes. Pizza is bread with a tomato sauce and cheese topping. Sausage or pepperoni, green pepper, and mushrooms may be added. This translates to bread, vegetable, and meat exchanges, with additional meat and vegetable exchanges. Exchange values have been published for items in popular fast-food chains.[39] The patient familiar with the exchange lists and with portion sizes can judge portions in relation to the menu pattern established and not feel obligated to eat everything. Many patients know the exchange lists well and can manipulate food choices within the menu pattern easily. A hamburger at McDonald's or Burger Chef counts as 1½ bread, 1 meat, and 1½ fat exchanges; a quarter-pounder, 2½ bread, 3 meat, and 1 fat exchanges. Exchange values for canned soups are available from the manufacturers. Exchange values for Southern ethnic foods have been published.[40] There are cookbooks

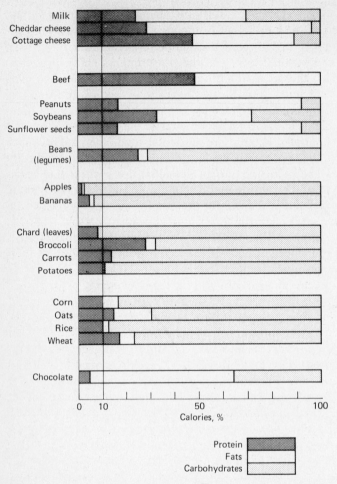

Figure 6-2 Calorie sources in common foods. (Note where protein contributes 10 percent or more of the caloric value.)

and pamphlets available which provide recipes and exchange list equivalents.

There is concern with arbitrary substitutions of one type of food for another solely on the basis of caloric value. Foods do differ in their vitamin and mineral contributions to the diet. This is illustrated in Fig. 6-4. The concentration of five vitamins and four minerals for the first food listed in each of the six 1976 exchange lists is shown. The black squares indicate that the food provides more than 20 percent of the recommended dietary allowance (RDA) figure for an adult; horizontal lines indicate 10 to 20 percent. Although the energy values of 1 cup of skim milk and 1 oz of medium-fat meat are similar (80 and 78 kcal), the nutrient contributions are quite different. The milk is rich in calcium and low in iron, while the meat is low in calcium and an important source of iron. If the patient does not drink milk or eat yogurt and will not use milk in food

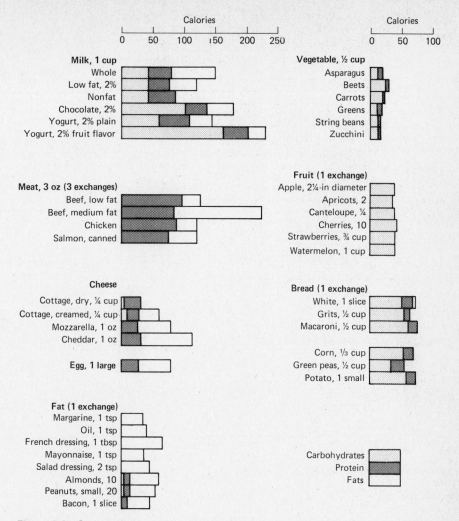

Figure 6-3 Carbohydrate, protein, fat, and calories in household portions of common foods.

preparation, an alternative source of calcium should be calculated into the diet pattern. This can be done by substituting 1 oz of cheddar cheese and 1 fruit exchange for 1 skim milk and 2 fat exchanges. Fractions of exchanges should be avoided unless the patient is comfortable with them.

When the exchange lists are used as the technique for meeting dietary goals, the patient should be given the meal pattern showing the exchange list and number of choices from each list for each meal or feeding. The dietitian should work together with the patient in defining the pattern. The system can be used when calorie control only is desired, when calorie and carbohydrate control is desired, or when calorie, protein, carbohydrate, and fat control is desired. The system has the advantage of being known and used throughout the

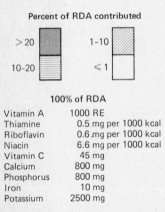

	Vitamins					Minerals			
	Vitamin A	Thiamine	Riboflavin	Niacin	Vitamin C	Calcium	Phosphorus	Iron	Potassium
Nonfat milk, 1 cup	10-20	>20	>20	>20	1-10	>20	>20		10-20
Asparagus, cooked, ½ cup	>20	1-10	>20	>20	>20	1-10	1-10	1-10	1-10
Apple, raw, 1 small	1-10	>20	10-20		>20	1-10	1-10	1-10	1-10
Bread, whole-grain or enriched, 1 slice		>20	>20	>20		1-10	1-10	1-10	1-10
Beef, lean, cooked, 1 oz		>20	>20	>20			1-10	1-10	1-10
Margarine, 1 tsp	1-10								

Percent of RDA contributed

> 20	▓	1-10 ▨
10-20	▤	≤ 1 □

100% of RDA

Vitamin A	1000 RE
Thiamine	0.5 mg per 1000 kcal
Riboflavin	0.6 mg per 1000 kcal
Niacin	6.6 mg per 1000 kcal
Vitamin C	45 mg
Calcium	800 mg
Phosphorus	800 mg
Iron	10 mg
Potassium	2500 mg

Figure 6-4 Vitamin and mineral contributions of foods. The first food in each exchange list in Table 6-9 is shown and the percent or the recommended dietary allowance (RDA) for each nutrient contributed by each food is indicated. As meat portions are usually larger than 1 oz, their contributions to diet are correspondingly greater. Any food contributing 10 percent or more of the RDA is considered a good source. (*Based on data from "Home and Garden Handbook," 72, USDA, 1977; and "Recommended Dietary Allowances," 8th ed., National Academy of Sciences.*)

country. This is helpful for patients who must travel or who change locations frequently.

Both sets of food lists for the exchange system are provided in Tables 6-9 and 6-10 at the end of this chapter. The lists can be adapted with relative ease for other dietary constraints, such as change in consistency (for surgery, dental problems, etc.), as illustrated in Table 6-4, and sodium restrictions. Modifications in amount and type of fat are easily handled by using the 1976 exchange lists.

Points System

Another technique for dietary management is the points system.[41] Foods are placed in four categories: calories, carbohydrate, protein, or fat. The total daily allowance of food may be written as a number of calorie points and a number of carbohydrate points, with meat, milk and/or fat to be included at each feeding. The most frequent use of this system is for calorie control or calorie and carbohydrate control. Advantages claimed for the system are (1) patients learn about nutrients, and (2) the technique offers something new.

Menu or Meal Plan

For the newly diagnosed patient or the patient confused and overwhelmed by demands, a very simple and rather rigid menu might be the best technique for dietary management, at least until difficulties are sorted out and the patient is ready for more variety in the diet and the responsibility of making his or her own food choices. The diet plan might well read: 4 oz orange juice, 1 cup cooked cereal, 1 slice of toast with 1 tsp butter, 8 oz (1 cup) of 2 percent milk, coffee, and so on. The menu, whatever the details, should conform to the dietary prescription and to the patient's preferences. When the patient is ready for more information and more freedom, exchange lists or another system can be introduced.

Percent of Carbohydrate System

Before exchange lists were developed, diet patterns based on the percent of carbohydrate in foods were used frequently. They are still used by many clinicians, and for the management of children. A sample for a 2800-cal diet used for children with diabetes is presented in Table 6-5. Fruits and vegetables are classified according to the grams of carbohydrate present in 100 g of the food; edible portion or portion size is varied so that the yield of carbohydrate is constant. For example, the dinner guide specifies 150 g of a 6 percent or 100 g of a 9 percent fruit or vegetable, since either would yield 9 g of carbohydrate.

Calculation of Dietary Intake by Patient

Diet calculation can be used by the patient who knows the concentrations of carbohydrate, protein, and fat in common foods. Such calculation is useful for insulin-dependent patients who may need a high degree of consistency in dietary intake. It allows a wider range of choices and provides social advantages for those eating often outside the home. Patients (and/or parents) may begin with the exchange system, which groups foods by calories and nutrients, and then move to the more complex method of diet calculation. Tables of food values are readily available from the government printing office[42,43] and are reproduced in many nutrition texts.

Table 6-4 Modification in Consistency

For a patient adhering to a diet prescription for diabetes mellitus: 2140 calories, 110 g protein, 100 g fat, 200 g CHO—(carbohydrate distribution: ⅓, ⅓, ⅓).

Food plan (usual guide)	Soft	Full liquid
Breakfast (exchanges)		
Fruit (1)	½ cup orange juice	½ cup orange juice
Bread (3)	½ cup oatmeal	1½ cup oatmeal gruel
	2 slices bread, white, enriched	
Meat (2)	2 poached eggs	2 eggs (in eggnog)
Milk (1)	1 cup milk	1 cup milk (in eggnog with saccharin and vanilla)
Fat (2)	2 tsp margarine	4 tbsp cream (in gruel)
Lunch (exchanges)		
Meat (2)	2 oz chicken	Pea soup (½ can diluted with 1 cup milk)
Bread (3)	3 slices bread	
Fat (2)	2 tsp margarine	
Vegetable A	½ cup tomato juice	
Fruit (1)	½ ripe banana	1 cup fruit nectar
Milk (1)	1 cup milk	½ cup milk
Supper (exchanges)		
Meat (6)	6 oz beef, tender	4 oz strained beef in broth
Vegetable A	½ cup green beans	1 cup vegetable puree
Vegetable B (2)	1 cup peas and carrots	
Bread (3)	1 cup mashed potatoes	1 cup cereal gruel
	1 slice bread, white, enriched	½ cup vanilla ice cream
Fat (2)	2 tsp margarine	(from ice cream)
Fruit (1)	½ cup canned peach, unsweetened	1 cup fruit juice or nectar, unsweetened
		1 cup skim milk with ⅓ cup skim milk solids

Source: Adapted from American Diabetes Association, Inc., American Dietetic Association, and Chronic Disease Program, U.S. Public Health Service, *Meal Planning with Exchange Lists* (Chicago: American Dietetic Association, 1950).

Note: Commercial products are available. The amounts to be used must be calculated to meet the dietary prescription. The majority of the products are milk-based. They can be purchased in drugstores and some grocery stores. In general they are more expensive. Some people find them unacceptable; others tire of them quickly. Examples:

	Calories	Protein, g	Fat, g	CHO, g
Sustagen, ⅔ cup + ⅔ cup water (concentrate for oral use)	330	20	3	63
Meritene, 1 oz in 1 cup milk	270	18	10	29
Dietene, 1 oz in 1 cup skim milk	188	18	T	29
Metracal, 8 oz	225	18	5	25
Meat-base formulas are also available				
Home-made mixture: 6 oz skim milk + ¼ to ⅓ cup dried milk solids (whole milk could be used as base)	182	18	1	25

Table 6-5 Measured Diet Using Percent of Carbohydrate
(2800-cal Diet)

Breakfast	Weight, g	Energy, cal	Lunch and dinner	Weight, g	Energy, cal
Milk	480	340	Milk	480	340
Choose one:			Choose one:		
Egg	100		Egg		
Egg and	50	154	Beef, veal, salmon, lamb, chicken,		
bacon	15		turkey, dried beef	80	
(cooked)			Pork, duck, luncheon meat,		
			weiners	60	
Choose one:			Liver (cooked)	85	
6% fruit	295		Fresh fish	100	161
9% fruit	200		Oysters and	100	
12% fruit	160	78	milk	135	
15% fruit	125		Liver (cooked) and	35	
Dried prunes	30		bacon (cooked)	15	
Banana	90		Egg and	50	
			bacon (cooked)	15	
Choose one:			Cottage cheese	150	
Cereal (prepared)	30	102	American cheese	40	
Cereal (cooked)	150	102			
Bread	60	160	Choose one:		
Butter or margarine	15	108	3% fruit or vegetable	150	
			6% fruit or vegetable	100	
			9% fruit or vegetable	70	
			Choose one:		
			6% fruit or vegetable	220	
			9% fruit or vegetable	150	
			12% fruit or vegetable	120	
			15% fruit or vegetable	95	62
			Banana	70	
			Dried apricots or prunes	22	
			Dates or raisins	20	
			Choose one:		
			18% fruit or vegetable	150	
			15% fruit or vegetable	190	
			12% fruit or vegetable	240	
			9% fruit or vegetable	—	
			Bread	45	
			Soda or graham crackers	30	120 A
			Sweet potato	75	
			Banana	135	
			Dried apricots or prunes	45	
			Dates or raisins	43	
			Macaroni, spaghetti, rice, dried		
			beans, or peas (cooked)	100	
			Noodles (cooked)	150	
			Choose one:		
			Bread	40	107
			Soda or graham crackers	25	107
			Butter or margarine	15	108

Source: Adapted from R. L. Jackson and S. W. Beckett, Dietary management of children with diabetes, *J.A.M.A.,* **32:**528–533, 1956.

Note: Energy values listed are average calories for each group of choices.

A Simplified System

What about the patient who finds the exchange system too much to handle? The Diabetes Teaching Program was developed at the University Hospitals of Cleveland for use with adult patients who have not completed high school and who find conventional written materials confusing. Although the patients are readers, the spoken word is the basic source of information. Programmed instructions with information on diet and other aspects of self-care for the diabetic patient have been developed.[44] The diet is a simplified version of the exchange system with the major priorities being control of caloric intake and consumption of a variety of foods (meat-milk, starch, vegetable-fruit) at each meal and for the evening snack. A dinner plate is color-coded for each of the three food types, as is a wall chart diagraming the meals for the day.

Standard Diets

Standard diets at various caloric levels have been calculated for every system described. They can be found in hospital and clinic diet manuals. They are not reproduced here because the diet plan, whatever the mechanics—exchanges, points, percent carbohydrate, or patient manipulation of nutrients—should be devised by the patient and dietitian in consultation to make it truly individual and "livable."

Written Instructions

Whatever mechanics are used to help the patient manage diet, the patient should be given written instructions which include the purpose of the diet, priorities, size, and choices for each meal or feeding, a list of foods that can be used in any amount, a list of foods which should be avoided, and directions for use of special foods important to the patient that might not appear on standard lists.

Written instructions should include information about extra food to be taken for unusual exercise and the use of food to prevent or treat hypoglycemia. Management of diet and insulin when ill should be written out as well, so that the insulin-dependent patient can avoid the complications of hypoglycemia.

The reader should recognize that all the systems described here maintain regular intake in definable limits. They do not ensure absolutely the same caloric, protein, carbohydrate, or fat intake for each meal or day. Absolute control is neither necessary nor practical. The variations are relatively small because of the food groupings. The different choices of meats, fruits, vegetables, and so on used through the week average out to meet the dietary prescription.

SPECIAL FOODS AND CONCERNS OF LIFE-STYLE

Questions about food and meal management for special events or activities should be expected whether the patient is newly diagnosed or experienced in managing diabetes. New foods are constantly introduced into the marketplace. Special dietary items and sugar substitutes are available and new items are being developed. In most families, at least one meal a day is eaten outside the home. Changes in work, social patterns, and life-style will affect choices in food.

Fortunately more information is available to staff and patients. Nutrition labels are useful, and food companies are becoming more responsive to questions about products. The dietitian should be asked to provide guidance for specific situations. The American Diabetes Association publishes *Diabetes Forecast,* a magazine many patients find helpful. Most issues have one or more articles about diet management and food preparation.

Nutrition Labels

Labeling regulations for packaged foodstuffs have changed, and the new nutrition labels provide a source of useful information for the patient and professional staff. The labeling program is voluntary for processors unless claims are made for nutritional value of the food. The label information is based on analysis of the product in the package.

The list of ingredients is not classified as part of the nutrition label. Items are listed in order by weight, largest quantities first. Sugar, sucrose, dextrose, corn-syrup solids, or corn sweetener on an ingredients list help the patient identify foods with simple sugars.

Samples of the information available from nutrition labels on food cans are given in Table 6-6. The label must include serving size and number of servings

Table 6-6   Nutrition Labels

	Pears		Peaches, heavy syrup	Pineapple juice	Tomatoes
	Water pack	Heavy syrup			
Serving size	½ cup	1 cup	1 cup	1 cup	1 cup
Servings per container	4	2	2	2½	2
Per serving:					
Calories	35	190	190	140	50
Protein, g	0	.1	1	1	2
Carbohydrate, g	9	49	50	35	11
Fat, g	0	0	0	1	0
Percent of U.S. recommended daily allowances					
Protein	*	*	*	*	2
Vitamin A	*	*	20	2	30
Vitamin C	4	4	15	10	60
Thiamine	*	*	*	10	8
Riboflavin	*	4	2	2	4
Niacin	*	2	8	2	10
Calcium	*	*	*	2	8
Iron	*	4	2	4	4

* Less than 2 percent of the RDA. These nutrients taken from labels of items in grocery store.

in the container. Unless specified otherwise, values include solids and liquids. Although the label for pears packed in water provides data for ½ cup of fruit and that for the pears packed in heavy syrup defines one serving as 1 full cup of fruit, the mathematics involved are simple enough that it can be determined that ½ cup of water-pack pears provides 35 cal in contrast to 95 cal for ½ cup of syrup-pack pears (or peaches). The fruit packed in heavy syrup is not the better choice because of the high caloric level for a ½-cup serving and because the additional calories come from sugar.

Most dietary instructions for diabetic patients urge the use of fresh fruit or fruits canned or frozen without the addition of sugar. A study of the consumption of fresh and processed pears by people with and without diabetes was conducted to determine if this restriction was necessary. Fresh, juice-pack, and light-syrup-pack pears in servings providing 35 g of carbohydrate were fed to fasting subjects. Blood samples were taken before and after consumption of the fruit and analyzed for glucose. Subjects with more severe diabetes had higher and more transient glucose levels. The study was limited to a small number of people and to pears as the sole item of intake. Response might differ if the pears were eaten as part of a regular meal. The data were interpreted to indicate that it might not be necessary to eliminate syrup-pack fruit from the diets of all diabetics.[45] Fruit packed in heavy syrup was not tested in this study. Frequently patients are instructed to eat syrup-pack fruit after washing off the syrup if no other choice is available.

The labels in Table 6-6 also demonstrate relative vitamin and mineral contributions to the diet. Of the five foods listed, tomatoes offer more nutritional value for the calories provided than any other item. Use of food labels can be of value to the patient and family in choosing foods of appropriate caloric and carbohydrate content. The information is adequate for the patient using the exchange system to make easy substitutions. Labels might also influence food choices related to total nutritional value. It is obvious from Table 6-6 that tomatoes provide more nutrients in relation to energy value than the other foods listed.

Special Foods and Sugar Substitutes

The diet does not require the use of special and costly food items. The use of special foods marked "dietetic" can lead to problems. These items may be low in sodium rather than sucrose. Many products may be low in sugar but high in calories because fat has been increased for palatable texture and flavor. Dietetic candies are expensive and not necessarily low in calories. Many use hexitols such as sorbitol or xylitol instead of sugar. Sugar alcohols are metabolized more slowly, thus limiting the peaks in blood glucose seen with sugar intake. Used in moderation, items made of hexitols provide some calories but probably not enough to cause concern. Used generously, they may produce diarrhea.

In the past, fruits canned without sugar were considered special diet items. Now juice-pack and water-pack fruits are frequently stocked beside syrup-pack fruits on store shelves. An increased variety of fruits frozen without additional sugar (or minimal sugar) is available in many stores.

Sugar substitutes are popular. Their value lies in providing a sweet flavor without the penalties of calories and blood glucose peaks associated with sugar intake. Although a study of the value of noncaloric sweeteners for diabetic patients demonstrated that adherence to the dietary prescription was independent of their use,[46] they are popular. Artificially sweetened drinks are used by a large portion of the public. Some contain appreciable sugar, so labels must be checked.

Twice within a decade the safety of artificial sweeteners has been questioned. Cyclamate was banned in 1969, and saccharin may be banned depending on further studies of cancer risk. In one report of public reaction to the proposed saccharin ban, 30 percent of the respondents called saccharin "absolutely essential" for those who must restrict sugar intake.[47] A recent regulation requires risk warning labels on products containing saccharin.

The public is not accepting the proposed saccharin ban quietly. Cohen has proposed a risk/benefit analysis which compares the risk of a person getting cancer from ingesting saccharin versus the risk of ingesting additional calories that cause excess body weight. He concludes that a person overweight by 10 percent has a risk of decrease in life expectancy of 9 s from ingesting one diet drink or one additional kilocalorie. "If ingesting a diet drink inhibits ingestion of more than 1 kilocalorie, its benefits exceed its risks."[48] There is no evidence that diet drinks reduce caloric intake (water relieves thirst too), and the calculation is based on many assumptions. This calculation is included to demonstrate public reaction.

Although saccharin was available as a noncaloric substitute for cyclamate in 1969, there is no compound available to replace saccharin. Sorbitol yields about the same calories as the sugar it replaces and is less sweet than sucrose. Fructose has been suggested. It is generally sweeter than sucrose, so smaller amounts could be used for sweetening, and it does not require insulin for certain metabolic steps. However, it does yield calories and it can be converted to glucose in the liver. Fructose is being tested, but it does not seem to offer any real advantage.

A recent cookbook published for people with diabetes or those who wish to limit caloric intake uses neither sugar nor saccharin. A "basic sweetener" made of equal measures of water and raisins blended until smooth is used in the recipes. The mix yields about 17 cal/tbsp, a little less than one-half a fruit exchange. The recipes were all tested, and caloric values, as well as exchange values, are provided.[49] A variety of similar cookbooks have been published.[50-52] In addition, most local diabetes associations have a variety of materials available, including materials for diet management. If there is no local association, the national offices may be contacted directly.[53,54]

The need for special sweeteners is being challenged.[55] Sucrose has not been allowed in traditional diets because it is considered a "fast" carbohydrate that gives rise to hyperglycemia and because it provides energy without providing essential nutrients. The caloric value of sugar is the most important reason for limiting intake for the majority of people with diabetes, since most are maturity-onset with obesity or weight-control problems. There is a general assumption that patients miss the sweet taste and need substitutes. Many of the products designed as special for the diabetic diet and without sugar (sucrose) contain high amounts of fat and/or alternate sources of carbohydrate and calories. An emphasis on control of sugar intake rather than caloric intake misleads many patients into believing that special dietary items may be used freely.

For the child or lean adult diabetic, regular inclusion of items such as a doughnut or a soft drink as part of a meal or snack in the total diet plan may prove the best answer. Regularity of intake from day to day and regularity of the composition of meals are priorities for management, as stated earlier. Children and lean adult diabetics generally have relatively high energy needs, and the volume of food to be consumed could be a problem. Including these foods as part of a diet that is coordinated with insulin activity may be useful in the management of certain patients.

Birthday Parties

One question that occurs frequently is that of birthday parties and cakes for the child. Some physicians allow ice cream and plain cake for special occasions. In the cookbooks previously mentioned, there are dessert recipes, many of which use artificial sweeteners. They all have energy value. One simple expedient is use of angel food cake. One (16-oz) package of angel food cake mix provides about 24 servings of cake at about 75 cal per serving. To provide variation, cocoa (¾ cup) can be added to the flour mixture in two-step mixes before folding in the egg whites. Check with the dietitian for suggestions that might be consistent with the management practices of the unit or supervising physician. For a diabetic child's birthday, the family can plan a party with refreshments provided for all the guests at the time regularly scheduled for the child's meal or snack. The menu can be based on the child's pattern, and feature favorite foods.

Alcohol

Alcohol is high in calories (7 kcal/g) and low in nutrient value. Beers and wines also contain carbohydrate (see Table 6-7). For most patients, occasional drinks are permitted, with fat calories traded for alcohol calories. If the patient wants an alcoholic beverage daily and the physician agrees, it may be considered in the calculation of the diet. Amounts should be small. Alcohol tends to promote hypertriglyceridemia. A combination of alcohol and insulin can potentiate hypoglycemia, so patients are usually advised to take the alcohol with food. Patients taking sulfonylureas (see Chapter 7) may experience symptoms such as flushing, tingling of the face, and palpitation.

Vegetarian Diets

For the patient who is a vegetarian, there are many choices. It is possible to use the exchange system. Those who use animal products such as milk, cheese, and eggs (lactovovegetarians) will find the lists easy to adapt.[56] Vegetable protein

Table 6-7   Alcoholic Beverages

Beverage	Carbo-hydrate, g	Protein, g	Fat, g	Calories, g
Gin, rum, vodka, whisky				
1 fl oz:				
80 proof	—	—	—	65
90 proof	—	—	—	74
100 proof	—	—	—	83
1 jigger (1½ fl oz):				
80 proof	—	—	—	97
90 proof	—	—	—	110
100 proof	—	—	—	124
Beer (4.5, 3.6%):*				
8-oz cup	9.1	0.7	0	101
12-oz can or bottle	13.7	1.1	0	151
Wine:				
Table (12.2, 9.9)*				
1 fl oz	1.2	T	0	25
Wine glass, 3½ oz	4.3	0.1	0	87
Dessert (18:8, 15.3):*				
1 fl oz	2.3	T	0	41
Wine glass, 3½ oz	7.9	0.1	0	141

* Percent alcohol content by volume, by weight.
Source: Nutritive value of American foods in common units, *Agriculture Handbook,* 456, USDA, 1975.
Note: T = trace.

products designed to substitute for meat are available in many grocery stores. They are made mostly from wheat or soy, and most contain egg-white protein in addition. Many can be substituted for meat with little change in the rest of the menu. Labels of the products a patient uses can be checked, and the items can be incorporated into the food lists.

For the patient who wishes to use nuts, legumes, and grains, the dietitian can work out a diet pattern and lists of alternative food choices that are based on the patient's preferences. Nuts and many seeds are rich in fat, so adjustment in fat exchanges is needed if they are substituted for meat. Legumes provide protein and starch (Fig. 6-2).

Planning is a little more difficult for patients who will use no animal products. The diet should be worked out by the dietitian and patient together to ensure nutritional adequacy. For meals, combinations of foods providing complete protein must be considered. In addition, the absence of milk and cheese from the diet means that calcium, riboflavin, and vitamin D needs must be met by other means. In this respect, dark-green and leafy vegetables are useful. Some foods not considered good sources of calcium because of the small amounts ordinarily consumed do serve as important sources for the vegetarian because the amounts consumed are large. For example, 1 lb of almonds contains 1061 mg of calcium, and also 2713 cal and 84.4 g of protein. Almonds are rich in fat, most of which is unsaturated. Since plant foods provide no vitamin

B_{12}, a supplement should be prescribed. The nutritional status of the patient using no animal foods should be monitored carefully, since absorption of nutrients, iron, for example, may be limited by the high fiber and phytate intake.

Camping and Backpacking

Summer camps for children and adolescents with diabetes have been organized to help both children and parents learn about the disease and the measures to maintain control. Children and parents find that seeing and meeting other young people with diabetes is the most important reason for attending.[57] The youngster learns to handle diet, insulin, changes in exercise, insulin reactions, and other aspects of personal management. Often these programs also help parents who need guidance in aspects of discipline. Fearful parents can impose unnecessary restrictions on a child; other parents may be unduly permissive. Dealing with an adolescent can be difficult for many parents. Anxiety is not eased when the child has a potentially life-threatening disease. Experiences at camps for the child with diabetes help the child accept the responsibility of management and gain confidence.[58,59]

Many children attend regular camps as well. This can be arranged by the family in consultation with the physician. The camp nurse should be told about the diet and medication schedule, as well as other aspects of management, so that help can be provided when needed. Many youngsters have found regular camps to be a happy experience.

Americans as a group are spending more and more of their leisure time in camping and other outdoor activities. For families using campers or staying in cabins or tents at the usual campsites, there is little difference in meal patterns other than a choice of foods prepared more simply. The meals are much like the meals at home, and little adjustment is needed. For those involved in more vigorous activities, such as hiking or backpacking, foods that are light in weight and keep well are important. Physical activity increases food requirements and may increase fluid needs. The following approach to planning the diet has been suggested by Labrenz:

1   To the patient's usual meal pattern, add a morning and afternoon snack, each of the same carbohydrate and protein value as the bedtime snack. If the patient is already eating snacks at these times, double the carbohydrate.

2   Figure the new daily total for carbohydrate by adding the total for carbohydrate of the three snacks to that of the three normal meals.

3   The new daily totals for protein and fat should each be approximately half that of the carbohydrate.

4   Breakfast, lunch and dinner should each contain approximately one-third and the bedtime snack approximately one-tenth of the total carbohydrate in the original diet. Each meal and snack should provide at least 8 to 10 gm. high-quality protein.[60]

As experienced campers and hikers know, planning daily menus and packing the food for each day in labeled bags is good technique whether one has special diet concerns or not.

Eating Out

People are eating meals away from home with increasing frequency. Sometimes it is necessary because of work, business, or school. The patient with diabetes has the same needs and desires for eating out for business or pleasure as anyone else. Knowledge of the meal plan, of individual responses (such as hypoglycemia), and a little discretion are all that is necessary.

The obese adult patient can plan for the meal by making adjustments in the total intake for the day, since total caloric intake is the major priority in diet management. Patients using insulin should maintain the schedule for meals and choose foods that fit the meal pattern.

When invited for a meal, patients can tell the host of their special needs. This presents no great problem to most hosts since the diet is the normal diet without concentrated sweets.

When ordering food in restaurants, the patient will usually find items on the menu that are suitable. When servings are large, the full portion should not be eaten. Meat, fish, and poultry can be roasted, baked, broiled, or boiled. Potatoes can be baked, boiled, or steamed. If vegetables are buttered, patients should use less butter on the bread. Vegetable salads can be ordered with dressing "on the side" so the patient can use the right amount. Appetizers can be chosen from vegetable juices, unsweetened or fresh fruit and juices, clear broth, bouillon, consommés, fresh vegetables such as celery and radishes, dill pickles, etc. Breads can be chosen keeping in mind the bread exchanges; and fats, the fat exchanges (see Tables 6-9 and 6-10 at the end of the chapter). For dessert, fresh fruits are pleasant. Plain cake, cookies, or a small scoop of ice cream may be used. If there is any doubt, patients should check with their physician. Ice cream is listed in the original exchange system (Table 6-10) as 1 bread and 2 fat exchanges. It is not listed in the revised system (Table 6-9). Beverages include coffee or tea, milk as listed in the diet plan, or diet-type soft drinks.

When a restaurant is patronized regularly, the server may remember how the patient wants food prepared. It may be useful for the patient to take menus from places visited regularly to the dietitian for assistance in choosing meals. If there are popular fast-food places in the area, some guidelines should be made available to patients and staff as well. Cafeterias usually offer enough flexibility in their menus that choosing food to meet the meal pattern is easy.

For the school child, diet counseling should include discussion of the lunch at school. The lunch may be the regular type-A pattern, cafeteria, or brown bag. Sufficient information should be provided so that the child can choose to carry lunch or buy it.

HYPOGLYCEMIA: MEAL DELAYS AND "SICK DAYS"

Insulin-dependent patients should have specific instructions for the use of food when meals are delayed or there is unusual exercise. Hypoglycemic episodes can result from too much insulin, too much exercise, delayed meals, or illness with anorexia or vomiting. Food intake may be unpredictable in hospitalized patients because of surgery or other problems.

Insulin reaction occurs when the blood sugar falls. The patient may notice hunger, shakiness, sweating, fast heartbeat, and negative sugar in the urine. The family may notice that the patient is talking incoherently or acting strangely or cannot be awakened. Immediate treatment is essential. A readily available source of glucose should be given. This can be lump sugar, sugar in water, fruit juices, or a soft drink (*not* a diet drink). In using the juices or fluids, give the patient about one-half cup and wait for a while to see the response. Table 6-8 lists items providing 10 g of readily available carbohydrate. Candy or sugar should be carried by the child or patient with labile diabetes so that it can be taken when symptoms first appear. Some facilities use milk drinks made with sugar as the feeding for hypoglycemia.

When meals are unavoidably delayed, intake of 15 to 30 g of carbohydrate will usually protect the patient from hypoglycemia for 1 or 2 h. Crackers, fruit juice, or soft drinks can be used. When traveling, it is easy to carry cheese or peanut butter and crackers. These provide protein as well as carbohydrate. Milk can be carried in a thermos if desired.

Usually no extra food is required for moderate exercise. Extra carbohydrate intake of 10 to 50 g might be advised for unusual exertion, based on the vigor of activity and duration. West suggests 10 to 15 g/h for moderate activity such as golf and 20 to 30 g/h for vigorous activity such as basketball.[61]

Hypoglycemic episodes can be distressing to child, adult, family, and

Table 6-8   Foods That Provide 10 to 15 g of Carbohydrate

Food	Measure	Carbohydrate
Fruit juice:*		
Orange juice	½ cup	14
Apple juice	½ cup	15
Beverages:		
Cola type	½ cup	12
Ginger ale (pale, dry)	½ cup	12
Gelatin dessert	½ cup	17
Sugar:		
Gram	1 tbsp	12
Rectangles	2	10
Cubes	4	10
Packets	2	12
Candy:		
Marshmallows	2	12
Miniature	⅓ cup (not packed)	12
Hard	½ cup	14
Crackers:		
Graham	2 squares	11
Soda	5 squares	10

* See fruit exchange list also.
  Source: Nutritive value of American foods in common units, *Agriculture Handbook*, 456, USDA, 1975.

friends. The insulin-dependent patient should be taught how to avoid episodes if possible. This is particularly important for drivers, since there is potential danger involved as well as loss of the driver's license. Patient, family, and professionals should be prepared to handle the hypoglycemic episode calmly and swiftly when it occurs. If the episode is repeated, the physician should be called; an unconscious patient should be taken to the hospital. Some physicians suggest keeping a glucagon emergency kit in the home.

When the insulin-dependent patient is ill and appetite fails, foods should be distributed throughout the day. Sweets such as soft drinks, gelatin desserts, and juices may be used as ready sources of carbohydrate. Soups and milk may also be acceptable. Small, frequent carbohydrate feedings help protect against hypoglycemia and ketosis. Clearly written instructions for the use of food and insulin in illness should be provided as part of the education program. A common problem is that many people omit taking the insulin when ill in the mistaken belief that they do not need it because food intake is poor. Sometimes food intake is deliberately limited by the patient who is "dieting" via some popular method. Regular, predictable intake is more important to good management than the professional's idea of "good diet." There are many ways diet and medication patterns can be adjusted to fit the patient's life-style.

PREGNANCY AND DIET MANAGEMENT

In 1970 a committee of the National Academy of Science reviewed the literature on maternal nutritional status, management, and the effect on the outcome of pregnancy.[61] Guidelines for weight and dietary goals to help improve the well-being of mother and child were established. The diet should provide sufficient energy to meet the needs of mother and fetus, permitting a total weight gain of about 25 lb (range, 22 to 30 lb). The diet should provide protein, vitamins, and minerals generously, as indicated in Table 6-1. Neither energy nor sodium should be restricted. For the pregnant woman with diabetes, an additional factor is essential—control of the blood sugar level. This applies to the woman with gestational diabetes and to the woman diabetic before pregnancy. These guidelines, together with goals of fasting blood glucose concentrations under 100 mg/dL and postprandial levels approximating 120 mg/dL, nutrition counseling, and liberal antenatal hospitalization, have been used to produce striking improvements in fetal and neonatal outcome.[62]

It is essential that the nutritional needs of the patient be determined with particular attention to energy. A weight-reduction diet or starvation regimens are contraindicated during pregnancy for all patients including those with diabetes. Starvation ketosis, whether due to patient- or physician-imposed low caloric intakes, is undesirable. The pattern of weight gain serves as a useful guide to adequacy. Gain should be minimal in the first trimester (1 to 2 kg) then proceed in a regular pattern of about 0.4 kg per week to term. General guidelines for energy levels for the woman according to age are provided in Table 6-1 together with the recommendation that an average of 300 cal per day be added to meet fetal needs. This is about 36 kcal/kg of body weight. The basal needs and activity patterns of the individual should be assessed and pattern of weight gain monitored carefully to determine the adequacy of energy intake throughout pregnancy.

The distribution of calories from protein, carbohydrate, and fat already described is applicable during pregnancy. In order to provide protein generously for growth, the planned diet should probably allow 20 percent of the calories as protein; 30 to 35 percent of the calories as fat is appropriate, as was noted earlier, but the level selected should be acceptable to the patient. Carbohydrate can provide 40 to 50 percent of the calories, with emphasis given to the use of foods providing complex carbohydrate. Foods with naturally occurring sugars (milk, fruit, vegetables) are included. Since control of blood sugar, avoiding sharp elevations or falls, is one goal, refined sugars and sweets are not used and exchanges are not made between foods with complex carbohydrate and those with simple carbohydrate. This means that breads and fruits are not exchanged.

Distribution of food throughout the day and regularity of meal times and size are important. Four feedings per day with 25 percent of the total carbohydrate at breakfast, 25 to 30 percent at lunch, approximately 30 percent at dinner, and 15 percent at night is a pattern used successfully in the management of women with gestational or prepregnancy diabetes.[63] When a midafternoon snack is needed, the carbohydrate content of lunch is 25 percent. This regimen works well for the patient using split doses of combined intermediate- and short-acting insulins. When insulin is not needed, as for many patients with gestational diabetes, distribution of energy and carbohydrate intake throughout the day is still important.

Some patients with gestational diabetes do need insulin, although the majority do not. Many are overweight. Weight reduction or limitation of weight gain should be avoided. Weight reduction for the mother after delivery of the infant is desirable and should be part of the total care plan.

Restriction of sodium intake by women during pregnancy has been a common practice. Unless there are predisposing medical problems not related to the pregnancy itself, sodium intake should not be limited.

The diet plan should provide the range of foods that will supply vitamins and minerals liberally. Milk intake for adequate calcium is important and additional milk incorporated for teenage patients or mothers carrying multiple fetuses. Since many women have histories of low iron intake, it is common practice to provide 30 to 60 mg of iron as ferrous salts.

Schulman has worked extensively with pregnant women who are diabetic and has found that the demands for control of meal size, frequency, and day-to-day consistency are difficult because most women are unaccustomed to rigid control. Diet management is based on the measured diet, using the exchange lists and a meal plan carefully worked out by the nutritionist to meet the patient's preferences, usual patterns of intake and activity, and medical needs. Nevertheless it is a challenge for both nutritionist and patient. The recommended carbohydrate content of the evening snack (15 percent) is more than in the usual snack for the nonpregnant patient, yet it is important, especially when NPH insulin is used. The rather even distribution of carbohydrate for breakfast, lunch, and dinner (25, 25 to 30, and 30 percent) has worked well in at least one unit providing care for pregnant women with either gestational or prepregnancy diabetes.[64]

THE ELDERLY PATIENT

Diabetes is more frequent in older people in part because of the diminished carbohydrate tolerance associated with aging. Most commonly the patient is of the maturity-onset type with excessive body weight. There may be other factors such as cardiovascular disease, hypertension, gout, or dental problems to consider. The objectives of nutrition management should include realistic and acceptable levels of body weight, blood sugar, and serum lipids, with avoidance of hypoglycemia.[65] The principles already described apply to the elderly as well. Weight control has beneficial effects on serum lipids as well as blood glucose. Should dietary modifications be required for other clinical disease, they should be developed gradually as a program planned between patient and dietitian. Types of diet modification often needed in addition to control of calories and carbohydrate include changes in the amount and type of fat (for serum lipids) and sodium, and consistency (for chewing and swallowing problems). When a patient is on a regimen of calorie and sodium restriction with diuretic medication, electrolytic balance should be monitored and the diet checked for adequacy of potassium intake. It is not helpful to tell the overweight patient to eat lots of bananas and drink orange juice. The potassium-rich foods should be included in the diet plan as part of the calorie-controlled pattern. Regular supervision with opportunities for discussion of diet management with an interested and knowledgable professional is as important for the elderly patient as for the young. A large proportion of elderly patients can be managed without insulin or oral hypoglycemic agents.[66]

MODIFYING FAT IN THE DIET

Throughout this chapter the recommendation has been made that fat provide 30 to 35 percent of the energy, that intake of saturated fat be 10 percent or less, and polyunsaturated fat 10 percent or more of total calories. The revised exchange lists from the American Diabetes Association and the American Dietetic Association in Tables 6-3 and 6-9 are designed to permit this dietary manipulation. Reducing the proportion of fat in the diet increases the proportion of carbohydrate that is acceptable. Because fat is a concentrated source of energy, this change also provides a larger volume of food, which can be advantageous for the patient whose total caloric intake is limited.

For most people the modification requires reducing total intake of fat. The usual Western diet pattern is rich in fat, with 45 percent or more of calories coming from fat. Reducing fat intake requires only some rather simple changes in food choice. Most fat in the diet comes from dairy products, meats, and the fats and oils used in seasoning and cooking food. This means that one uses nonfat or low-fat milks, exercises care in the kinds and amounts of meats and cheeses used, and limits the fat and oils used in food preparation. The patient with diabetes has already limited intake of fat-rich foods such as cake, pie, cookies, and frozen desserts because of their sugar content. The contribution of fat calories by various common foods grouped according to exchange lists is shown in Fig. 6-3. The difference in fat content of various milks is obvious, as it is for various cheeses. Cheeses and meats are grouped as low-, medium-, and high-fat choices in the food exchange lists in Table 6-9. One can make a significant change in the fat contributed by meat, fish, and poultry by choosing items of lower fat concentration and by carefully trimming the separable fat from these foods before cooking them. The difference in the fat content of protein-rich foods and the effect of further trimming fat before cooking is shown in Fig. 6-5. The portions illustrated are 3½ oz, i.e., 100 g of the food cooked and ready to eat. Beef, lamb, ham, and pork contain significantly less fat when only the separable lean is used. Meats have traditionally been graded according to fat content, with the higher grades of meat higher in fat. Choice cuts are illustrated in Fig. 6-5; prime is the highest grade. Poultry and fish are

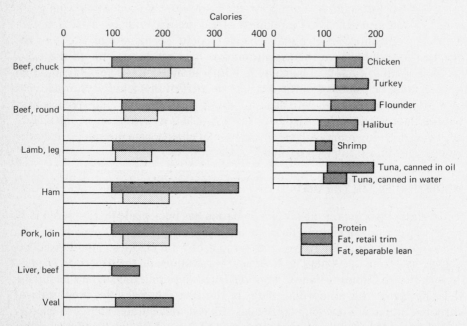

Figure 6-5 Fat in 3½-oz portions of protein-rich foods. Using only the separable lean of beef, lamb, pork, and ham will reduce caloric and fat levels. Using poultry, fish, and lean meats such as veal will also reduce fat intake. These measurements are for cooked, choice-grade meats to which no fat has been added in preparation. (*Based on data from USDA Food Composition Tables.*)

Table 6-9 Exchange Lists for Meal Planning, 1976

Milk exchanges (nonfat, saturated fat)

Nonfat fortified milk:		Low-fat fortified milk:		Whole milk:	
Skim or nonfat milk	1 cup	1% fat fortified milk	1 cup	Whole milk	1 cup
Powdered (nonfat dry, before		2% fat fortified milk	1 cup	Canned, evaporated whole	
adding liquid)	⅓ cup	Yogurt made from 2% for-		milk	½ cup
Canned, evaporated, skim milk	½ cup	tified milk (plain,		Buttermilk made from	
Buttermilk made from skim milk	1 cup	unflavored)	1 cup	whole milk	1 cup
Yogurt made from skim milk				Yogurt made from whole	
(plain, unflavored)	1 cup			milk (plain, unflavored)	1 cup

Vegetable exchanges

½-cup servings:

Asparagus	Greens:	Onions
Bean sprouts	Beet	Rhubarb
Beets	Chards	Rutabaga
Broccoli	Collards	Sauerkraut
Brussels sprouts	Dandelion	String beans, green or yellow
Cabbage	Kale	Summer squash
Carrots	Mustard	Tomatoes
Cauliflower	Spinach	Tomato juice
Celery	Turnip	Turnips
Cucumbers	Mushrooms	Vegetable juice cocktail
Eggplant	Okra	Zucchini
Green pepper		

Raw vegetables (use as desired):

Chicory	Endive	Lettuce	Radishes
Chinese Cabbage	Escarole	Parsley	Watercress

Fruit (raw or unsweetened)

Apple	1 small	Dates	2	Orange	1 small
Apple juice	⅓ cup	Figs, fresh	1	Orange juice	½ cup
Applesauce	½ cup	Figs, dried	1	Papaya	¾ cup
Apricots, fresh	2 medium	Grapefruit	½	Peach	1 medium
Apricots, dried	4 halves	Grapefruit juice	½ cup	Pear	1 small
Banana	½ small	Grapes	12	Persimmon, native	1 medium
Berries:		Grape juice	¼ cup	Pineapple	½ cup
Blackberries	½ cup	Mango	½ small	Pineapple juice	⅓ cup
Blueberries	½ cup	Melon:		Plums	2 medium
Raspberries	½ cup	Cantaloupe	¼ small	Prunes	2 medium
Strawberries	¾ cup	Honeydew	⅛ medium	Prune juice	¼ cup
Cherries	10 large	Watermelon	1 cup	Raisins	2 tbsp
Cider	⅓ cup	Nectarine	1 small	Tangerine	1 medium

Cranberries may be used as desired if no sugar is added.

Bread exchanges (includes starchy vegetables)

Bread (low-fat):		Rye wafers, 2 × 3½ in	3
White (including French and Italian)	1 slice	Saltines	6
Whole wheat	1 slice	Soda, 2½-in sq	4
Rye or pumpernickel	1 slice	Dried beans, peas, and lentils:	
Raisin	1 slice	Beans, peas, lentils (dried and	½ cup
Bagel, small	½	cooked)	
English muffin, small	½	Baked beans, no pork (canned)	¼ cup
Plain roll, bread	1	Prepared food (count as 2 fat	
Frankfurter roll	½	exchanges also):	
Hamburger bun	½	Potato or corn chips	15
Dried bread crumbs	3 tbsp	Cereal (low-fat):	
Tortilla, 6 in	1	Bran flakes	½ cup
Crackers (low-fat):		Other ready-to-eat unsweetened	¾ cup
Arrowroot	3	cereal	
Graham, 2½-in sq	2	Puffed cereal (unfrosted)	1 cup
Matzoth, 4 × 6 in	½	Cereal (cooked)	½ cup
Oyster	20	Grits (cooked)	½ cup
Pretzels, 3⅛ in long × ⅛-in diam	25	Rice or barley (cooked)	½ cup

Pasta (cooked), spaghetti, noodles, macaroni	½ cup	Pumpkin	¾ cup
		Winter squash, acorn, or butternut	½ cup
Popcorn (popped, no fat added)	3 cups	Yam or sweet potato	¼ cup
Cornmeal (dry)	2 tbsp	Prepared foods (count as 1 fat exchange also):	
Flour	2½ tbsp		
Wheat germ	¼ cup	Biscuit 2-in diam	1
Starchy vegetables (low-fat):		Corn bread, 2 × 2 × 1 in	1
Corn	⅓ cup	Corn muffin, 2-in diam	1
Corn on cob	1 small	Crackers, round butter type	5
Lima beans	½ cup	Muffin, plain small	1
Parsnips	⅔ cup	Potatoes, french fried,	8
Peas, green (canned or frozen)	½ cup	length 2 to 3½ in	
Potato, white	1 small	Pancake, 5 × ½ in	1
Potato (mashed)	½ cup	Waffle, 5 × ½ in	1

Lean meat exchanges

1 oz	Beef: baby beef (very lean), chipped beef, chuck, flank steak, tenderloin, plate ribs, plate skirt steak, round (bottom, top), all cuts rump, spare ribs, tripe
1 oz	Lamb: leg, rib, sirloin, loin (roast and chops), shank, shoulder
1 oz	Pork: leg (whole rump, center shank), ham, smoked (center slices)
1 oz	Veal: leg, loin, rib, shank, shoulder, cutlets
1 oz	Poultry: meat without skin of chicken, turkey, cornish hen, guinea hen, pheasant
1 oz	Fish: any fresh or frozen
¼ cup	Canned salmon, tuna, mackerel, crab, and lobster
5 (1 oz)	Clams, oysters, scallops, shrimp
3	Sardines, drained
1 oz	Cheeses containing less than 5 percent butterfat
¼ cup	Cottage cheese, dry and 2 percent butterfat
½ cup	Dried beans and peas (omit 1 bread exchange)

Medium-fat meat exchanges

1 oz	Beef: ground (15 percent fat), corned beef (canned), rib eye, round (ground commercial)
1 oz	Pork: loin (all cuts tenderloin), shoulder arm (picnic), shoulder blade, Boston butt, Canadian bacon, boiled ham
1 oz	Liver, heart, kidney, and sweetbreads (these are high in cholesterol)
¼ cup	Cottage cheese, creamed
1 oz (3 tbsp)	Cheese: mozzarella, ricotta, farmer's cheese, neufchatel, parmesan
1	Egg (high in cholesterol)
2 tbsp	Peanut butter (omit 2 additional fat exchanges)

High-fat meat exchanges

1 oz	Beef: brisket, corned beef (brisket), ground beef (more than 20 percent fat), hamburger (commercial), chuck (ground commercial), roasts (rib), steaks (club and rib)
1 oz	Lamb: breast
1 oz	Pork: spare ribs, loin (back ribs), pork (ground), country style ham, deviled ham
1 oz	Veal: breast
1 oz	Poultry: capon, duck (domestic), goose
1 oz	Cheese: cheddar types
4½ × ⅛ in slice	Cold cuts
1 small	frankfurter

Fat exchanges (polyunsaturated, other)

Margarine, soft, tub or stick*	1 tsp	Butter	1 tsp
Avocado (4-in diam)†	⅛	Bacon fat	1 tsp
Oil, corn, cottonseed, safflower, soy, sunflower	1 tsp	Bacon, crisp	1 strip
		Cream, light	2 tbsp
Oil, olive†	1 tsp	Cream, sour	2 tbsp
Oil, peanut†	1 tsp	Cream, heavy	1 tbsp
Olives†	5 small	Cream cheese	1 tbsp
Almonds†	10 whole	French dressing‡	1 tbsp
Pecans†	2 large whole	Italian dressing‡	1 tbsp
Peanuts:†		Lard	1 tsp
Spanish	20 whole	Mayonnaise‡	1 tsp
Virginia	10 whole	Salad dressing,	
Walnuts	6 small	mayonnaise type‡	2 tsp
Nuts, other†	6 small	Salt pork	¾-in cube
Margarine, regular stick	1 tsp		

Other (not limited)	
Diet calorie-free beverage	Nutmeg
Coffee, tea	Lemon
Bouillon without fat	Mustard
Unsweetened gelatin	Chili powder
Unsweetened pickles	Onion salt or
Seasonings:	powder
Salt and pepper	Horseradish
Red pepper	Vinegar
Paprika	Mint
Garlic	Cinnamon
Celery salt	Lime
Parsley	

* Made with corn, cottonseed, safflower, soy, or sunflower oil only.

† Fat content is primarily monounsaturated.

‡ If made with corn, cottonseed, safflower, soy, or sunflower oil, can be used on fat modified diet.

Source: Adapted from American Diabetes Association, Inc., American Dietetic Association, and National Institutes of Health, U.S. Public Health Service, *Exchange Lists for Meal Planning* (Chicago: American Dietetic Association, 1976).

Table 6-10   Meal Planning with Exchange Lists, 1950

Foods that need not be measured (insignificant carbohydrate or calories)

Coffee	Gelatin (unsweetened)	Saccharin
Tea	Rennet tablets	Pepper and other spices
Clear broth	Cranberries (unsweetened)	Vinegar
Bouillon (fat free)	Mustard (dry)	Seasonings
Lemon	Pickle (unsweetened)	

Chopped parsley, mint, garlic, onion, celery salt, nutmeg, mustard, cinnamon, pepper and other spices, lemon, saccharin, and vinegar may be used freely.

List 1: Milk exchanges

One exchange of milk contains 8 g of protein, 10 g of fat, 12 g of carbohydrate, and 170 calories. This list shows the different types of milk to use for 1 exchange.

Whole milk (plain or homogenized)	1 cup	Powdered skim milk (nonfat dried	
Skim milk*	1 cup	milk)*	¼ cup
Evaporated milk	½ cup	Buttermilk (made from whole milk)	1 cup
Powdered whole milk	¼ cup	Buttermilk (made from skim milk)*	1 cup

One type of milk may be used instead of another, for example, ½ cup of evaporated milk in place of 1 cup of whole milk.

List 2: Vegetable exchanges, group A

Group A contains little protein, carbohydrate, or calories. One cup at a time may be used without counting it.

Asparagus	Chard†	Cauliflower	Pepper†
Broccoli†	Collard†	Celery	Radishes
Brussels sprouts	Dandelion greens†	Chicory†	Sauerkraut
Cabbage	Kale†	Cucumbers	String beans, young
Escarole†	Mustard†	Lettuce	Summer squash
Eggplant	Spinach†	Mushrooms	Tomatoes†
Beet greens†	Turnip greens†	Okra	Watercress†

List 2: Vegetable exchanges, group B

Each exchange contains 2 g of protein, 7 g of carbohydrate, and 35 calories; ½ cup of vegetable equals 1 exchange.

Beets	Onions	Pumpkin	Squash, winter‡
Carrots‡	Peas, green	Rutabagas	Turnip

List 3: Fruit exchanges

One exchange of fruit contains 10 g of carbohydrate and 40 calories. This list shows the different amounts of fruits to use for 1 fruit exchange.

Apple (2-in diam)	1 small	Grapes	12
Applesauce	½ cup	Grape juice	¼ cup
Apricots, fresh	2 medium	Honeydew melon	⅛ medium
Apricots, dried	4 halves	Mango	½ small
Banana	½ small	Orange§	1 small
Blackberries	1 cup	Orange juice§	½ cup
Raspberries	1 cup	Papaya	⅓ medium
Strawberries§	1 cup	Peach	1 medium
Blueberries	⅔ cup	Pear	1 small
Cantaloupe (6-in diam)§	¼	Pineapple	½ cup
Cherries	10 large	Pineapple juice	⅓ cup
Dates	2	Plums	2 medium
Figs, fresh	2 large	Prunes, dried	2 medium
Figs, dried	1 small	Raisins	2 tbsp
Grapefruit§	½ small	Tangerine§	1 large
Grapefruit juice§	½ cup	Watermelon	1 cup

List 4: Bread exchanges

One exchange contains 2 g of protein, 15 g of carbohydrate, and 70 calories. This list shows the different amounts of foods to use for 1 bread exchange.

Bread	1 slice	Flour	2½ tbsp
Biscuit, roll (2-in diam)	1	Vegetables:	
Muffin (2-in diam)	1	Beans and peas, dried, cooked	½ cup
Cornbread (1½-in cube)	1	(Lima, navy, split pea, cowpeas, etc.)	
Cereals, cooked	½ cup	Baked beans, no pork	¼ cup
Dry, flake, and puff types	¾ cup	Corn	⅓ cup
Rice, grits, cooked	½ cup	Popcorn	1 cup
Spaghetti, noodles, cooked	½ cup	Parsnips	⅔ cup
Macaroni, etc., cooked	½ cup	Potatoes, white	1 small
Crackers		Potatoes, white, mashed	½ cup
Graham (2½-in sq)	2	Potatoes, sweet, or yams	¼ cup
Oyster (½ cup)	20	Sponge cake, plain (1½-in cube)	1
Saltines (2-in sq)	5	Ice cream (omit 2 fat exchanges)	½ cup
Soda (2½-in sq)	3		
Round, thin (1½-in diam)	6		

These foods are measured carefully because they contain significant amounts of carbohydrate.

List 5: Meat exchanges

One meat exchange contains 7 g of protein, 5 g of fat, and 75 calories. This list shows the different amounts of foods to use for 1 meat exchange.

Meat and poultry (medium fat)		Fish: haddock, etc.	1 oz
beef, lamb, pork, liver, chicken, etc.,		Salmon, tuna, crab, lobster	¼ cub
cooked	1 oz	Shrimp, clams, oysters, etc.	5 small
Cold cuts (4½ × ⅛ in)		Sardines	3 medium
salami, minced ham, bologna, liver-		Cheese:	
wurst, luncheon loaf	1 slice	Cheddar type	1 oz

| Frankfurter (8–9 per lb) | 1 | Cottage | ¼ cup |
| Egg | 1 | Peanut butter¶ | 2 tbsp |

List 6: Fat exchanges

One fat exchange contains 5 g of fat and 45 calories. This list shows the different foods to use for 1 fat exchange.

Butter or margarine	1 tsp	French dressing	1 tbsp
Bacon, crisp	1 slice	Mayonnaise	1 tsp
Cream, light	2 tbsp	Oil or cooking fat	1 tsp
Cream, heavy	1 tbsp	Nuts	6 small
Cream cheese	1 tbsp	Olives	5 small
Avocado (4-in diam)	⅛		

* Skim milk and buttermilk have the same food values as whole milk, except that they contain less fat. Two fat exchanges are added when 1 cup of skim milk or buttermilk made from skim milk is used in place of whole milk calculated in a diet pattern.

† These vegetables contain a lot of vitamin A.

‡ These vegetables contain a lot of vitamin A.

§ These fruits are rich sources of vitamin C.

¶ Peanut butter is limited to 1 exchange a day unless the carbohydrate in it is allowed for in the calculated diet pattern.

Source: Adapted from American Diabetes Association, Inc., American Dietetic Association, and Chronic Disease Program, U.S. Public Health Service, *Meal Planning with Exchange Lists* (Chicago, American Dietetic Association, 1950).

generally lower in fat content, as are liver and veal. To lower total fat intake from protein-rich sources, most people should reduce their intake of beef and other meats and use poultry and fish more frequently as the main course in meals. With use of dairy and animal products lower in fat, there is also reduction in the amount of fats and oils used in food preparation.

Changing the type of fat in the diet so that a smaller proportion comes from saturated fat and a larger proportion comes from polyunsaturated fat requires a relatively minor change in food choice in addition to the changes in use of dairy and animal products. The fats and oils used to prepare and season foods and the spread used on bread should be those higher in polyunsaturated fat. The fatty acid content of different food fats is shown in Fig. 6-6. Since the goal is to decrease intake of saturated fat and increase intake of polyunsaturated fat, the foods of choice are those relatively lower in total saturated fat and higher in linoleic acid. Oleic acid is a monounsaturated fat. With this goal in mind, it becomes obvious that the spread of choice is a soft margarine. Many margarine labels provide information about fat. This is helpful to the shopper. The oils from corn, safflower, cottonseed, and soy are preferred as cooking fats. Cost should be taken into account in making recommendations to the patient, since there may be quite a difference between products. Meats are higher in saturated fats than most poultry or fish, as well as being higher in total fat. Moderate portions are used to reduce total fat intake. Fish and poultry are used more frequently than meats because of their lower fat content and higher proportion of linoleic acid.

In general, fat from plant sources is lower in saturated fat than that from animal sources. Plant fats may be hydrogenated to increase stability for storage

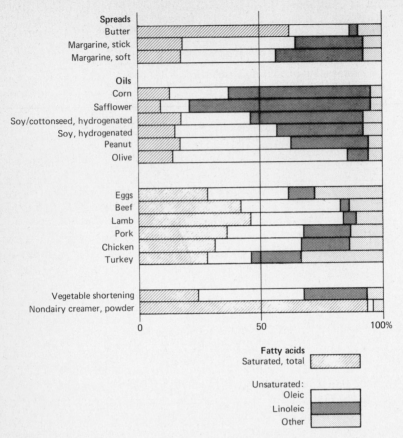

Figure 6-6 Fatty acid content of food fats. The usual modification requires reducing intake of fats relatively high in saturated fat, such as butterfat and meat, and increasing intake of foods high in linoleic acid (polyunsaturated). (*Based on data from "Home and Garden Handbook," 72, USDA, 1977.*)

and cooking. Two common plant fats are vegetable shortening and the substitutes for cream. Vegetable shortenings are hydrogenated oils; they are lower in saturated fat than butter or lard and lower in polyunsaturated fat than corn or soy oils. When a solid fat is needed and the soft margarines are unacceptable, vegetable shortenings or stick margarines may be preferable. The substitutes for coffee cream, sour cream, and whipped topping are usually quite high in saturated fat, as shown in Fig. 6-6. Many people are confused about these items, believing them to be low in calories, low in fat, and low in saturated fat. Check the labels carefully before using them.

When the total fat is reduced to about one-third of the calories and foods are chosen to reduce saturated fat and increase polyunsaturated fat proportions, the dietary cholesterol intake is reduced as well. Dietary cholesterol is found associated with the fat of animal foods and in eggs and liver. Since eggs and liver are rich sources of high-quality protein, vitamins, and minerals, they are valuable in any diet pattern. However, they should be used in moderation.

OTHER DIET MODIFICATIONS

The patient with diabetes has minor illnesses just as anyone else does. Often appetite falters, but soft or liquid foods can be substituted for the regular diet, as was already discussed. Those who have been hospitalized may have experienced the practice of liquid replacements for food not eaten on the regular tray. Providing the patient with written guidelines for meal management during illness will help avoid problems. For the insulin-dependent patient, instructions about insulin and food during minor illness are particularly important. Menu suggestions such as those outlined in Table 6-4 can be planned by the patient and professional together as part of the total education program. It has been suggested that some patients might ingest significant sugar in various prescription and nonprescription drugs.[67] This source of calories might be investigated if there are special problems with no readily apparent explanation in management of minor illness.

For the majority of obese maturity-onset patients, reduction of weight brings improvement in blood glucose, blood lipid, and blood pressure levels. Hypertriglyceridemia in the obese individual responds to restricted caloric intake if the patient does or does not have diabetes. Fat modification is frequently an integral component of the regular dietary prescription and for that reason was discussed in a separate section. There is general agreement on the advisability of lower fat intake (35 percent of calories), with a lower saturated fat and cholesterol intake if acceptable to the patient. Despite the lack of firm evidence, such a dietary stance will delay or prevent complications such as atherosclerosis.[68-70] When hyperlipidemia persists in the patient with weight and blood glucose under control, a fat-modified diet may be prescribed for control of blood lipid.

High-carbohydrate diets have also been suggested by some workers as appropriate for adults with mild diabetes. In one report, a diet with 75 percent of calories from carbohydrate with generous dietary fiber was tested and found satisfactory in a small group of men observed for a short period of time.[71] Testing of carbohydrate levels, with generous use of starches and fibers, is being conducted in many research and treatment centers.

What about dietary modifications in addition to those already prescribed for the patient as part of the treatment program for diabetes? In its report, the Diabetes Commission noted that complications of diabetes still develop even with the best of care and include impaired kidney function and peripheral blood flow, loss of peripheral nerve sensation, and increased periodontal disease.[72] Common problems include renal failure, congestive heart failure, and gastrointestinal disorders including ulcers. Gluten intolerance (celiac disease) has been seen; some children with cystic fibrosis of the pancreas develop diabetes. Diet manuals provide information about the types of foods to use or avoid when these modifications are required.

One of the most frequent modifications prescribed is sodium restriction. With potent hypertensive drugs now available, severe limitations of sodium are rarely prescribed. A mild or moderate sodium restriction (1 to 2 g) enhances the effectiveness of the drug and limits potassium depletion aggravated by high salt intakes. Some attention to intake of potassium is important since continuous use of diuretics may lead to chronic depletion. The diet should be reviewed to ensure use of potassium-rich foods. Potassium supplements may be prescribed but may produce unpleasant symptoms. These symptoms may be reduced by taking the supplement with meals. Fruits and vegetables are good sources of potassium and should be provided as generously as the caloric levels of the diet permit.

Chronic renal failure requires more complicated dietary management. Limitation of protein intake, control of sodium and potassium intakes, and sufficiently high caloric intake to avoid catabolism of body muscle, together with an adequate supply of vitamins and minerals, are dietary goals. The diet is low in protein and high in starch. The limitation in protein means that intake of foods not ordinarily considered good protein sources must be limited, as review of Figs. 6-2 and 6-3 reveals. Furthermore, the protein provided should be of high biologic value.

Careful dietary control and management to meet patient nitrogen and nutrient needs is part of hemodialysis therapy as well. With transplantation, restrictions on protein, salt, etc. may not be necessary. Patients with diabetes are now being accepted as candidates for hemodialysis and transplant. Since chronic renal failure has become the leading cause of death in patients with juvenile-onset diabetes,[73] use of these treatment modalities may increase. Chronic renal failure and chronic hemodialysis pose special long-term management problems, including bone disease. Patients are followed closely in dialysis centers by teams of physicians, nurses, and dietitians.

Modifications in consistency of diet may be needed when the patient is to undergo surgery, when there is difficulty in chewing or swallowing, or when dental work is done. Liquid or soft diets are standard in hospitals, but the ambulatory patient needs some help in making appropriate choices.

Bland diets may be prescribed for patients with gastrointestinal problems. There is considerable controversy about the value of bland diets, although there is general agreement that alcohol, pepper, mustard, and caffeine contribute to distress and should be limited. Frequently the diet order is "as tolerated." Careful questioning of the patient helps identify those foods which cause discomfort. These are limited, and the diet is adjusted to ensure nutritional adequacy.

It is not particularly difficult to adjust the diet prescription to another condition when one is a trained health professional. However, it is difficult for the patient. Consultation and guidance in planning menus and fitting the patient's new food needs to family patterns are important.

ROLE OF THE DIETITIAN

The primary resource person for dietary counseling and guidance is the registered dietitian.* The person's title may be dietitian, nutritionist, or some variation such as nutrition consultant.

In collaboration with the physician, the dietitian prescribes a diet which meets patient needs and which the patient is willing and able to follow. The questions asked in the section "Dietary Management" provide a basis for dietary planning. It is essential that a careful, quantitative dietary history be taken to provide basic information about patient habits, resources, caloric intake, and preferences. The history should include usual eating patterns (when, where, what, and how much is eaten), use of supplements, daily activity and work patterns, history of special diets and/or changes in pattern, family situation, budget, facilities for food preparation and storage, and food preferences and avoidances. Different techniques may be used, including self-administered questionnaires, but this will depend on the patient's ability to read and write English and other factors such as anxiety. These techniques facilitate but do not replace the interview.

Often it is useful to ask the patient to keep a diary of food intake and activity. This not only provides basic information for counseling but also makes the patient aware of food habits. It is not unusual for a patient to bring the diary back with a list of changes to be made.

The dietitian should evaluate the history and/or record for nutritional adequacy of protein, vitamins, and minerals as well as for caloric, fat, and carbohydrate intake. When the diet prescription is determined, the current pattern should be reviewed to identify the food habits which should be reinforced and those which need to be changed. The dietitian and patient together should establish goals for meeting the prescription. It is unrealistic to expect the patient to make major adjustments in living patterns overnight. Dietary counseling should include guidance for changes to be taken as the patient can manage them. For example, a patient used to eating 3000 cal or more cannot immediately reduce intake to 1000 cal. Long-term compliance and benefit might be better realized by making gradual changes. For example, the patient may agree that a realistic dietary goal for the next visit might be to reduce the four slices of bread carried in the lunch bag to two. When this new habit is formed, another goal can be set. Much can be accomplished by taking one small step at a time. This must be coordinated with medication for the insulin-dependent patient, which is not that difficult.

Regular follow-up sessions are essential for checking results, identifying problems the patient may be having, and providing additional information, encouragement, and support. Periodically dietary histories and/or diaries

---

* The title *registered dietitian* (RD) indicates the individual has met national standards of educational preparation in the field, has passed a national examination, and meets requirements for continuing education. Registration is confirmed annually.

should be obtained and evaluated, with appropriate counseling provided as needed.

The dietitian may participate in classes or group sessions provided for patient education. The dietitian also may be involved in home visits.

Moreover, the dietitian should be aware of the patient's use of commercially prepared foods, artificial sweeteners, dietetic foods, and supplements. The dietitian can determine the composition of food products and restaurant items patients wish to use and show the patient how these can be included in the diet pattern. Since there are regional differences in foods available and in the ingredients of many nationally advertised products, a listing of the items popular in the area should be maintained.

The dietitian can identify books, pamphlets, and other audio or visual aids useful to patients, check them for content and appropriate use, and make them available. New ones can be developed to meet the needs of the group. Since control of portions is essential, food models and other visual aids for teaching portion size are particularly useful.

Special problems related to restrictions on food choice or intake for religious observances or other reasons should be referred to the dietitian to work out with the patient. When another dietary modification must be imposed, consultation is important. As mentioned previously, complications such as diabetic nephropathy, hyperlipidemia, or hypertension may occur and require dietary changes.

In the hospital setting, the dietitian should be involved in the assessment of the patient's nutritional and dietary needs; his or her nutritional care, including the in-house diet and education for diet management at home; the maintenance of records and reports; and the provision of written instructions for the patient (and/or family) and referral agency or other facility for follow-up care. In outpatient settings, records and written instructions are also important, as in continued follow-up of the patient with periodic assessments of dietary management and changes in need associated with growth, pregnancy, aging, and life-style. In either setting, the nurse will be identifying patient needs for dietary counseling as part of the nursing care assessment.

RESOURCES FOR THE PATIENT

Many sources of information for the patient have been mentioned already, such as *Diabetes Forecast*, special cookbooks, nutrition labels, and food composition tables. Diabetes associations offer a variety of educational materials and classes, and the opportunity to meet other people with diabetes. There is a tendency to overlook the tremendous amount of help and emotional support patients can offer each other.

Dietary counseling is especially important for the patient with diabetes. If no dietitian is available for consultation in the office or unit providing health care for the patient, a source of such help should be identified for the patient. There are dietitians in private practice who will work with patients referred by physicians. Some state and local health departments and visiting nurse associations provide service. Local diabetes associations may have staff or volunteer dietitians. Hospital dietary departments may be able to provide assistance under special circumstances for the outpatient, but their first responsibility is to the patient population admitted to the institution or enrolled in its clinics. Many patients who have been hospitalized used the hospital menus as a guide for home.

The American Diabetes Association, Incorporated, the Juvenile Diabetes Foundation, and the American Heart Association have national offices and local units. Check the telephone book or write the national offices for the address of the nearest unit.* Many of the state and local units have materials prepared specifically for people in the area. Many offer workshops, classes, and lectures for patients and families.

Local and state health departments are also resources. Because diabetes is common, most public health units have educational materials available. These departments should also be able to supply information about special programs, camps, health benefits and services available, food stamps, Meals-on-Wheels, or other special food programs for the elderly or ill.

The American Dietetic Association can provide educational materials and information about dietary services.† In many areas of the country, dietitians provide a free public information service, Dial-a-Dietitian. The service does *not* provide therapeutic dietary prescriptions or counseling for the obvious reason that the necessary teamwork between physician, dietitian, and patient is impossible over the telephone. But the service will provide information about food composition, sources of information, nutritional needs, and so on. Check the telephone book or local newspaper to see if Dial-a-Dietitian is available in the patient's area. The national office can also provide addresses of state and local dietetic association officers who can then be contacted to identify local resources.

In recent years there has been a proliferation of materials including games, books, teaching tapes, slide/tape units, and films. Some are available through regular channels such as bookstores; others must be ordered from private units or producers. Drug companies frequently offer booklets and standard diet forms. The physician, nurse, or dietitian should check these materials carefully before recommending them. The information should be accurate and appropriate for the patient. The recommendations for medication, diet, and hygiene should be consistent with the recommendations given the patient in the clinic, hospital, and/or physician's office. Use of standard diet forms is questionable since they obviously are not tailored to meet individual needs nor is the patient involved in planning the management program.

---

* American Diabetes Association, Inc., 1 West 48th Street, New York, New York 10020. Juvenile Diabetes Foundation, 26 East 26th Street, New York, New York 10010. American Heart Association, 7320 Greenville Avenue, Dallas, Texas 75231.
† American Dietetic Association, 420 North Michigan Avenue, Chicago, Illinois 60611.

Games have been developed to teach nutrient content of foods, meals planning, food budgeting, weight control, and food exchange lists. Most are based on bingo, rummy, or common board games. Games and other audiovisual materials are listed and/or reviewed in the *Journal of the American Dietetic Association* and the *Journal of Nutrition Education*.* Puzzles can be fun and instructive. Crossword and the "seek and find" types are popular. Since one learns by developing the game, patients could be encouraged to create games or puzzles for each other.

A variety of books have been written and published in hardcover and paperback. The local diabetes association or health agency may have annotated lists of books available. Any library or bookstore should have the trade volumes *Books in Print* and *Paperback Books in Print*, which list all books on the market by author, publisher, and subject matter.

The federal government is a rich source of materials. Several agencies including the National Institute of Health (NIH), the Public Health Service, and the Department of Agriculture have materials on food, nutrition, budget, diet management, diabetes, and other health subjects. Usually one copy of an item will be sent without charge to a person who writes directly to the Office of Information in care of the unit such as Agriculture, NIH, and so on. Since addresses in Washington change frequently, ask the local librarian for the current listing. A book of federal agencies and addresses is published annually. Catalogs of books, pamphlets, films, and slides published by federal agencies are readily available from the U.S. Government Printing Office, with listings based on subject matter.† Write to that office specifying the kinds of information sought. Many items are available in large easy-to-see print, an important consideration for patients with vision problems. Some items are available in Spanish.

There are many resources available to the patient with diabetes. Many patients will not know about them without guidance from the nurse, dietitian, or health educator. So much is available that care should be exercised in selecting materials that will be truly helpful to the patient.

REFERENCES

1   Bierman, E. L., et al. Principles of nutrition and dietary recommendations for patients with diabetes mellitus: 1971, *Diabetes,* **20:**633–634, 1971.
2   West, K. M. Diabetes mellitus, in H. A. Schneider et al. (eds.), *Nutritional Support of Medical Practice* (Hagerstown, Md.: Harper & Row, 1977), chap. 17.
3   National Center for Health Statistics. *Characteristics of Persons with Diabetes, United States, July 1964–June 1965,* Public Health Service Publication no. 1000, series no. 40, Washington, D.C., 1967.

* Society for Nutrition Education, 2140 Shattuck Avenue, Suite 1110, Berkeley, California 94704.
† Superintendent of Documents, U.S. Government Printing Office, Washington, D.C. 20402.

4 Levine, R. Newer knowledge of diabetes management in adults, in A. M. Beeuwkes (ed.), *Institute on the Education of the Diabetic and His Family,* Continuing Education Series 138 (Ann Arbor, Mich.: Univ. of Michigan Press, 1966).

5 West, K. M. Diet therapy: an analysis of failure, *Ann. Intern. Med.,* **79:**425–434, 1973.

6 Etzwiler, D. D. Who's teaching the diabetic? *Diabetes,* **16:**111–117, 1967.

7 Wood, F. C., Jr. and Bierman, E. L. New concepts in diabetic dietetics, *Nutrition Today,* **7:**4–10, 1972.

8 Ibid.

9 University Group Diabetes Study Program. A study of the effects of hypoglycemic agents on vascular complications in patients with adult-onset diabetes, *Diabetes,* **19:**747–815, 1970.

10 Food and Nutrition Board, National Research Council. *Recommended Dietary Allowances,* 8th ed. (Washington, D.C.: National Academy of Sciences, 1974).

11 Knowles, H. C., et al. Diabetes mellitus: the overall problem and its impact on the public, in S. S. Fajans (ed.), *Diabetes Mellitus,* DHEW Publication no. NIH-76-854, Washington, D.C., 1976, chap. 2.

12 Bierman et al. Loc. cit.

13 West. Diabetes mellitus.

14 University Group Diabetes Study Program. Loc. cit.

15 West. Diabetes mellitus.

16 Kalkhoff, R. K. Diet and diabetes mellitus, in S. S. Fajans, (ed.), *Diabetes Mellitus,* DHEW Publication no. NIH-76-854, Washington, D.C., 1976, chap. 22.

17 Beal, V. A. The nutritional history in longitudinal research, *J. Am. Diet. Assoc.,* **51:**426–532, 1967.

18 Bray, G. A., et al. Eating patterns of massively obese individuals. Direct vs. indirect measurements, *J. Am. Diet. Assoc.,* **72:**24–27, 1978.

19 Food and Nutrition Board, National Research Council. Loc. cit.

20 West. Diet therapy.

21 Bierman et al. Loc. cit.

22 Caso, E. K. Calculation of diabetic diets: report of the committee on diabetic diet calculations, American Dietetic Association, *J. Am. Diet. Assoc.,* **26:**575–583, 1950.

23 Diet and coronary heart disease. A joint statement of the Food and Nutrition Board, National Academy of Sciences' National Research Council and the Council on Foods and Nutrition, American Medical Association, July 1972, *Nutr. Rev.,* **30:**223–225, 1972.

24 U.S. Senate Select Committee on Nutrition and Human Needs. *Dietary Goals for the United States,* 2d ed., Washington, D.C., 1977.

25 Farinaro E., et al. Plasma glucose levels: long-term effect of diet in the Chicago Coronary Prevention Evaluation Program, *Ann. Intern. Med.,* **86:**147–154, 1977.

26 West, K. M. Prevention and therapy of diabetes mellitus, *Nutr. Rev.,* **33:**193–198, 1975.

27 Perrett, A. D., et al. Blood lipids in treated diabetics, *Diabetologia,* **10:**115–118, 1974.

28 Maruhama, Y., et al. Dietary intake and hyperlipidemia in controlled diabetic outpatients, *Diabetes,* **26:**94–99, 1977.

29 Siperstein, M. D., et al. Control of blood glucose and diabetic vascular disease (editorial). *N. Engl. J. Med.,* **296:**1060–1063, 1977.

30 West. Diabetes mellitus.

31 West. Diet therapy; and Diabetes mellitus.

32 Holland, W. M. The diabetes supplement of the National Health Survey. III. The patient reports on his diet, *J. Am. Diet. Assoc.*, **52**:387–390, 1968.

33 Traisman, H. S. *Management of Juvenile Diabetes Mellitus*, 2d ed. (St. Louis: Mosby, 1971).

34 American Diabetes Association, Inc., American Dietetic Association, and Chronic Disease Program, U.S. Public Health Service. *Meal Planning with Exchange Lists* (Chicago: American Dietetic Association, 1950).

35 American Diabetes Association, Inc., American Dietetic Association, and National Institutes of Health, U.S. Public Health Service. *Exchange Lists for Meal Planning* (Chicago: American Dietetic Association, 1976).

36 American Diabetes Association, Inc., and American Dietetic Association. *A Guide for Professionals: The Effective Application of "Exchange Lists for Meal Planning"* (Chicago: American Dietetic Association, 1977).

37 Kaufmann, R. L., et al. Plasma lipid levels in diabetic children. Effect of diet restricted in cholesterol and saturated fats, *Diabetes*, **24**:672–679, 1975.

38 Levy, R. I. Dietary management of hyperlipoproteinemia, *J. Am. Diet. Assoc.*, **58**:406–416, 1971.

39 Fuchs, H., and Midgley, W. Fast food restaurants. Are they for you? *Diabetes Forecast*, **29**:6–11, 1976.

40 Goldsmith, M. P., and Davidson, J. K. Southern ethnic food preferences and exchange values for the diabetic diet, *J. Am. Diet. Assoc.*, **70**:61–64, 1977.

41 Stucky, V. The meal plan, in D. W. Guthrie and R. A. Guthrie (eds.), *Nursing Management of Diabetes Mellitus* (St. Louis: Mosby, 1977).

42 *Nutritive Value of Foods*, Home and Garden Bulletin no. 72, Revised, Consumer and Food Economics Institute, Agriculture Research Service, U.S. Department of Agriculture, Washington, D.C., 1977.

43 *Nutritive Value of American Foods in Common Units*, Agriculture Handbook no. 456, Agriculture Research Service, U.S. Department of Agriculture, Washington, D.C., 1975.

44 *New Century*, Educational Division, Meredith Corporation, 400 Park Avenue South, New York, New York 10016.

45 Odell, A. C., et al. Effect of processed pears on glucose tolerance in diabetes, *J. Am. Diet. Assoc.*, **63**:410–412, 1973.

46 Farkas, C. S., and Forbes, C. E. Do non-caloric sweeteners aid patients with diabetes to adhere to their diets? *J. Am. Diet. Assoc.*, **46**:482–484, 1965.

47 Parham, E. S. Comparisons of responses to bans on cyclamate (1969) and saccharin (1977), *J. Am. Diet. Assoc.*, **72**:59–62, 1978.

48 Cohen, B. L. Relative risks of saccharin and calorie ingestion, *Science*, **199**:983, 1978.

49 James, J., and Kraus, B. *Better Meals for You with Low Calorie Gourmet Recipes* (Cleveland, Ohio: Diabetes Association of Greater Cleveland, 1977).

50 Behrman, Sister M. *A Cookbook for Diabetics* (New York: American Diabetes Association, 1959).

51 Jones, J. *The Calculating Cook* (San Francisco: 101 Productions, 1974).

52 Revell, D. *Diabetes Control Cookery* (New York: Diabetes Control Cookery, 1975).

53 American Diabetes Association, Inc., 1 West 48th Street, New York, New York 10020.

54 Juvenile Diabetes Foundation, 26 East 26th Street, New York, New York 10010.

55 Arvidsson Lenner, R. Specially designed sweeteners and food for diabetics—a real need? *Am. J. Clin. Nutr.*, **29**:726–733, 1976.

56 *Vegetarian Diet Manual,* rev. ed., 1974, Seventh Day Adventist Dietetic Association, Box 75, Loma Linda, California 93252.

57 Prater, B. M. Why diabetic children go to summer camp, *J. Am. Diet. Assoc.*, **55**:584–587, 1969.

58 Etzwiler, D. D., et al. Wilderness camping for the diabetic, *Diabetes,* **14**:676–681, 1965.

59 McCraw, R. K., and Travis, L. B. Psychological effects of a special summer camp on juvenile diabetics, *Diabetes,* **22**:275–278, 1973.

60 Labrenz, J. B. Planning meals for the backpacker with diabetes—nutritional values of freeze-dried foods, *J. Am. Diet. Assoc.*, **61**:42–48, 1972.

61 West. Diabetes mellitus.

62 Committee on Maternal Nutrition, Food and Nutrition Board, National Research Council. *Maternal Nutrition and the Course of Pregnancy* (Washington, D.C.: National Academy of Sciences, 1970).

63 Rodman, H. M., et al. The diabetic pregnancy as a model for modern perinatal care, in M. I. New and R. H. Fiser, Jr. (eds.), *Diabetes and Other Endocrine Disorders during Pregnancy and in the Newborn,* vol. 10, *Progress in Clinical and Biological Research* (New York: Alan R. Liss, 1976), pp 13–32.

64 Schulman, P. Personal communication.

65 Hillman, R. W. Sensible eating for older diabetics, *Geriatrics,* **29**:123–132, 1974.

66 Hadden, D. R., et al. Maturity-onset diabetes mellitus: response to intensive dietary management, *Br. Med. J.,* **2**:276–278, 1975.

67 Bosso, J. A., and Pearson, R. E. Sugar content of selected liquid medicinals, *Diabetes,* **22**:776–785, 1973.

68 Bierman et al. Loc. cit.

69 Traisman, H. S., and Friedeman, C. Dietary treatment of juvenile diabetes mellitus, in H. S. Traisman (ed.), *Management of Juvenile Diabetes Mellitus,* 2d ed. (St. Louis: Mosby, 1971).

70 Kaufmann, R. L., et al. Loc. cit.

71 Kiehm, T. G., et al. Beneficial effects of a high carbohydrate, high fiber diet on hyperglycemic diabetic men, *Am. J. Clin. Nutr.*, **29**:895–899, 1976.

72 Maugh, T. H. Diabetes commission: problem severe, therapy inadequate, *Science,* **191**:272–274, 1976.

73 Kussman, M. J., et al. The clinical course of diabetic nephropathy, *J. Am. Med. Assoc.*, **236**:1861–1863, 1976.

Management of Diabetes by Pharmacologic Agents

Marti Sachse

Medical science has come a long way since ancient civilizations first described diabetes mellitus. At that time, the understanding of the disease went no farther than its description as "a melting down of the flesh and limbs into urine," and knowledge of its treatment was nonexistent. Those afflicted were victims of a "disgusting and painful" short-lived disease, and it was expected that "at no distant term they expire."

Knowledge of the disease has expanded tremendously from this basic description of symptoms to an ever-increasing understanding of the etiology, pathophysiology, and multiple long-term effects of the disease. These advancements have had a dramatic impact on the treatment of diabetes, particularly since the discovery of insulin by Banting and Best. Although this was a major breakthrough and meant survival and increased longevity for the diabetic, more recent investigations have shown that insulin, even with the new modifications and therapeutic approaches, does not duplicate normal glucose homeostasis.

Diabetes is no longer considered merely a disorder of carbohydrate metabolism in which the patient has an absolute or relative lack of insulin. It is now believed that diabetes may in fact be a bihormonal disease involving not only a deficiency of insulin but also an excess of glucagon, a hormone secreted by the alpha cells of the pancreas. Research is currently being done on methods for controlling hyperglucagonemia, which also characterizes the diabetic state.

Current therapeutics in diabetes have had a remarkable effect on life expectancy for these patients. Relatively few die from diabetic coma today, and many live relatively productive lives. However, even with controlled diabetes, a number of other disease processes can afflict the diabetic who is especially prone to them. These patients may be on multiple drug regimens in addition to their diabetic therapy. Increasing the number of medications a patient must take also increases the likelihood of drug interactions and the development of problems with control. Practitioners are now giving closer attention to these potential problems, particularly in diabetic patients with concurrent complications.

Much is still being learned in relation to the long-term effects of agents used to lower blood glucose. With use of insulin and the oral hypoglycemics over a substantial period of time, problems with therapy and individual toxicities are being identified. These observations have been directly responsible for continued research and dedication in the search for an ideal treatment or cure for diabetes.

Increased emphasis has been placed on research in diabetes involving pharmacologists in every part of the world. As more is discovered on the cellular level, attempts at developing pharmacologically active agents to work at specific sites in the disease process are being made. Involvement of clinical pharmacists in this area has contributed a great deal to advancements in diabetes therapy. The testing of agents, the gathering of data on the effects of current therapy, the developing of bioavailability and pharmacokinetic data, and the study of long-term effects, as well as their role in therapeutic consultations with primary care physicians and nurses and in patient education and monitoring, are some of the areas in which clinical pharmacists are helping to expand knowledge and affect the care of diabetic patients.

The management of diabetes is not as simple as a "shot a day" or a "tablet bid." It should be kept in mind that effective management can be achieved only inasmuch as the patient understands his or her disease and is willing to accept responsibility for his or her own care. Compliance problems arise primarily from either nonacceptance or not realizing the seriousness of the disease. Noncompliance with diet is most frequently seen, as patients admit to "cheating occasionally" or express a real concern over their problems in adjusting to new dietary habits. With pharmacologic agents, noncompliance may result from fear, inconvenience, or complaints of troublesome side effects.

The evolution of diabetic management from the preinsulin era to the present has been quite striking. No longer do patients endure the old starvation diets which were actually effective on a short-term basis only. Insulin therapy marked a new era for the diabetic in 1921; but since it was unperfected, it still posed problems of control and adjustment to acute complications. In 1950 when the oral hypoglycemics were introduced, convenience and better control were afforded the symptomatic, maturity-onset diabetic who could not be satisfactorily controlled on diet alone and was unable or unwilling to inject insulin. The use of these agents has increased greatly over the years in this category of patients. In spite of the recognition of increased cardiovascular mortality, it is still difficult to dampen the enthusiasm over the "oral insulins."

Since 1921, medical and pharmaceutical technology have been working continually to improve on existing treatment modalities in diabetes mellitus. Insulin has undergone quite a transformation in the past 50 years, with the development of purer forms that have fewer associated complications. New agents are currently being developed and tested for the control of diabetes and its associated biochemical effects at several different levels.[1,2]

These advances are very promising, yet unproven. Management of diabetes with current therapy at best is still imperfect.

PHARMACOLOGY

Understanding the pharmacology of agents used in treating diabetes is basic to understanding the rationale for individualized therapeutic approaches. The agent's mechanism of action and the pharmacokinetics are critical in this discussion.

Pharmacology of Insulin

The formation of insulin occurs initially in the beta cells of the pancreas with the synthesis of proinsulin. This insulin precursor is transported to storage granules in the Golgi apparatus and is secreted in response to an elevation in blood glucose. Proteolytic enzymes convert proinsulin from the single polypeptide chain by removing the C chain, or central portion of the molecule. The remaining A chain and B chain, linked by disulfide bonds, becomes the double-chained polypeptide, insulin. Even though all three peptides, proinsulin, the C chain, and insulin, are secreted, the only biologically active molecule in controlling glucose homeostasis is insulin (see Fig. 4-7).

The exact mechanisms of insulin's activity is still under investigation in spite of the more than 50 years' experience with insulin in successfully controlling hyperglycemia.

Some tissues and organ systems in the body are known to be insulin-independent, utilizing glucose efficiently in spite of insulin deficiency. These include the brain, renal medulla, pancreatic beta cells, gut epithelial cells, and hepatic cell erythocytes.[3,4] In contrast, muscle and fat tissues do require insulin to efficiently utilize glucose as a major energy source. Here, insulin determines the cellular membrane transport of glucose or the rate in which glucose is transported across the cell membrane. By attaching to specific receptor sites on the cell, a signal or chemical mediator is emitted which permits accelerated entry of glucose (see Fig. 4-1).

When blood glucose is elevated by an exogenous source of carbohydrate, insulin is normally secreted to handle the increased availability of glucose in the blood. In accordance with the bihormonal theory, secretion of glucagon by the alpha cells is reduced as a result of the inhibitory action of insulin. The resulting metabolic process in addition to glucose utilization includes storage of glucose as glycogen, fat, and protein. The hepatic microenzyme system is responsible for conversion of glucose (via phosphorylation by the enzyme glucokinase) into glucose 6-phosphate, the product which enters into a number of metabolic pathways. Release of glucose by the liver is slowed, and an increased synthesis of glycogen occurs. Glucose is also stored in adipose tissues as glycogen, to some degree, and triglycerides, primarily. In muscle, glucose is utilized for protein synthesis and is stored as glycogen and fat.

The interrelationship of activities which occur in the presence of insulin can essentially be described as a decrease in glycogenolysis and gluconeogenesis, a decrease in lipolysis or conversion of fat and triglycerides to fatty acids and glycerol, and an increase in protein synthesis.[5]

To emphasize an important point with respect to insulin's antilipolytic effect, insulin, in lower levels than those necessary to control glucose activity, can prevent breakdown of fat and triglycerides. This phenomenon might explain why in maturity-onset diabetics, obesity is a commonly associated factor, as is "ketosis resistance."[6,7]

Description Insulin is a protein composed of 51 amino acids and having a molecular weight of approximately 6000. It is available commercially in this country and is derived from beef and pork pancreas. In comparison to human insulin, pork insulin bears the highest resemblance, differing in only one amino acid on the B chain. Insulin preparations may be a combination of beef and pork or pure beef or pork.[8]

A number of modifications have been made in insulin since 1921, and these modifications have given greater flexibility in the management of diabetes.[9-11]

Regular insulin (CZI) is a pure crystalline form of the first commercially available amorphous insulin with the same activity. It is composed of a clear solution of zinc-insulin crystals with a pH of 3.5, giving it a rapid absorption from subcutaneous sites, rapid onset of action, and short duration. Acid regular insulin (ARI) has nearly been replaced with neutral regular insulin (NRI), which was developed as a result of the increased purification process and elimination of precipitation which occurred if the pH was above the acid range with the former. An advantage of the neutral product was increased stability, allowing for maintenance of 95 percent potency for 12 months at 37°C as opposed to 25 percent loss of potency in ARI under the same conditions. The activity of the two regular insulins is the same pharmacologically.

The first modification to acid regular insulin was the addition of a basic protein, protamine, yielding a protamine-insulin complex (pH 7.4) that was quite insoluble at body pH. This accounts for the extended activity of protamine zinc-insulin suspension (PZI), which is slowly released from the depot site. It therefore has a longer onset, peak, and duration.[12-14]

Globin insulin, which combines the protein globin (rather than protamine) with insulin, is considered an intermediate-acting insulin. Since globin insulin does not provide coverage for 24 h, the insulin is seldom used clinically. Burroughs-Wellcome is currently the only manufacturer.

Neutral protamine hagedorn (NPH) insulin, generically called isophane-insulin suspension, was developed following clinical investigations of potential modifications for an intermediate-acting insulin. It was observed that a mixture of regular insulin and protamine-zinc insulin in a ratio of 2 : 1 yielded an activity similar to protamine given in smaller doses with supplements of regular insulin, affording an intermediate action. The proportion of insulin to protamine in this mixture is near 1:1 versus a larger proportion of protamine in the PZI. In addition to its advantage as an intermediate-acting insulin, NPH lends itself to addition of more regular insulin without losing activities of either regular or NPH. This is so because no excess protamine is available to bind with the regular insulin. A combination of regular plus PZI in a ratio of less than 1:1 results in an activity characteristic of PZI alone.[15-17]

Ultralente and *semilente insulins* were discovered in 1951 when rather than adding a modifying protein, the zinc concentration of the suspension was increased and an acetate buffer was substituted for phosphate. The result was a preparation insoluble at body pH. Ultralente is basically a crystalline form, and semilente, microcrystalline. Logically, the microcrystalline form has greater solubility than the former, thus a shorter onset, peak, and duration. Ultralente is classified as a long-acting insulin with PZI, while semilente, a fast-acting insulin, closely approximates regular insulin in onset and peak, but with an intermediate duration of action.

Lente insulin is a mixture of 30 percent semilente and 70 percent ultralente. This insulin and NPH have almost identical intermediate activities and are the most frequently used of all currently available insulins.

All the insulins, with the exception of regular insulin, are stable (maintains potency) at room temperature for 24 months. Regular insulin, the only insulin solution, is less stable, as previously noted.

The trend in current utilization of insulin in diabetic therapy is toward the U-100 concentration. Though still available, U-40 and U-80 strengths are on the decline. The advantages of the U-100 are, obviously, less volume to be injected and easier metric conversions; in addition, it is a more purified form of insulin that results in less complications with repeated injections.

The new, purer insulin preparations currently marketed by Lilly in the United States and by Nova in Denmark are single-peak and single-component. *Single-peak insulin* is 70 to 75 percent pure insulin and 25 to 30 percent desamino insulin. *Single-component insulin* is 99 percent pure insulin; it must be specially ordered. The use of both these preparations is discussed later in the section on insulin allergy.

Mixtures of insulin are commonly used to achieve control in some diabetics. The principles for mixing insulins and the stability of various preparations are as follows:[18]

Neutral or acid regular insulin and PZI in a 1:1 ratio equal PZI alone; in a 2:1 ratio they equal NPH; and in a 3:1 ratio they equal NPH plus regular. There is really no advantage to any of these combinations, and because of stability problems, they should be mixed just prior to injection.

Acid regular and lente should not be mixed in a proportion greater than 1:1. Differences in pH may cause unpredictable time-action curves. Therefore, mixing just prior to injection is recommended.

Neutral regular and NPH or lente may be mixed in any proportion and may be mixed 2 to 3 months prior to injection.

Lentes (semilente, lente, or ultralente) may be mixed in any proportion and are stable indefinitely upon premixing.

For diluted insulins when very small doses are needed, regular insulin with insulin diluting fluid has an advantage over normal saline, affording greater stability. Any proportion may be mixed; however, if normal saline is used, the preparation should not be premixed any longer than 2 to 3 h before use.

Pharmacokinetics Pharmacokinetic properties of the insulins are important factors in managing the diabetic. Knowledge of the onset, peak, and duration of each insulin enables the practitioner, working with other health professionals, to coordinate the diet and exercise prescriptions accordingly. Timing is the key in balancing these three basics in diabetic management. In summary, DIET is the mainstay in diabetes: D, diet; I, insulin; E, exercise; T, timing.

A number of sources have categorized the insulins according to short acting, intermediate acting, and long acting, and specific data regarding onset, peak, and duration vary from reference to reference. Table 7-1 gives ranges for each classification which should be considered as general guidelines in predicting insulin activity in each individual patient.[19,20]

In discussing the bioavailability and pharmacokinetics of exogenously administered insulin, researchers include absorption, distribution, metabolism, and excretion, as well as a comparison of results by route of administration. In diabetics there are significant alterations in the pharmacokinetics of insulin as compared with normal individuals. Factors such as insulin antibodies, pancreatic reserve, receptor site affinity for insulin, etc., make basing therapeutic approaches on standard pharmacokinetic data extremely complex and difficult. Therefore, the discussion of problems of bioavailability encountered in diabetic patients appears to have greater significance and relevance to patient management than do present data obtained by investigators from normal subjects.

Table 7-1 Characteristics of Insulin Preparations

Insulin	Onset, h	Peak, h	Duration, h
Regular (CZI)	½–1	2–3	5–7
Semilente	½–1	4–7	12–16
Lente	1–4	8–12	18–24
NPH	1–2	8–12	18–24
Ultralente	4–8	16–18	36
Protamine zinc (PZI)	4–8	14–20	36

Insulin Absorption   The *absorption of insulin* from subcutaneous injection sites can vary significantly depending on the size of dose, location, and type of insulin being administered.[21] Absorption occurs more rapidly with the injection of larger volumes of regular insulin, while conversely, with NPH insulin or other insulin suspensions, the larger the volume, the slower the absorption. Insulin is absorbed more rapidly from the arm than the thigh under normal conditions. During leg exercise, however, absorption is accelerated, presenting an increased risk of hypoglycemia. Injecting in the arm or abdomen reduces this likelihood. Absorption of insulin is also slower when injection is into the buttocks, because of less peripheral circulation and a proportionately higher amount of fatty tissue.

Another very important factor affecting insulin absorption is related to rotation of injection sites. When repeated injections into the same area result in hypertrophy, absorption can be delayed or erratic. This points up the importance of stressing regular rotation of injection sites in patient education.

All diabetics develop antibodies to insulin in varying degrees within 2 to 3 months of initiation of therapy.[22] These insulin-binding antibodies may be responsible for delayed absorption and release into the tissues.

Following absorption, exogenous insulin is rapidly *distributed* into extracellular fluids. The half-life in plasma is normally 6.5 to 15 min and may be prolonged up to 13 h in diabetics.[23]

Metabolism occurs in the liver, kidneys, and muscle tissue, primarily in the liver by the enzyme, glutathione insulin transhydrogenase.[24]

Renal excretion is an important factor that can affect the activity of insulin. Insulin is filtered in the glomerulus, and approximately 98 percent is reabsorbed in the proximal tubules, 40 percent returning to venous blood and the remainder undergoing metabolism in the proximal convoluted tubules. Renal impairment, which may be coexistent with diabetes, renders the patient insensitive to insulin by some unknown mechanism. With the progression of renal disease, insulin requirements decrease. This has been explained by several factors which occur during this stage of renal disease. First, since the kidney is a site for insulin metabolism, this process is diminished and the plasma half-life is increased. In addition, substances have been identified in the plasma of uremic patients which promote glucose utilization. Finally, food intake is usually diminished in such patients.[25]

Measurement of Insulin   Methods for determining insulin concentrations in plasma have been developed utilizing in vivo and in vitro assay techniques.[26,27] The early in vivo method proved to be very limited in accurately determining levels of insulin, and thus in vitro assays currently provide the best approach. The *biological assays* include the rat diaphragm method and the rat epididymal fat pad method of measuring glucose uptake.

Comparison of these two methods yields higher values for the second method because of the presence of noninsulin factors in fat with insulin-like activity. The former method can yield variable results upon dilution of the serum, which results in a dilution of insulin inhibitors.

Since both biological assays are based on the observation of the *results* of insulin activity rather than a direct measurement of insulin itself, the *radioimmunoassay* was developed. This method, heralded as the most satisfactory in vitro method, measures the amount of free insulin as well as the amount of insulin bound to antibody.

The development of insulin assay techniques has been a major advancement in understanding how insulin secretion is regulated and what stimuli are responsible for insulin activity. Researchers compared plasma insulin and glucose levels after administration of glucose by oral and intravenous routes and discovered the insulin response was much greater following orally administered glucose. This led to isolation of factors in the intestinal tract which enhance insulin secretion. Such factors include secretin, pancreozymin-cholecystokinin, gastrin, and "gut glucagon" (a glucagon-like substance). The 10 essential amino acids were also found to enhance insulin secretion, working synergistically with glucose. Further studies have identified substances such as oxytocin, vasopressin, potassium ion, ACTH, and TSH as insulin stimulators.[28] The clinical importance of these discoveries lies in the assessment of these factors in relation to degrees of severity in the diabetic.

Pharmacology of the Oral Hypoglycemics

Contrary to the belief of some lay people, the oral hypoglycemic agents are not oral forms of insulin. These agents, chemically related to sulfa antibacterials and known as the *sulfonylureas*, are pharmacologically active in their effect of stimulating the release of insulin from the beta cells in the pancreas. In order to achieve the desired therapeutic effect in controlling hyperglycemia, it is necessary that beta cells in the islets of Langerhans possess some functioning capacity. For this reason, growth-onset diabetics will not respond to these agents.

The sulfonylureas are not capable of restoring normal function to these cells. However, some researchers feel that there is a generation of new beta cells as a result of therapy with oral hypoglycemics.[29]

Beyond this simple explanation of the mechanism of action for the sulfonylureas, other mechanisms have been proposed as contributing to control of blood glucose. It has been suggested also that sulfonylureas facilitate the ability of glucose to stimulate insulin release. Plasma glucagon levels may also be suppressed, inhibiting glucagon-stimulated glucose production in the liver. Finally, after chronic use it appears that endogenous insulin becomes more effective.[30]

The primary action of the oral hypoglycemics, to stimulate insulin release, should be a consideration in management of the obese diabetic. Theoretically, the release of more insulin in such patients who are already hyperinsulinemic could lead to even further weight gain. As mentioned earlier, insulin has a lipogenic activity.

The only classification of oral hypoglycemics currently used are the sulfonylureas. In the past few years, there has been much controversy over a second class, the *biguanides,* of which *phenformin* (DBI, Meltrol) was the single agent then on the market. It was removed from the therapeutic regimens of many diabetics upon its recall by the Food and Drug Administration. Because of the high incidence of lactic acidosis associated with phenformin, and because of inadequate monitoring and control of these patients, phenformin was felt to be unsafe in treating diabetes. Phenformin was used widely for control of the obese diabetic based on its unique pharmacologic property not characteristic of the sulfonylureas. Its primary mechanism of action (MOA) was in decreasing absorption of glucose from the gastrointestinal tract. In addition, its hypoglycemic activity was enhanced by inhibition of hepatic gluconeogenesis and increased glucose utilization by anaerobic glycolysis.

Pharmacokinetics Currently, there are four sulfonylureas on the market. Each varies somewhat in pharmacokinetic activity, even though therapeutic responses are quite similar.

All sulfonylureas are absorbed readily from the gastrointestinal tract, but again various resources differ in their assignment of absorption times, peak actions, and duration. Table 7-2 lists the generally accepted ranges for these agents.[31,32] The major differences among the sulfonylureas can best be explained by discussion of each individually with regard to metabolism and excretion.[33,34]

Tolbutamide, the first of the group to be used clinically, has a rapid absorption time and the shortest duration of action. It is protein-bound and rapidly metabolized via oxidation to carboxytolbutamide and hydroxytolbutamide in the liver. These inactive metabolites are then excreted in the urine within 24 h.

Tolazamide is the most recent addition to the sulfonylurea hypoglycemic agents and, like acetohexamide, has generally an intermediate activity. It is more slowly absorbed, however, than any of the others and may have a shorter duration than acetohexamide. It is metabolized in the liver to six metabolites of which three are active (possess hypoglycemic properties). However, none of these are as active as the parent. Eighty-five percent of an administered dose is recoverable in the urine.

Acetohexamide, classed as the earliest intermediate-acting sulfonylurea, is rapidly absorbed and metabolized to hydroxyhexamide. This agent deserves

Table 7-2   Characteristics of Sulfonylureas

	Onset, h	Peak, h	Duration, h	$T_{1/2}$, h	Dose, g
Tolbutamide (Orinase)	½–1	3–5	6–12	4–5.6	0.5–2.0
Acetohexamide (Dymelor)	1	3	10–24	5–8	0.25–1.5
Tolazamide (Tolinase)	4–6	15	10–15	6–8	0.1–1.0
Chlorpropamide (Diabinese)	1	72	40–72	35	0.1–0.5

Sources: L. Young and M. A. Kimble, *Applied Therapeutics for Clinical Pharmacists* (San Francisco: Applied Therapeutics, Inc., 1975); and T. W. Boyden, The proper place of oral hypoglycemics in diabetes management, *Drug Therapy,* March 1978, pp. 66–77.

particular consideration since its metabolite possesses hypoglycemic activity up to three times greater than the parent compound. If this were not the case, the half-life of acetohexamide would be approximately 1.6 h. Considering the activity of hydroxyhexamide, the combined half-life is approximately 5.3 h. Following metabolism by the liver, the drug is excreted primarily via the kidney, with 15 percent by biliary excretion.

The longest-acting sulfonylurea is *chlorpropamide*. Following rapid absorption, it is highly bound to plasma protein, a factor which could be largely responsible for its prolonged effect. It was originally believed that very little (less than 1 percent) chlorpropamide was metabolized and that the drug was excreted unchanged via the kidney. This is no longer felt to be the case; it is now suggested by advanced analytical techniques that as much as 80 percent of the drug undergoes metabolism, with 20 percent excreted unchanged. The rate of metabolism is perhaps much slower than with the other agents, accounting for its prolonged activity. It is important to keep in mind that there is a wide range of activity with chlorpropamide, and these values can vary markedly from patient to patient.

Dosage Based on their pharmacokinetic properties, dosage of these agents is usually consistent with half-life and duration. Tolbutamide is usually administered two to three times a day in a maximum daily dose of 3.0 g, with the usual range being 0.5 to 2.0 g/day. Acetohexamide and tolazamide can be given in single doses, with the advantage of better patient compliance, but they are often administered twice daily. Recommended dosages include 0.25 to 1.5 g daily (1.5 g maximum) for acetohexamide and 0.1 to 1.0 g (0.75 to 1.0 g maximum) for tolazamide. Because of the prolonged effect of chlorpropamide, a single daily dose is recommended. The range is 0.1 to 0.5 g daily, with 0.5 g being the maximum. Maximum doses are considered to be quite important in therapeutic management, since any amount in excess of these will produce no further hypoglycemic activity and will increase the likelihood of side effects.

With tolbutamide as the least potent (mg potency ratio = 1), acetohexamide is approximately 2½ times as potent, and tolazamide and chlorpropamide have 5 times the potency.[35]

Just as there are individual variations in response to these agents and thus variations in the pharmacokinetics from patient to patient, there are also certain prominent factors which affect the pharmacokinetics. These are critical in the management of patients on oral hypoglycemics.

Appropriate adjustments must be made when renal dysfunction, hepatic disease, or old age becomes a part of the clinical picture in patients on the sulfonylureas. In the case of renal disease, accumulation of chlorpropamide, acetohexamide, and tolazamide is likely to occur since active drug or metabolites are dependent on the kidney for elimination. This results in a prolonged effect of the drug and, without alteration of dose, may result in prolonged hypoglycemia. Tolbutamide, since it is completely metabolized to an inactive compound prior to elimination, would be the best choice of agent in these patients.

Liver disease poses a serious problem in the administration of any of the sulfonylureas. Since metabolism occurs primarily in the liver, it would stand to reason that drug levels would be prolonged, resulting in extended hypoglycemia. Alteration of dosage is essential and careful monitoring imperative in patients with liver dysfunction concurrently on a sulfonylurea.

Chlorpropamide was once thought to be the agent of choice in hepatic disease, but since it has been recognized that it too is metabolized by the liver, the theory no longer holds. Whether or not the already prolonged half-life is markedly affected by liver metabolism is questionable.

In elderly patients, response to any pharmacologic agent is usually exaggerated as a result of a number of factors, foremost of which is a decrease in hepatic enzyme activity. Lower doses are usually necessary to prevent the occurrence of hypoglycemia. Particularly with the oral hypoglycemics, it is important to encourage regular food intake since appetite seems to decrease in elderly patients.[36]

Problems associated with oral hypoglycemics and insulin therapy will be considered later in the chapter.

MANAGEMENT OF ACUTE AND CHRONIC DISORDERS OF DIABETES

Goals of Management

Specialists in diabetes management have yet to resolve the controversy over the degree to which diabetes control should be achieved. It is universally agreed that, ideally, diabetic control should aim for *normoglycemia*, the restoration of carbohydrate abnormality toward a more physiologic state, and that a diabetic should be encouraged to live a full and useful life, carrying out normal activities with family and career. Generally, the treatment goals emphasized by a number of practitioners include:

1 Normal fasting blood glucose and postprandial blood glucose as close to normal as feasible
2 Normal or slightly below normal body weight
3 Little or no glycosuria
4 Normal lipids
5 Freedom from ketoacidosis and hypoglycemic episodes
6 Prevention of macrovascular and microvascular disease
7 Healthy mental attitude toward diabetes and an acceptable life-style.

These goals may often be difficult to achieve in some diabetics, and the question arises, "Is strict control absolutely essential if it means sacrificing the diabetic's emotional stability in coping with an obligatory regimentation?"

Herein lies the controversy. Supporters of "tight" or "rigid control" believe that this practice results in a patient who feels better; is not troubled with the symptoms of polyuria, polydipsia, and nocturia; has fewer infections and more normal lipid metabolism; and enjoys a delay in or lack of vascular complications. They claim that "loose control," on the other hand, results in 24-h hyperglycemia with associated symptoms, chronic intracellular dehydration, visual disturbances, retinopathy, cataracts, greater incidence of infection, neuropathy, and early vascular disease.[37]

If control is too tight, the patient is likely to experience severe hypoglycemic episodes, which could lead to mental deterioration. This appears to be the major concern of those with a liberal attitude toward control. They contend that strict control is difficult to achieve because of patient errors in medication and diet regimens; the inadequacy of periodic urine and occasional blood glucose tests in properly assessing control; the inadequacy of current treatment methods for glucose control; the unavailability of drugs to control gluconeogenesis, lipolysis, proteolysis, glucagon secretion, and growth hormone levels; and finally, the problems of acceptance by family and peers which strict regimentation might impose.[38]

Retrospective studies have failed to delineate clearly a direct relationship between control and the occurrence of vascular complications. However, there is increasingly more evidence being brought forth to support the strict control theory.[39] In order to prove this theory, however, a definitive prospective study is needed. Unfortunately, because of the complexity of such a study and the financial cost it would entail, it is not feasible at the present time. Two other considerations are whether strict control can actually be achieved with current pharmacologic agents and whether blood glucose is the critical measurement for assessment of control.

Dr. David Kudzma of New York stated, "Nobody has ever shown that hyperglycemia is good for you; but there are indications that normalization may prevent or postpone diabetic complications."[40] Dr. Howard Goldstein of the Joslin Clinic summed it up by saying, "Control of diabetes goes beyond the elimination of acute signs and symptoms of high blood glucose all the way to normalization of the metabolism whenever possible. This goal is difficult to attain because of the foibles of human nature and because the means at hand are imperfect. Nevertheless, this goal is held out to the patient since to do less is to encourage indifferent compliance . . . and is less than the best that present medicine has to offer."[41]

Criteria for Control

Specific criteria for control with respect to blood and urine glucose have been established by a number of diabetologists. The Joslin Clinic considers the blood glucose values listed in Table 7-3 as desirable for the insulin-dependent and non-insulin-dependent diabetic. In addition, Table 7-4 illustrates three categories of control based on amount of urine glucosuria.[42] Runyan describes the following specific goals for the growth-onset diabetic and maturity-onset diabetic, with subclassifications for the latter.

Table 7-3 Joslin Clinic Criteria for Control of Blood Glucose Concentrations

Time after food, h	Blood glucose, mg/100 mL	
	Diet/oral hypoglycemics	Insulin
Fasting	80–100	80–120
1	180	200–220
2	120	140
3	100	120
4	80–100	80–120

Expect wide swings in both blood sugar (80–275 mg%) and urinary sugar. However, attempt to get urine free of sugar once or twice per day in the labile type. Encourage regularity in food intake and insulin administration. Patient and family should be taught to increase or decrease insulin dosage depending upon degree of control. Establish rapport with patient and family in clinic and by home visit. Emphasize positives in dealing with the patient and family. Most problems in the juvenile are psychological. Hypoglycemic episodes occurring in late afternoon can be prevented by regularly having a snack such as milk and a half of a sandwich or cereal in mid afternoon. A single low blood sugar may not mean that insulin should be lowered particularly if hypoglycemic episodes are infrequent. A snack prior to strenuous exercise may prevent hypoglycemia.[43]

In the same work, Runyan also describes goals for three classes of maturity-onset diabetics:

Middle-Aged, Obese

1   Random blood glucose level below 200 mg per 100 mL and above 100 mg per 100 mL.

2   Urine glucose negative.

3   Reminders about diet and weight loss.

4   Ideal control is possible, but dietary indiscretion remains a problem in some.

Middle-Aged, Normal Weight

1   Random blood glucose level usually below 200 mg per 100 mL and above 100 mg per 100 mL.

2   Urine glucose negative unless patient is subject to hypoglycemia; may spill sugar occasionally.

Table 7-4 Joslin Clinic Criteria for Control of Glycosuria

24-h Urine glucose*	
< 5% of daily CHO intake	Excellent control
<10% of daily CHO intake	Good control
>10% of daily CHO intake	Not controlled

* Adjust values for low renal threshold if necessary.

3 Diet should be consistent in amount and timing, with less emphasis on restriction, especially if patient is subject to reactions.

4 Stable diabetes is achievable for this category; however, some remain unstable.

Elderly

1 Random blood glucose level below 250 mg per 100 mL and above 125 mg per 100 mL; when sugars run high without urinary sugar, contact physician.

2 To lessen possible hypoglycemia, occasional glycosuria (trace, 1+) is preferred.

3 Weight loss is a goal if patient is obese; correct dietary idiosyncracies when possible.

4 Control should neither be absolutely strict nor extremely loose; patient should be active and comfortable.

The maturity-onset diabetic, in particular the obese patient, requires a greater emphasis on diet control as opposed to high doses of insulin or the oral hypoglycemics. This approach is attempted primarily to prevent peripheral hyperinsulinism and resulting lipogenesis. Weight reduction is often all that is necessary to bring the patient's diabetes under control. Addition of oral agents which stimulate release of more insulin will increase levels in patients who already have hyperinsulin states and result in increased food intake and weight gain. Administration of increasingly large doses of insulin tends to provoke the same type of consequence.

Maintenance of an adequate pancreatic reserve of insulin is another consideration in the management of the maturity-onset diabetic. Causing excessive release of insulin from insulin storage sites may eventually "wear out" the patient's capability of producing and releasing endogenous insulin. This might possibly be one mechanism of eventual failure on oral agents. Ensuring an adequate hepatic supply of insulin is important, however, in maintaining appropriate enzymatic control in carbohydrate metabolism and storage of glycogen.

In establishing individual goals, it is important to realize that such goals are more likely to be achieved in working *with* the patient. It is not realistic to require every diabetic to follow the same patterns universally. Just as every diabetic responds differently to the disease, so should each regimen be planned accordingly. Personality and patient understanding play important roles in management. Rather than impose a complete change in life-style, every attempt should be made to devise a therapeutic regimen which the patient can fully understand and cope with. In the case of young diabetics, Guthrie believes that "the key to adolescent control is complete honesty, inclusion, and flexibility." Understanding diabetes allows the patient to comprehend why certain restrictions may be necessary and accept these with greater ease.

Criteria for Selection of Specific Therapy

It would seem that selection of specific therapy for the diabetic patient would be relatively simple: insulin for the juvenile diabetic who lacks the capacity for endogenous insulin production and either diet, oral agents, or sometimes insulin for the adult diabetic who develops relative insulin-deficiency states.

However, diabetic treatment protocols are not always so simple. The juvenile diabetic poses a greater problem in control than most adults. Usually juvenile diabetes is much more severe, nutritional requirements are greater and the change in these is constant, activity is more varied, and the patient's emotional character takes wide swings, particularly during adolescence. Control is especially critical to ensure normal growth and development. Although insulin will always be required through the adult years, the variability is much less once growth is complete. The appropriate balance of insulin, exercise, and diet is much more difficult for the juvenile diabetic to achieve than for the adult-onset diabetic (who may require only small amounts of insulin).

Insulin requirements vary according to the severity of the insulin deficit, which is exemplified by associated symptomatology and the duration of the disease. The symptoms associated with juvenile diabetes are usually quite severe, indicating a severe insulin deficiency. However, in the adult-onset group, symptoms are not quite so pronounced and may actually be unnoticed or related to another medical problem (e.g., blurred vision). Insulin is thus not necessary for control in such patients, but may be required later in the course of the disease if control becomes inadequate with oral hypoglycemics.

The diabetic condition is one factor, but consideration of the total patient is equally important in planning a treatment protocol. The patient's age and age at onset of the disease have already been discussed. Other patient factors to take into account are weight, activity, occupation, compliance estimate based on personality, any underlying disease states, and contraindications. The latter two areas will be discussed later.

Weight Weight is a particular problem for the obese, maturity-onset diabetic. In such patients, care should be taken to emphasize the diet prescription and the problems of overmedication. Especially if insulin is needed, large doses can make it difficult for the patient to lose weight. Small doses should be given, with emphasis on the goal of weight reduction for effective control of blood glucose.

Activity The patient's level of activity will be reflected in weight and blood glucose. The sedentary adult will need to restrict food intake to a greater degree and may perhaps require larger initial doses of insulin or oral hypoglycemics. The young, insulin-dependent diabetic who is very active logically will have higher caloric requirements and thus greater food intake. Insulin will need to be adjusted accordingly. See Chapter 6 for further discussion about food and activity.

Occupation The patient's occupation should be taken into account in planning a regimen that coincides with work patterns, since a major goal of diabetic therapy is to allow the patient "to live a full and useful life carrying out normal activities with family and career." Planning for the most active times of the day or night to avoid hypoglycemia is crucial.

Personality   Personality is oftentimes overlooked in the diabetic patient. How well is the patient dealing with his or her diagnosis? Does he or she have a fear of injections? What does the patient feel about the social acceptability of his or her disease? These questions and others may affect how readily the patient adapts to a life-style that now involves a diabetic regimen and complies with treatment. Some patients are slower in adapting than others, so treatment plans should be made to gradually include patient self-care. There is also a physical element which sometimes limits the patient's capabilities, and unless "someone does it for them," it will not be done.

Medication Therapy: Recommended Protocols

The most common treatment associated with diabetes mellitus is insulin. However, exogenous insulin is not always required, as the preceding sections have revealed.

Insulin is an absolute necessity for the juvenile, growth-onset diabetic who demonstrates the classical symptoms of the diabetic syndrome and who has had ketoacidosis at some time during the disease. Usually patients before age 40 will require insulin. In addition, any patient in diabetic coma from ketoacidosis or one who has nonketotic hyperosmolar type of coma will require insulin.

Under certain conditions, any diabetic patient may require the administration of insulin on an intermittent basis.[44] These conditions include unstable diabetes, thinness in older diabetics, inadequate control on oral hypoglycemics, failure of diet therapy, pregnancy, febrile illnesses and infections, and major surgery. If an elderly patient is both thin and has unstable diabetes, he or she will likely require insulin on a continuous basis, as would a juvenile, insulin-dependent patient.

There are a number of factors which affect the dose of insulin needed by each individual patient. Already mentioned were increased food intake, decreases in exercise, fever, infections, pregnancy, surgery, and ketoacidosis (requiring an increase in insulin dose.) An in-depth discussion of concomitant disease states and medications will follow later in the chapter.

Individual response to a single dose of intermediate-acting insulin has been described by Hallas-Møller and classified into three types.[45] Type A is characterized by hyperglycemia in the early morning, evening, and throughout the night, with hypoglycemia occurring during the remainder of the daytime hours. Type C responders are hyperglycemic during the day and hypoglycemic during the waking hours and evening, suggesting a delayed response via serum protein binding. The type B patient responds ideally, maintaining normoglycemia for a 24-h period. This patient can be managed simply on one dose of insulin a day. Types A and C will probably require therapy utilizing a combination of insulins and appropriate timing of a "split dose."

Insulin Dosing for the Juvenile Growth-Onset Diabetic   Initiating therapy for the juvenile diabetic presenting with classical symptoms of polyuria, polydipsia, polyphagia, weight loss, and perhaps ketoacidosis will require large doses of insulin and possibly fluid and electrolyte replacement if ketoacidosis is present. This type of patient, the moderately severe diabetic, is perhaps best brought under control in a hospital setting where she or he can be monitored more frequently.

There is no question that patients with severe ketoacidosis should be hospitalized. However, there are differing opinions regarding treatment settings for patients with mild ketonemia. This is largely the decision of the physician. Whether a patient is hospitalized or therapy is initiated on an outpatient basis depends on the needs of the patient and family and the existing programs available for diabetic patient education. Many hospitals provide in-depth teaching in diabetes, and some outpatient clinics and private physicians are able to provide much the same for their patients.

A number of methods for initiating therapy are currently used. Rather than present a standard, these several methods are outlined below.

Sliding scale or *rainbow schedule* is a method used frequently for initiating therapy, but many feel it is not a rational approach and should not be recommended. However, use of this method in certain other instances has proven helpful, such as in poorly controlled, difficult to evaluate diabetics, in obstetrical procedures and delivery, in preoperation and postoperation periods, and following ketoacidotic and hyperosmolar coma.[46-48]

Administration of a dose of insulin is based on frequent urine glucose determinations using the copper-reduction (Clinitest) test on urine samples that are double voided (the patient empties his or her bladder ½ to 1 h before obtaining a second specimen to be tested). This procedure is done four to five times daily in some practices. More frequently, however, patients test their urine before meals and before bedtime. Clinitest is preferred over Tes-Tape because it is *quantitatively* more accurate.

The number of units of regular insulin (CZI) for each "plus" obtained by Clinitest should be specified by the physician. Usually, the amount given is 4 to 5 U. Thus for 4+, 20 U are given; for 3+, 15 U; for 2+, 10 U; and for 1+, 5 U. If acetone is present in the urine, an additional 5 U are administered. The dose is given ½ to 1 h (some recommend 1 to 1½ h) before a meal. It has been recommended by Bressler that administration of insulin by the sliding scale occur every 6 h rather than every 4 h, as had been common practice previously.[49] Since maximum hypoglycemic activity may not be seen for up to 10 h in some patients, it would seem logical to delay administration of the next dose until the previous dose has had its full effect. Urine samples obtained before 4 h would not appropriately reflect the insulin requirement for the following period. The delay in action and prolongation of regular insulin is probably due to the development of insulin antibodies in patients previously treated with insulin.

The purpose of the sliding-scale method is to determine as closely as possible the 24-h insulin requirement. When the patient's fasting blood glucose is within normal limits (which may require several days), the total 24-h requirement for the previous day is the basis for calculating the NPH or lente (intermediate-acting insulin) to be given that morning. Usually two-thirds to three-fourths of the total is administered. If urine glucose indicates the dose to be insufficient, supplemental regular insulin is administered before meals as needed. Usually the amount of supplemental insulin is less (approximately 3 U for each "plus" reading), but again, this must be specified by the physician.

An alternate approach is to administer *a second dose of intermediate insulin* before the evening meal based on the level of fasting blood glucose (FBG) that morning. For every 10 mg per 100 mL increment above normal, 1 U of insulin is given, e.g., for an FBG of 200 mg per 100 mL (normal = 100 percent), 10 U of NPH or lente are given. Two-thirds of this dose is added on to the next morning's dose, and this is repeated until the subsequent FBG is within normal limits. This method assumes that the sliding scale is utilized for only 1 day and not until a normal FBG is achieved with regular insulin. It is believed by some diabetologists that more than 1 day of sliding-scale doses of regular insulin is a waste of time, and that intermediate insulin should be administered on the morning after diagnosis or after recovery from ketoacidosis.[50] When intermediate-acting insulin is initiated early, the recommended starting dose is 0.5 to 1.0 U/kg daily, adjusted accordingly.

Once a patient is on NPH or lente with one dose in the morning, obtaining a 4 P.M. blood glucose level to determine the insulin effect at peak activity is valuable in identifying potential hypoglycemia or inadequacy of dose.

A method based on *caloric needs and standard insulin dose* is described by Jackson and Guthrie. This method emphasizes nutritional needs in the diabetic child in the postacidotic stage.[51]

During this period, the insulin requirement is approximated at 2.0 U/kg daily. Because of food intolerance, 30 to 40 kcal/kg during the first 24 h is prescribed until the patient is able to tolerate more.

Four doses of regular insulin are administered (every 6 h) with four small meals for the first few days, and adjustments are made in both insulin and diet based on urine tests and patient response.

If over the 6-h period following the first dose, urine contains 3 percent glucose consistently, then insulin is increased by several units. Likewise, if urine is glucose-free, then insulin is decreased by several units, and 50 to 100 kcal are added if the patient has tolerated the previous meal. If only small amounts of glucose appear in the urine during the second 6-h period and the patient's hunger is not satisfied, the insulin dose remains the same and another 50 to 100 kcal are added. The total of the four doses for the first 24-h period will approximate the next day's requirement.

During this recovery period while the child is repleting nutritional stores, requirements for calories and other nutrients will be higher, as will insulin need, than those necessary for maintenance.

Following the first few days of recovery with the administration of regular insulin, the patient is switched to a 2:1 mixture of NPH and regular insulin (usually premixed in a sterile vial for convenience). Two-thirds of the daily requirement is given $^1/_2$ h before breakfast and one-third before the evening meal.

Since diet plays an important role in this method of initiating insulin therapy, the recommended division of calories is $^4/_{18}$ at breakfast, $^2/_{18}$ for a midmorning snack, $^5/_{18}$ at the noon meal, $^1/_{18}$ for a midafternoon snack, $^5/_{18}$ at the evening meal, and the remaining $^1/_{18}$ for a bedtime snack. This schedule provides calories needed during active times of the day and "coverage" for the peak activity of insulin.

Based on urine glucose, insulin is adjusted either upward or downward at a rate of approximately 3 U per day. With adequate and early treatment of the child, insulin requirements will approximate 0.3 U/kg per day. Jackson and Guthrie have determined that young patients whose treatment is not carefully planned and controlled in this manner and who have been taking only one injection a day will have a higher insulin requirement of 0.7 to 1.5 U/kg per day.

Methods for Uncomplicated, Nonketotic Diabetics Patients who do not present with the serious symptoms of "total" diabetes are much better managed on an outpatient basis. Initiating therapy in this manner allows the patient a regulation period that is consistent with normal daily activities.

Goldstein from the Joslin Clinic recommends that initial doses be 12 to 16 U of intermediate-acting insulin in a single dose for adults and $^1/_4$ U/1b of ideal body weight for children.[52] The dose is increased each day by 10 to 25 percent until an acceptable blood glucose range is achieved. Dose effectiveness is evaluated by random second-voided urine specimens before meals and at bedtime, 24-h urines, and fasting blood glucose determinations. Less emphasis is placed on the 2-h postprandial blood glucose since premeal hypoglycemia can result if attempts are made to normalize glucose at this time. Once a patient is stabilized, the 2-h postprandial blood glucose is often normalized with only one injection a day.

Another method, which requires weekly blood glucose tests and fractional urines four to five times daily before meals and at bedtime for daily adjustments of dose, begins with an initial dose of 10 to 20 U of NPH or lente.[53] If urine glucose readings obtained with the copper-reduction test (Clinitest) range from 3+ to 4+ for the day, the next day's dose should be increased by 4 U; if 0 to 2+ (not all 0), then the insulin dose remains the same. When values obtained are between 0 and 1+, the dose should be decreased by 4 U. Schedules for daily adjustment of insulin doses are often individually devised by the physician. One such schedule used in an outpatient pediatric clinic is as follows:[54]

Three out of four tests negative, decrease insulin 4 U.
Four out of four tests negative, decrease insulin 8 U.
Three out of four tests positive (2+ to 4+), increase insulin 2 U.
Four out of four tests positive (2+ to 4+), increase insulin 4 U.

When the insulin requirement reaches 50 to 60 U and the patient is still not controlled, splitting the dose is advisable. Two-thirds of the daily dose is given in the morning before breakfast and the remaining one-third before the evening meal. This schedule provides better control for the patient who remains hyperglycemic in the evening or has a persistent elevated fasting blood glucose. For patients whose morning postprandial glucose is elevated consistently, the addition of 4 to 6 U of regular or semilente insulin to the morning dose is recommended.

Dr. Peter Chase of the University of Colorado Medical Center has successfully started young, early-diagnosed diabetics on intermediate-acting insulin, giving 0.5 to 1.0 U/kg per day.[55] It is his belief that a 50% ultralente, 50% semilente mixture provides more benefit than lente insulin (70% ultralente and 30% semilente) for children, reducing the chance for nighttime or early morning hypoglycemia.

Insulin Therapy for the Brittle Diabetic The greatest therapeutic challenge in diabetes management is posed by the labile, brittle diabetic. This syndrome is characterized by wide fluctuations in blood glucose despite careful balancing of food, exercise, and insulin dose.[56]

Molnar et al. has suggested that regular insulin be given every 6 h around the clock or every 5 h during the day, with semilente for nighttime coverage.[57] Corresponding with insulin activity, meals and snacks may be needed 4 to 6 times a day.

Before instituting a regimen of this sort, an investigation of factors which could affect control should be done. Irregular feeding and exercise, diseases, infections, emotional status, insulin-administration techniques, and insulin antibodies may contribute to the instability found in the brittle diabetic.

Adjustment of Insulin Therapy for Maintaining Control "The earlier the diagnosis is made, the lower the insulin requirement and the easier it will be to attain and maintain a high degree of control with little risk of hypoglycemia." In treating the diabetic child, Jackson and Guthrie have observed that if insulin is instituted early, undue serious advancement in the disease is avoided and the patient can be maintained on a lower dose of insulin for longer periods of time.[58] In contrast, the patient with total diabetes (the advanced stage of diabetes) will require larger doses and more strict self-discipline. Jackson and Guthrie recommend that the juvenile diabetic remain on a permanent schedule of two injections a day, a more physiologic approximation of insulin need with less likelihood of hypoglycemic episodes. After the initial period of carbohydrate intolerance, insulin requirements may decrease within only a few weeks or months. This remission or honeymoon period in which 10 percent of patients require no insulin is usually of short duration, and within 2 to 3 years such patients become severe diabetics.

The consensus among diabetologists is to maintain insulin therapy (which may be as little as 2 to 4 U per day) during the remission regardless of duration. Bressler and Galloway give several reasons for this policy.[59] First, and perhaps most important, the patient realizes that his or her diabetes is a lifelong disease and that insulin administration will always be a part of daily life. There are no false hopes that the diabetes will "go away." In addition, the psychological impact of reinstituting insulin when carbohydrate tolerance deteriorates might be interpreted as a worsening of the patient's condition. Another important reason for maintaining insulin during this period is the reduced likelihood of developing insulin allergy or resistance, which can occur when insulin is stopped and restarted.

It is expected that insulin requirements will change in correlation with physical growth, rising in prepuberal years with more difficulty in control, decreasing after puberty, and remaining relatively constant during adult life.[60]

Patients who are regulated in the hospital may require a change in dose upon returning home and back to daily activities. A reduction in dose of 4 to 6 U is usually made prior to discharge, with further adjustments being made as needed on an outpatient basis.[61]

Most patients are well controlled on a single morning dose of intermediate-acting insulin. However, as previously mentioned, some patients develop a transient (type C) or delayed (type A) response to insulin which results in problems with control. Consequently, adjustments in therapy must be made.[62,63]

With the type C responder who is hyperglycemic during the day and normoglycemic to hypoglycemic at night, insulin absorption is slower and response is thus delayed. If this condition is marked, severe nocturnal hypoglycemia can occur. Rebound hyperglycemia (Somogyi phenomenon) and headache are usually present upon awakening (see Chapter 8). The solution to this type of response is to decrease the dose of intermediate insulin, since an increase would result in even more severe nocturnal hypoglycemia. For adequate daytime control, regular insulin is added to the morning dose, and if necessary, regular insulin is given before the evening meal as well. The usual proportion of NPH or lente to regular insulin is a 2:1 ratio, affording successful control. With supplemental regular insulin, the dose of NPH or lente is reduced and nocturnal hypoglycemia avoided.

Goldstein recommends adding 4 to 6 U to the morning dose to control the "postbreakfast tide" of hyperglycemia and afford satisfactory control throughout the day, advocating the avoidance of fixed ratios to provide day-to-day flexibility.[64]

When a transient type A response occurs, the intermediate insulin is absorbed rapidly, reaching peak activity by midafternoon. This shortens the duration of coverage to less than 24 h. The fasting postbreakfast, prelunch, postsupper, evening, and nighttime glucose levels are high, while in the afternoon and before the evening meal, normoglycemic or hypoglycemic situations are present. Increasing the morning dose of intermediate insulin would only serve to intensify the afternoon hypoglycemia without affecting the fasting glucose.

This problem is best handled, Goldstein feels, by decreasing the dose by 10 percent and splitting the amount between morning and evening: 70 percent of the total daily dose before breakfast and 20 percent at bedtime (or before the evening meal if bedtime sugars are consistently positive). If this does not control the patient effectively, then regular insulin (4 to 6 U) can be added to either morning and/or evening injections depending on urine tests before the noon meal and at bedtime. In contrast, Bressler and Galloway recommend that two-thirds of the total daily dose be given in the morning and one-third before the evening meal.[65] The morning dose is a 2:1 mixture of regular (CZI) to NPH or lente and a 1:1 ratio for the evening dose, resulting in a greater amount of short-acting insulin in the total daily dose.

Alternatives to the two daily dose regimens include a mixture of lente and ultralente in a single morning dose for the type A transient responder and a mixture of lente and semilente for the type C delayed responder.

Illness   Illness is often responsible for disrupting balance in the diabetic's control. During sick days, insulin requirements usually increase, and insulin should not be eliminated on such days. The relative requirements do need to be adjusted and individualized, however, based on food tolerance and patient response. Urine should be checked more frequently for glucose and ketones. The amount of regular insulin administered is usually greater than the amount of intermediate-acting insulin given such periods.

Jackson and Guthrie have devised general guidelines for treatment of the child during sick days.

1   Insulin requirements usually increase, provided the child continues to tolerate food. Both morning and evening doses will be greater, and supplemental doses of regular insulin may be required at noon and in the late evening.

2   If urine glucose is 3 percent or greater (without acetone) 30 min before lunch, regular insulin in a dose of one-sixth the morning dose should be administered. If acetone is also present, the regular insulin dose should be one-third the morning dose.

3   With 3 percent or greater glycosuria in the late evening (11 P.M.), a dose one-fourth of the evening dose should be given. If acetone is also present, a dose one-half of the evening dose should be given.

4   If ketonuria persists, regular insulin should be given before four small meals every 6 h.[66]

Therapy for the Non-Insulin-Dependent, Maturity-Onset Diabetic   In contrast to the juvenile-onset diabetic, the maturity-onset diabetic is not absolutely dependent on exogenous insulin for survival and has several potential treatment options depending on the severity of the condition.

There is little dispute over the philosophy that attempts to manage diabetes by strict diet control and weight reduction as the foundation of therapy. Often the condition is mild and asymptomatic, and with adherence to diet and dedication to keeping weight within ideal limits, no further therapy is needed.

Oral hypoglycemic agents are less effective in treating the overweight diabetic than is diet control. However, if diet fails to keep the fasting blood glucose below 130 mg per 100 mL and the patient asymptomatic, additional measures are often needed. An adequate trial on diet alone would be 2 to 3 months—less if the patient becomes severely symptomatic. Again, severity of the disease will determine the choice between insulin and oral hypoglycemics.

Dr. Karl Sussman, professor of medicine and leading diabetologist in Denver, Colorado, follows a logical progression in the management of maturity-onset diabetes. The patient is placed on a prescribed diet. If the diet is followed and good control is maintained, there is no change in therapy. If, however, the diet is followed but the patient remains poorly controlled, the choice between oral hypoglycemics and insulin is made. When an oral hypoglycemic is used and control is poor after a 1-month trial, insulin is considered. If control with the oral agent is good, then the drug is stopped in an attempt to determine if diet therapy alone will adequately control the patient's blood glucose.[67] If patient fails again on diet alone, oral agents are restarted. If the diet is not followed, then insulin or an oral agent and behavior modification are instituted (see Fig. 7-1).

The recommended indication for oral hypoglycemic agents posed by the Food and Drug Administration is that such agents "should be used only in patients with symptomatic adult-onset diabetes mellitus who cannot be adequately controlled by diet alone and who are not insulin dependent." Included in the label warning is the following statement:

> Diet and reduction of excess weight are the foundations of inital therapy of diabetes mellitus. When the disease is adequately controlled by these measures, no hypoglycemic drug therapy is indicated. Because of the apparent increased cardiovascu-

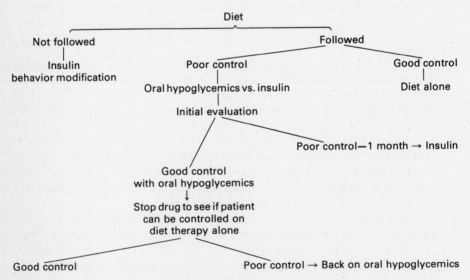

Figure 7-1 Sussman plan for management of maturity-onset diabetes.

lar hazard associated with [the use of oral hypoglycemic agents,] they are indicated in adult-onset, nonketotic diabetes mellitus only when the condition cannot be adequately controlled by diet and reduction of excess weight alone, and when, in the judgment of the physician, insulin cannot be employed because of patient unwillingness, poor adherence to injection regimen, physical disabilities such as poor vision and unsteady hands, insulin allergy, employment requirements, and other similar factors.[68]

The American Diabetes Association recommends that "trial with appropriate diet should come first. If this does not establish satisfactory control, insulin is to be preferred to other therapeutic agents because it is more uniformly effective in controlling hyperglycemia and the UGDP study indicates that it may be safer."[69,*]

There are opinions on both sides regarding the benefits and hazards of oral hypoglycemic agents, and these will be discussed under "Oral Hypoglycemics."

Several patient factors are associated with successful response to the oral hypoglycemics:[70,71]

1   Adult-onset diabetes, diagnosis made after age 30 or 40
2   Duration of diabetes for less than 10 years
3   Ketosis resistance, no episodes of ketoacidosis
4   Insulin requirement of less than 30 to 40 U/day
5   Nonobese

Tolbutamide (Orinase) 0.5 to 2.0 g per day in divided doses is usually the agent used initially. Up to 3.0 g per day may be tried if response is inadequate to 2.0 g. However, 2 g is probably just as effective as 3 g, with less chance for side effects.

Second-line choices are acetohexamide (Dymelor) or tolazamide (Tolinase). These are given once or twice a day, depending on patient response (see dosage ranges in Table 7-2). Finally, chlorpropamide (Diabinese) is tried when the patient fails to respond to other agents.

With all the sulfonylureas, initiation of therapy should be gradual, starting with small doses and titrating upward until the patient responds adequately. This is particularly critical in elderly patients with poor eating habits who are placed on chlorpropamide (in whom prolonged hypoglycemia may be a potential risk).

If response to oral hypoglycemic agents fails and the patient is no longer adequately controlled, insulin therapy may then be required.

---

*The UGDP (University Group Diabetes Program) study was a controlled clinical investigation of the effectiveness of tolbutamide (and later, phenformin) in patients of 12 medical centers. Beginning the study in 1961, the researchers reported in 1970 that cardiovascular deaths were more frequent (12.7 percent) in those treated with tolbutamide than in those treated with insulin or diet (6.2 percent or less).

Failure to Respond to Oral Hypoglycemic Therapy   Failure to respond to oral hypoglycemic therapy is classified as either primary failure or secondary failure. *Primary failure* occurs when the patient is not adequately controlled on a particular agent with maximum dosage after a 1-month trial. *Secondary failure* refers to the patient who no longer responds after a month or more of successful treatment. Before secondary failure is diagnosed, other factors that can cause loss of control should be ruled out. These include acute infection, dietary indiscretion, increased weight, change in exercise, pregnancy, emotional stress, addition or deletion of medications, medication errors, or a combination of several factors.

Several alternatives for the treatment of secondary failure are available.[72,73] However, increasing the oral agent to greater than maximum recommended doses increases the likelihood of toxic effects without the benefit of lowering blood glucose and should not be considered a valuable course of action.

Institution of a brief period of insulin to reestablish metabolic control and than a return to oral agents may be sufficient in 50 percent of cases. The theory postulated for ineffectiveness of oral agents relates to a plasma factor present during uncontrolled diabetes which results in resistance to therapy. Once control is achieved with insulin, resistance may subside and the patient may once again be sensitive to an oral agent within 1 to 2 weeks.

The procedure for switching the patient from insulin to oral agents is as follows. Patients requiring 20 U or less may be placed directly on an oral agent (usually tolbutamide), and insulin may be discontinued. When the insulin requirement is between 20 and 40 U, a 30 to 50 percent reduction in insulin dose can be tried initially, with a concurrent oral hypoglycemic agent. Further daily reduction of insulin is made as response to the oral agent is observed. More than 40 U of insulin necessitates only a 20 percent reduction on the first day, with further reduction on a gradual basis until response to the oral agent is observed. If manipulating the dose of the oral agent does not prove adequate and other sulfonylureas are tried, also without success, the usual course is insulin therapy as a final and lifelong mode of treatment.

If the patient develops ketosis, elevation of blood glucose, or other complications 24 h after withdrawal of insulin, withdrawal of the oral agent and reinstitution of insulin should be followed.

Careful monitoring of blood and urine glucose is important during transitions of therapy, as well as close observation of the patient for episodes of hypoglycemia.

Caution is encouraged in starting, stopping, and restarting insulin therapy at some later time, since this procedure has been associated with the development of insulin allergy and resistance.

Treatment of Ketoacidosis   Ketoacidosis, and the potential shock which may ensue, requires immediate hospitalization and medical treatment. This condition, with its critical life-threatening nature, has been a subject of serious consideration as diabetologists have questioned and evaluted what constitutes adequate treatment to effectively reverse this complicated metabolic disorder.

Two methods of insulin administration are currently advocated, both of which have been successful. These include the conventional method and the more recent continuous low-dose insulin-infusion method. Variations in dosage schedules have been described in both methods.

Conventional methods of treatment involve administration of regular insulin exclusively, by the subcutaneous route, by intravenous bolus, and recently by the intramuscular route. Often as many as 300 to 500 U of insulin total are needed to reverse ketoacidosis.

One method utilizes the *10 percent rule*.[74] This procedure requires an initial dose equal to 10 percent of the patient's blood glucose concentration in milligrams per 100 mL (e.g., blood glucose = 700 mg per 100 mL, dose = 70 U of regular insulin). Half this dose is given by intravenous bolus and half by the subcutaneous route. The rule applies only to adults. If the adult patient is unconscious, then 100 U administered in the same manner is an accepted alternative.

Initial doses recommended on the basis of *age and severity of the condition* are:[75,76]

Adults (conscious) and children over 10 years old	25–50 U
(doubled when blood glucose is 600 mg per 100 mL)	
Children under 10 years old	10–20 U
Adolescents with strongly positive ketonemia	50 U
Children less than 10 years old with strongly positive ketonemia	25 U
Infants with strongly positive ketonemia	10 U

Following the initial dose, the administration schedule is as follows. In 2 h, if the blood glucose level falls by 25 percent, then no insulin is given. If the blood glucose level is not decreased by 25 percent, then the 10 percent rule is followed. This schedule is repeated every 2 h until the blood glucose level is 250 to 300 mg per 100 mL or lower.

This method emphasizes control based on blood glucose levels, which may not adequately reflect the degree of ketoacidosis present. Some juvenile diabetics may be severely ketoacidotic at lower blood glucose concentrations than might be seen with an adult with hyperosmolar ketosis (refer to Chapter 5).

When results of *serum ketones* provide the basis for administration of insulin, the initial dose may be much higher, ranging from 100 to 400 U. Duncan and Gill describe a method for determining insulin dosage based on serum acetone levels.[77] A serum acetone reading of 4+ (undiluted specimen) would require approximately 100 U for an adult. If the specimen is diluted 1:2 and reads 4+, 200 U should be given; if 1:4 and 4+, 300 U; if 1:8 and 4+, 400 U. Extreme caution should be taken in recommending 400 U, because this may be very high and possibly greater than needed initially unless there is a previously known insulin resistance. Severe hypoglycemia may result.

For children or young adolescents with a 4+ plasma acetone reading in an undiluted specimen, 50 U are given; if 1:2 dilution, 100 U; if 1:4, 150 U; if 1:8, 200 U, one-half of the adult requirement. One-half the amount again is given for each dilution if the child is less than 10 years old, and for infants, 10, 20, 30, and 40 U are given, respectively, for each dilution showing 4+ acetone. Subsequent doses are given based on 1-h or 2-h glucose and acetone determinations.

A number of other alternatives which have been used are illustrated in Table 7-5.[78] The method of utilizing the intramuscular route was advocated since the half-life of insulin in the muscle is 2 h as opposed to 4 h if it is administered subcutaneously. The effect of a dose is thus observed sooner and control is achieved earlier.

Table 7-5   Methods of Determining Insulin Dosage in Ketoacidosis

Joslin Clinic

Immediate dose
  25–50 U intravenously plus 20–50 U subcutaneously if patient is conscious
  50–100 U intravenously plus 50–100 U subcutaneously if patient is unconscious; also when blood glucose level is less than 300 mg per 100 mL
In 1 h
  Blood glucose > 300   20–50 U intravenously; 20–50 U subcutaneously (conscious)
                         50–100 U intravenously; 50–100 U subcutaneously (unconscious)
  Blood glucose > 600   100–150 U intravenously; 100–150 U subcutaneously (conscious)
                         150–200 U intravenously; 150–200 U subcutaneously (unconscious)
  Blood glucose >1000   150–200 U intravenously; 150–200 U subcutaneously (conscious)
                         200–300 U intravenously; 200–300 U subcutaneously (unconscious)
Subsequent doses (every 4 h):
  Based on blood glucose values obtained every 2 h.

Steinke, Thorn

Serum acetone, strongly and with dilution	Initial dose (subcutaneous)
1:4	50 U
1:8	100 U
1:16	150 U
<1:16	200 U

Bongy

Intravenous regular insulin (50–100 U) until patient improves.

Hockaday, Alberti

Plasma Ketostix	Insulin	
	Intravenous	Intramuscular
Strongly + (1:4)	120	180
Strongly + (1:2)	80	120
Strongly + (undiluted)	40	60
Weakly + (undiluted)	Await blood glucose	

Williams, Porte

100 U intravenously or subcutaneously initially. 50–100 subcutaneously every hour.

Alberti

(Small intramuscular doses)
16 U initially, 5–10 U intramuscular every hour
Cumulative dose: 100 U over 24 h

Sources: T. M. Boehm, Advantages of continuous low dose insulin infusion in diabetic ketoacidosis, *Resident and Staff Physician,* May 1975, pp. 123–128; and K. G. Alberti, T. D. Hockaday, and R. C. Turner, Small doses of intramuscular insulin in treatment of diabetic coma, *Lancet,* **8**:515–522, 1973.

Some drawbacks of the conventional methods have been described as follows by Dr. Timothy Boehm of the Walter Reed Army Medical Center:[79]

1 Serum acetone and serum glucose may not necessarily correlate. In the case of the severely ketotic individual whose blood glucose is not grossly elevated, a substantial risk of hypoglycemia exists when dose is based on serum acetone alone.

2 Mobilization of insulin from subcutaneous sites may be more difficult in patients who are volume-depleted. The rate of absorption is slow, variable, and unpredictable. When tissue perfusion improves in the course of treatment, release of insulin stores may result in hypoglycemia.

3 Intravenous insulin has a serum half-life of 4 to 5 min. Dosing every hour leaves a substantial amount of time when the patient has no circulating insulin.

4 Intravenous bolus doses of 100 U of insulin provide more than is required for maximal cellular glucose uptake.

5 Alternate intravenous/subcutaneous methods may create gaps in adequate serum insulin concentrations.

6 When dosing is based on serum glucose and results are not readily available, intervals without insulin are likely.

The continuous low-dose insulin-infusion method is also described by Boehm, who lists seven advantages:[80]

1 Continuous intravenous infusion avoids peaks and valleys created by boluses and subcutaneous injections.

2 Serum insulin levels attained by this method more closely approximate those in nondiabetic subjects and do not exceed maximum levels for glucose uptake (approximately 200 μU/mL).

3 It is more physiologic.

4 The rate of decrease of serum blood glucose is fairly constant, allowing better anticipation of hypoglycemia. If the rate of fall is too rapid, signs of hypoglycemia may occur when the patient's glucose is still above normal.

5 Since less insulin is required than for conventional methods, fewer problems with insulin antibodies are encountered.

6 Hypokalemia may be less of a problem.

7 Convenience is characteristic and fewer decisions are needed on a trial and error basis.

Two protocols for continuous low-dose infusion are given in Table 7-6. Both methods for continuous low-dose infusion are relatively similar in procedure. There are pros and cons with respect to the addition of albumin to the solution. Some claim it is absolutely necessary, while others claim the adsorption of insulin to tubing and glass is a minor problem and effective results are achieved with or without addition of albumin. However, it is recommended that the solution be renewed every 4 h if albumin is not used.

Hofeldt described another protocol which essentially entails giving a load-

Table 7-6   Protocols for Continuous Low-Dose Infusion

Genuth
200 U of regular insulin are added to 1000 mL of 5% dextrose in water (0.2 U/mL). 50 mL are given by intravenous push (10 U insulin). Infusion is started at rate of 1 mL/min (10 to 12 U/h) until blood glucose reaches 250 mg per 100 mL.

Boehm
5 mL of 25% albumin (to prevent adsorption of insulin to bottle and administration set) are added along with 100 U of regular insulin to 500 mL normal saline or ½ normal saline (0.2 U/mL). If patient is severely ketoacidotic, 10 U (50 mL) are given by intravenous push. Infusion is started at 50 mL/h (10 U/h) until blood glucose reaches 250 mg per 100 mL. At this point, intravenous infusion may be discontinued, and subcutaneous insulin, given every 6 h, or the rate of infusion may be decreased to 5 mL/h (1 U/h).

Sources: S. M. Genuth, Constant intravenous insulin infusion in diabetic ketoacidosis, *J.A.M.A.*, **223**:1348–1351, 1973; Current concepts of insulin therapy in diabetic ketoacidosis, in *Diabetes in Review: Clinical Conference 1976* (Boston: American Diabetes Association, 1976); and T. M. Boehm, Advantages of continuous low dose insulin infusion in diabetic ketoacidosis, *Resident and Staff Physician*, May 1975, pp. 123–128.

ing dose of 10 to 20 U of regular insulin intravenously (10 U is usually sufficient).[81] Fifty units of regular insulin are added to 500 mL of ½ normal saline (0.1 U/mL). Infusion is started at 0.1 U/(kg·h) (70 mL for a 70-kg patient), which is expected to decrease the blood glucose by 10 percent per hour.[82] When 250 mg per 100 mL blood glucose is reached and if acidosis is not corrected, then 5% dextrose in water should be added to maintain blood glucose at 250 to 300 mg per 100 mL while insulin infusion is continued.

Treatment of ketoacidosis is not sufficiently accomplished merely by administration of insulin. Defects in fluid, potassium, sodium, chloride, magnesium, and phosphate also occur, and it may take up to 12 days to restore complete metabolic and electrolyte balance.

Although the patient admitted with ketoacidosis may have normal or high potassium levels, the need for potassium replacement will be necessary once the blood glucose falls and fluid therapy is initiated. Hypokalemia may occur as early as 1 h after treatment is begun, resulting from dilution by administered fluids and reentrance into the cell facilitated by administered insulin. Potassium requirement also increases when bicarbonate therapy is instituted. Because the rate of fall in blood glucose is more efficiently controlled with continous low-dose infusion, hypokalemia is less likely to occur.

Fluid and electrolyte losses are estimated as 10 percent of body weight in water, 7 meq/kg sodium, 5 meq/kg chloride, and 5 meq/kg of potassium. For correction of dehydration, approximately 1 to 2 L/h of normal saline can be administered until clinical improvement is shown. Caution should be exercised in avoiding too rapid hydration, particularly in patients with cardiac disease and previous history of heart failure.

Sodium bicarbonate is recommended if the patient's bicarbonate level is less than 10 meq/L, but is perhaps best reserved for those patients with arterial pH < 7.1 and $HCO_3^- < 5$ meq/L. Estimation of the amount for replacement is determined by multiplying the total bicarbonate reduction from normal by 50 percent of body weight in kilograms.

Dr. Leonard R. Madison of Dallas, Texas has pointed out the importance of phosphate therapy in the treatment of ketoacidosis and the potential problems associated with bicarbonate therapy. He cites the discovery in 1939 by Guest and Rapoport of the decrease in RBC 2,3-diphosphoglycerate (2,3-DPG), an organic polyphosphate of red blood cells in diabetic ketoacidosis (DKA) and evidence of marked phosphaturia and phosphate depletion. This state causes a shift in the oxygen dissociation curve to the left, resulting in tissue anoxia. In acidosis a shift to the right occurs which counterbalances the effect of low phosphate, and thus tissue oxygenation is uncompromised. The problem arises with administration of bicarbonate (alkalinizing solution). This causes a shift of the oxygen dissociation curve to the left, compounding the effect of low inorganic phosphate, and results in tissue anoxia and aggravation of cerebral edema.

Madison states, "It has taken about 35 years for the medical profession to realize the clinical importance of severe hypophosphatemia and phosphate depletion and to return to a previously used therapy. . . . Since slow recovery of RBC 2,3-DPG is related to the hypophatemia that occurs during and after treatment of DKA, rational therapy dictates the early use of phosphate replacement and the exclusion of bicarbonate whenever possible."[83]

In addition to potential cerebral and tissue hypoxia, acute worsening of hypokalemia and production of paradoxical cerebrospinal fluid acidosis may result from bicarbonate therapy (see Chapter 5). Madison recommends administration of potassium phosphate, since phosphate depletion and potassium deficiency go hand in hand.

Problems Associated with Diabetic Therapy

Insulin Reaction   The major acute problem associated with insulin therapy is hypoglycemia or insulin reaction, which results when too much insulin is actively circulating in the blood and there is insufficient glucose to counterbalance the effect.[84,85] In hypoglycemia, blood glucose falls below normal, usually less than 40 to 50 mg per 100 mL, although symptomatology is not always correlated with actual glucose levels. Insulin reaction may be precipitated by a number of factors. Insulin overdose and increased unanticipated exercise without additional caloric intake are probably the most common causes. Improper injection techniques (e.g., failure to agitate the vial before withdrawing insulin), injecting into atrophic areas, and improper measurement can result in excessive dosages or erratic release of insulin from a depot site.

Hypoglycemia may also appear in conjunction with renal disease (e.g., Kimmelstiel-Wilson lesions) because of increased reabsorption of insulin from the kidneys.

Liver dysfunction, hypoadrenalism, hypopituitarism, and specific hepatic enzyme defects such as glycogen storage disorders are additional metabolic disorders likely to precipitate hypoglycemia. Extrapancreatic tumors or pancreatic acinar carcinoma and insulinomas are also associated with increased abnormal levels of insulin.

In addition, a number of drugs can interact with insulin and potentiate hypoglycemia (see Table 7-7).

Symptoms The symptoms of hypoglycemia can be related to two factors. The physiologic response to a fall in blood glucose is the release of epinephrine, resulting in sympathetic nervous system activity which accounts for tachycardia, sweating, chills, weakness, hunger, trembling, irritability, nervousness, and pallor. Because there is a decrease in the amount of glucose available to the brain, mental confusion, psychiatric symptoms, neurologic manifestations (numbness and tingling of lips and tongue), headache, blurred vision, diplopia, incoherent speech, loss of temper, and fatigue may result. Behavior is often interpreted as alcohol intoxication.

The rate at which blood glucose falls determines which symptoms are likely to be manifested. With a rapid fall, symptoms related to epinephrine release are seen, while a slow drop in blood glucose is associated with cerebral symptoms. The former usually occurs with rapid-acting insulin or from strenuous exercise. Intermediate or long-acting insulins are more likely to cause a slower reaction.

The occurrence of hypoglycemia is most likely to correlate with peak activities of the particular insulin a patient is on (refer to Table 7-1).

To adequately prevent episodes of hypoglycemia, adjustments are made in either insulin regimen or caloric intake. Snacks just prior to the peak activity of insulin are recommended, as is advising the patient to increase food intake if he or she plans to engage in strenuous activity.

Treatment Treatment of hypoglycemia or insulin reaction should be immediate upon recognition of symptoms to prevent serious progression to shock and loss of consciousness. "Quick" sugar is recommended, such as fruit juices, sugar, regular soft drinks, honey, hard candy, etc. Candy bars should be avoided since their sugar content is absorbed much more slowly. Getting sugar into the blood as quickly as possible is critical. Commercially available products which may also be used include Instant Glucose and Reactose. For patients who experience severe hypoglycemic reactions, glucagon injection is recommended. The kit provided by Lilly contains 1 mg of glucagon, the usual dose needed to counteract hypoglycemia. If no response is felt, a second dose may be given in 10 to 15 min.

Following initial treatment, 25 g of carbohydrate should be consumed to prevent relapse into recurrent hypoglycemia from depleted glycogen stores.

Insulin Allergy Insulin allergy poses another problem with therapy in some patients.[86-89] Allergic responses to insulin are rarely life-threatening, but they are a source of bother to the patient. Antibodies to insulin may be of two types, those which bind with insulin and block the effect on glucose utilization and those which produce allergic symptoms.

Cutaneous allergic reactions may be localized as a wheal or "knot" at the site of injection. This type is usually seen in patients receiving insulin for the first time or patients in which insulin is reinstituted. The probable cause of this reaction is the modifying proteins in insulin preparations rather than the species source.

A generalized reaction resulting in hives, with possible systematic symptoms of itching, gastrointestinal complaints, and sometimes hypotension, is another type of allergic response.

Treatment Treatment involves ruling out possible improper injection techniques and using 91 percent isopropyl alcohol in place of 70 percent (less irritating impurities). If local reactions do not subside spontaneously, an oral antihistamine may be given 2 h prior to insulin injection. Such reactions have become less frequent with the newer purified insulins. Consideration of species source as the culprit is recommended if cutaneous reactions fail to subside. Pork insulin is generally effective in bringing about improvement in such patients.

Rarely does insulin allergy manifest as generalized anaphylaxis, but since insulin is not exempt from this possibility, appropriate measures should be taken to effectively treat such a reaction.

If it is determined by skin testing that the diabetic patient is allergic to all sources of insulin, *desensitization* may be necessary. This procedure utilizes pork insulin since it is the least antigenic and most clearly resembles human insulin. Single-component insulin also affords a much purer preparation and is also less antigenic. However, single-peak pork insulin is recommended by researchers at Lilly for desensitization because it is easier to obtain and its use results in desensitization to minor contaminants which may be present in all batches of single-peak pork insulin.[90] Insulin allergy desensitization kits containing the various dilutions needed are available from Lilly.

Desensitization is accomplished by the following schedule with 0.1-mL subcutaneous injections:

Day 1: $^{1}/_{1000}$, $^{1}/_{500}$, $^{1}/_{250}$, $^{1}/_{100}$ U
Day 2: $^{1}/_{100}$, $^{1}/_{50}$, $^{1}/_{25}$, $^{1}/_{10}$ U
Day 3: $^{1}/_{10}$, $^{1}/_{5}$, $^{1}/_{2}$, 1 U
Day 4: 1, 2, 4, 8 U

Injections should be given every 4 h. If an allergic reaction occurs, the next two injections should be given with dilutions of the two previous injections.

The procedure, hopefully, will allow the patient to tolerate therapeutic doses of insulin. However, low-grade allergy may persist, requiring antihistamines or low-dose prednisone.

Insulin Resistance *Insulin resistance* is defined as an insulin requirement of 200 U or more daily for a period longer than 2 days in the absence of infection or other diabetogenic factors and coma.[91-93] There are patients who require greater than 100 U of insulin daily. Consequently, the same mechanisms present in insulin resistance may also be present in these insulin-insensitive patients.

The mechanisms of insulin resistance are not completely known. However, two types have been reported. The *immune type* involves the development of antibodies which bind insulin and prevent effective activity in controlling glucose homeostasis. The *nonimmune type* results from obesity or various medical problems.[94] Such conditions include pheochromocytoma, Cushing's syndrome, hyperthyroidism, surgical stress, hepatic disease, acromegaly, pregnancy, hemochromatosis, infection, and lipoatrophic diabetes.

It is not uncommon for all diabetics to develop insulin antibodies. Within 6 weeks to 3 months after insulin therapy is begun, antibodies appear in the serum. The binding of insulin which results is usually less than 10 U/L, and such patients can still be well controlled on average doses of insulin.

Periods of insulin resistance may last only a few weeks, during which time the patient may be asymptomatic. In this case, no treatment is required and the patient will be continued on the high dose necessary to maintain control.

Diabetics who become extremely difficult to control despite unusually large doses present the real therapeutic problem. Since the condition is self-limiting, some physicians question the benefit of adjunctive therapy. When patients require several thousand units of insulin to prevent ketacidosis, it is more realistic to attempt control with the aid of additional agents rather than subject the patient to prolonged hypoglycemia or analphylaxis, the hazards of increasingly large doses of insulin by the intravenous route.

Treatment   Agents used to treat insulin resistance are varied, ranging from insulin from different species sources to steroids.[95] Least successful in most severe cases has been the pork-derived insulin, in spite of its known property of causing the least antigenicity. Agents which have been tried include 2,3-dimercaptopropanol, nitrogen mustard, pork insulin, tolbutamide, phenformin, and adrenocortical steroids. The most consistent in altering insulin resistance have been the adrenal steroids and ACTH. The rationale for ACTH therapy is to suppress antibody formation. The proposed mechanisms by which steroids exert their effect are (1) by decreasing the binding of insulin to the antibodies; (2) removal of antigen-antibody complexes at a rate more rapid than that for gamma globulin; (3) direct facilitation of glucose entry into cells; (4) increase in capillary permeability, thereby allowing more "bound" insulin to reach interstitial fluids; and (5) effect on plasma-nonimmune insulin antagonists.

Treatment with steroids is considered rational and probably beneficial for patients who require high doses of insulin over a prolonged period or whose course is characterized by unstable fluctuations between ketoacidosis and hypoglycemia, who have a history of insulin allergy (especially if intravenous insulin is necessary), or who develop frequent sterile abscesses or other reactions at the injection site.

Initiation of steroid therapy, when advisable, begins with prednisone 60 to 80 mg per day in divided doses. The dose is gradually reduced once response is observed, and a daily maintenance dose of 5 to 10 mg is continued. Treatment with steroids beyond a month is not recommended. Return to an insulin-sensitive state is often achieved in about 75 percent of cases.

Lipodystrophy Primarily a cosmetic complication of insulin therapy, lipodystrophy may occur usually during the first 6 months to 2 years in 28 to 35 percent of children, adult females, but rarely in adult males.[96]

Changes in the subcutaneous fat at the injection site may be either of two types, lipoatrophy or hypertrophy. *Lipoatrophy* results in "dimpling" or "denting" of the skin from a "melting away" of fat tissue, leaving the skin to rest on underlying muscle. *Hypertrophy* is characterized by the development of large masses of fibrous, avascular scar tissue which results from repeated trauma to a particular injection site or sites. Injections into these areas become rather painless and are therefore self-perpetuating. Absorption of insulin from these sites is variable and unpredictable and may result in erratic control.

Several theories in the treatment of lipodystrophy have been proposed.[97] Since remission of lipoatrophy is rare as opposed to spontaneous remission of hypertrophy with frequent site rotation, attempts to treat atrophy have been considered to a larger extent. Successful "filling in" of atrophic areas has been seen in patients who injected purified insulins, single-peak and single-component, into areas of atrophy. Resolution occurred over a period of 1 to 2 years. Guthrie recommends that the insulin be injected daily in a "circular fashion," starting at the perimeter of the area and working toward the center. This method has shown remarkable results in resolution by the time the final injection into the area is given. Areas that have filled in may need to be injected every 2 to 4 weeks to prevent recurrence of atrophy.

Atrophy appears to be less of a problem with the U-100 insulins than with previous U-40 and U-80 strengths, which were felt to contain impurities with lipolytic capabilities. Although no definitive studies have been done, insulin kept at room temperature rather than injected cold may result in less trauma at the injection site and a decrease in hypertrophy.

Oral Hypoglycemics Therapeutic problems associated with oral hypoglycemic agents often result from side effects patients may experience or from toxic effects which have been brought to light by the UGDP study.

Like insulin, all the sulfonylureas are capable of producing severe hypoglycemia. Reactions have occurred after a single dose, after several days of therapy, and after as long as several months of therapy. The likelihood of hypoglycemia is especially greater if too high a dose is given, if the patient does not eat properly, or if, because of liver or kidney dysfunction, the drug is not properly metabolized or excreted. Chlorpropamide, with its long duration of action, has been associated with severe hypoglycemia which may last several days. Following initial treatment, the patient should be watched closely for several days for recurrence of hypoglycemia.

Other side effects which may occur are allergic skin reactions (erythema, pruritis, urticaria, and maculopapular or morbilliform rash), gastrointestinal complaints, and hematological disorders.[98] Cutaneous reactions are usually transient, but withdrawal of the agent may be necessary if the condition persists. Gastrointestinal complaints are often alleviated when the agent is taken with meals or the dose reduced. Reaction with alcohol producing an antabuse-like effect is very likely with chlorpropamide. Rarely do blood dyscrasias occur with the sulfonylureas, but there have been reported cases of leukopenia, thrombocytopenia, agranulocytosis, and aplastic anemia.

Hepatotoxicity (jaundice from cholestasis) and nephrotoxicity have been associated with phenformin to a greater degree than with sulfonylureas. In addition, a major factor resulting in the withdrawal of phenformin from the market was the high incidence of lactic acidosis, sometimes fatal, in patients whose use of this agent was not carefully monitored.

An additional problem with chlorpropamide not seen with the other sulfonylureas is water retention and dilutional hyponatremia.[99-102] The effect results from chlorpropamide's ability to potentiate endogenous antidiuretic hormone activity both in hypothalamic-pituitary release and on the renal tubular level. In patients with congestive heart failure and cirrhosis of the liver, administration of chlorpropamide should be avoided.

Following the conclusion of the UGDP study, the potential for cardiovascular mortality became a serious concern in the treatment of adult, maturity-onset diabetics.[103] Although an initial decline in the use of the sulfonylureas resulted, their use continues to be considerable today.

The results of the UGDP study have been challenged and the study design closely scrutinized by a number of groups.[104,105] The Biometric Society concluded that "suspicions of cardiovascular mortality caused by tolbutamide and phenformin could not be dismissed," considering the evidence of harmfulness "moderately strong."[106]

Dr. James M. Moss of Georgetown University, after careful consideration of the study, concluded:

> No amount of statistical manipulation can compensate for the erroneous conclusions that result when one-third of the patients did not have the disease under study, three-fourths should not have been given the drug under study, the wrong dose of drug was used and the treated group had twice as much pre-existing cardiovascular disease than did the control group. The value of any therapeutic agent should be judged by the benefits that are obtained when it is used properly and not by the harm that results when it is used indiscriminately."[107]

Despite absolute evidence, the use of oral hypoglycemics in the treatment of maturity-onset diabetes is recommended only for selected patients, and diet and insulin are recommended for first attempts at control in patients not responding to diet alone.

Patients with juvenile diabetes, renal failure, hepatic failure, pregnancy, and ketosis-prone conditions should not receive these agents. Patients with allergy to sulfa drugs are likely to show cross-allergenicity to the sulfonylureas as well.

If one were to include the results of the UGDP study, patients with concurrent cardiovascular disease should also be excluded from use of these agents.

Some diabetologists prefer treatment with insulin versus oral hypoglycemics when a patient has coexisting long-term diabetic complications, i.e., retinopathy, neuropathy, etc.

Drug Interactions with Diabetes Therapy

Complications with multiple drug regimens are a far greater problem in management of the diabetic patient than many recognize. The response to medications is affected not only by other concurrent medications, but also by the patient's disease state. Where a patient has several medical problems and is on a number of medications, the interrelationship of diseases and therapeutic regimens has the potential for multiple drug-drug and drug-disease interactions.

Previously discussed were disease states and conditions which alter response to antidiabetic agents—renal and liver disease, hyperthyroidism, pregnancy, surgery, infections, hypopituitarism, hypoadrenalism, and so on.[108] Other medical problems which may be involved in aggravating diabetes or increasing the likelihood of hypoglycemia by virtue of the medications used in their treatment are hypertension, gout, arthritis, hypothyroidism, and conditions requiring anticoagulant, antibiotic, or hormonal therapy, to mention a few.

Table 7-7 is a listing of medications reported to have been implicated in episodes of hypoglycemia or hyperglycemia.[109–115] Some of the most significant of these are included in the following discussion.

Table 7-7 Medications with Effects on Blood Glucose

Hypoglycemia	Hyperglycemia
Acetaminophen	Acetazolamide
Alcohol	Alcohol
Allopurinol	Amphetamines
Anabolic steroids	Arginine HCl
Clofibrate	Asparaginase
Chloramphenicol	Barbiturates
Chlorpromazine and orphenadrine	Dextrothyroxine
Dicumarol	Diazoxide
EDTA (and insulin)	Epinephrine
Fenfluramine	Glycerin/glycerol
Guanethidine	Glucagon
Isoniazid	Glucocorticoids
Magnesium (and insulin)	Glucose
MAO inhibitors	Levodopa
Oxyphenbutazone	Marijuana
Oxytetracycline (and insulin)	Nicotinic acid
Pentamidine	Narcotics
Phenylbutazone	Oral contraceptives
Phenyramidol	Phenothiazines
Probenecid	Phenytoin
Propranolol	Potassium depletion
Salicylates	Sympathomimetics
Sulfinpyrazone	Thiazide diuretics
Sulfonamides	
Theophylline	

The Diabetic Patient with Hypertension The thiazide diuretics (hydrochlorthiazide, chlorthiazide, etc.), as well as ethacrynic acid, furosemide, and acetazolamide, may lead to hyperglycemia and glycosuria in patients who have a predisposition to diabetes and sometimes aggravate carbohydrate tolerance in established diabetes. High doses are not required to cause this effect, which may occur 3 to 7 days after therapy is started.

Elevations of blood glucose are usually minimal and appear more frequently with concurrent use of oral hypoglycemic agents. Patients on insulin are usually not affected. The mechanisms for this occurence are believed to be potassium depletion or inhibition of insulin release by the thiazides.

The diuretics are essential in controlling high blood pressure and do not represent a contraindication in patients on oral hypoglycemics. Ensuring that adequate potassium levels are maintained and (perhaps a slight) modification in dose of antidiabetic agents will allow satisfactory control.

Diazoxide (Hyperstat), a thiazide but not a diuretic used in treating malignant hypertension, exhibits diabetogenic activity by blocking insulin release. This drug is also used in treating malignant insulinomas.

The thiazides are not the only problem in the diabetic hypertensive patient. One of the oral hypoglycemics, chlorpropamide, has an activity uncommon to the other sulfonylureas which can create a problem in the management of hypertension and cardiovascular disease (congestive heart failure and angina pectoris). Fluid retention induced by chlorpropamide as a result of inappropriate secretion of antidiuretic hormone (ADH) is undersirable in such patients. The results are increased systolic hypertension and aggravation of congestive heart failure and nocturnal angina. When chlorpropamide is part of the therapeutic regimen of patients with these conditions or renal or hepatic disease, peripheral and pulmonary edema and hepatomegaly may occur.

Before chlorpropamide is prescribed for the diabetic, the potential hazard of hyponatremia (which is compounded when thiazides are given) and water intoxication should be considered, particularly when the patient has cardiovascular, hepatic, or renal disease. Another sulfonylurea should be prescribed since this syndrome is associated only with chlorpropamide. Chlorpropamide has been used in the treatment of diabetes insipidus, a disorder involving deficiency in pituitary secretion of ADH.

Other antihypertensive therapy, e.g., guanethidine, monoamine oxidase (MAO) inhibitors, and propranolol, have been associated with hypoglycemic episodes in diabetics. Mechanisms involve depletion of tissue catecholamines for guanethidine, beta-adrenergic stimulation by some of the MAO inhibitors, and suspected antagonistic action to catecholamines and an ability to stimulate insulin release for propranolol. Patients on propranolol should be monitored carefully, since this drug may prevent the symptoms of hypoglycemia from manifesting.

The Diabetic Patient with Arthritis and Gout Antiinflammatory agents used in the treatment of arthritis which will likely require an adjustment in therapy with the oral hypoglycemics include phenylbutazone (Butazolidin,

Azolid), oxyphenbutazone (Oxalid, Tandearil), salicylates, acetaminophen, and corticosteroids. The sulfonamides and aspirin may enhance the hypoglycemic response by displacing sulfonylureas from plasma-protein binding sites, while phenylbutazone and oxyphenbutazone may inhibit the excretion of sulfonylureas. Downward adjustment of oral hypoglycemic dose may be necessary. Acetaminophen in large doses may also enhance the hypoglycemic effect.

Corticosteroids are notorious for their diabetogenic effect, and a condition known as steroid diabetes is not uncommon following systemic administration. Several mechanisms have been postulated—primarily the increase in glucose production by the liver from gluconeogenesis. In addition, mobilization of fatty acids, antagonism to insulin by growth hormone, and decreased utilization of glucose by the tissues may contribute to the features of steroid diabetes.

The picture corresponds to the usual diabetic state except that acidosis and acetonuria are absent, even with marked hyperglycemia, and serum pyruvate levels are elevated. The condition is reversed when steroids are withdrawn. However, its appearance may be indicative of early diabetes.

In addition to the potential hypoglycemic effect of salicylates, research is currently being done by the Veterans' Administration Cooperative Study on what effect this agent with antiplatelet activity may have on preventing the progression of vascular disease in diabetes.[116]

In patients who are being treated with allopurinol (Zyloprim) for gout, a tendency toward hypoglycemia, particularly with concurrent chlorpropamide therapy, has been noted. Allopurinol inhibits metabolism and prolongs the half-life of chlorpropamide in the blood. Sulfinpyrazone (Anturane) and probenecid (Benemid) may also potentiate the sulfonylureas.

The Diabetic Patient on Hormonal Therapy   The oral contraceptives, synthetic hormonal steroids, have resulted in diminished glucose tolerance in some patients with a family history of diabetes. Patients with a history of gestational diabetes (diabetes occurring with pregnancy) are more likely to develop irreversible diabetes on oral contraceptives.

Dextrothyroxine (Choloxin), an antilipemic agent, and L-thyroxine, for the treatment of hypothyroidism, may necessitate an increase in dose of insulin or oral agents.

Anabolic steroids, such as methandrostenolone (Dianabol), may cause hypoglycemia via inhibition of oral hypoglycemic metabolism and result in enhanced activity.

The Diabetic Patient on Antibiotic Therapy   Most significant is the potential interaction between the sulfonamide antibacterials and the oral sulfonylureas. Occurrence seems to be mainly with tolbutamide therapy and concurrent antibiotic therapy with sulfaphenazole (Sulfabid) and sulfisoxazole (Gantrisin). Competition for excretion and displacement from plasma-protein binding are thought to be the mechanism of interaction resulting in hypoglycemia.

Chloramphenicol inhibits metabolism of oral hypoglycemics, and a reduction of dose may be necessary to prevent hypoglycemia from occurring.

The antitubercular agent, isoniazid (INH), with a structure similar to the MAO inhibitors, may also reduce blood glucose during concomitant tolbutamide therapy.

Oxytetracycline (Terramycin) therapy has been shown to enhance the effect of insulin, and reduction in dose is sometimes indicated.

The Alcoholic Diabetic   Alcohol can be a difficult problem in the diabetic, particularly when the tendency toward alcoholism is recognized. Problems result from interaction with antidiabetic therapy and, additionally, from characteristic dietary neglect.

In nondiabetics, hypoglycemia from alcohol can result following a 2- to 3-day fast, and in diabetics who are particularly susceptible (with little or no glycogen reserve), hypoglycemia can result from alcohol at levels which normally produce only mild intoxication. Hypoglycemia can be a critical situation in such patients. The unknowing observer may think the person is merely drunk and not recognize the total situation. If the patient goes into shock, he or she will likely be left alone to ''sleep it off'' and can die. Insulin-dependent diabetics have died in irreversible hypoglycemic coma following alcoholic binges.

Hyperglycemia may result from alcohol ingestion in well-nourished individuals (increase in blood glucose by 10 percent). However, hypoglycemia is more common and the major problem.

Mechanisms proposed are several: the ability of alcohol to inhibit gluconeogenesis and to increase the amount of insulin released in response to glucose, in addition to the ''intrinsic hypoglycemic activity'' of alcohol itself. In some but not all cases, alcohol *decreases* the half-life of tolbutamide. With chlorpropamide, an antabuse-like reaction is possible when alcohol is ingested even in small amounts.* This is not as likely with the other sulfonylureas.

The combination of alcohol and insulin seems to be especially dangerous with respect to severity of hypoglycemia. It is recommended that if the patient insists on social drinking, adequate carbohydrate be taken along with the alcohol. If the patient on chlorpropamide continues to drink in spite of recommendations to the contrary, the drug should be discontinued.

Miscellaneous Drugs Affecting Diabetic Control   Fenfluramine (Pondomin), an appetite suppressant which has intrinsic hypoglycemic activity, increases glucose uptake by the skeletal muscle. Its potential as an antidiabetic agent has been considered.

Amphetamines may have hypoglycemic or hyperglycemic activity. The former is possible if less is actually eaten and hypoglycemia is potentiated by subnormal potassium levels. Glucose utilization is increased by an increase in

---

* This reaction may include such symptoms as subjective sensation of warmth, headache, lightheadedness, nausea, and shortness of breath, as well as objective signs of flushed skin and tachycardia.

metabolism. Hyperglycemia may result from a breakdown of glycogen in the liver and increase in plasma glucose.

Marijuana use seems to increase the craving for food, sweets in particular. Impairment of glucose tolerance is still questionable.

"Phenothiazine diabetes" has been noted with increased frequency, most often following chlorpromazine therapy, 100 mg per day for several months. Concurrent use of sulfonylureas rather than insulin is associated with a higher incidence of interaction with phenothiazines.

Clofibrate (Atromid-S), a cholesterol-lowering agent, can increase the half-life of chlorpropamide by competition for renal tubular secretion.

Anticoagulant therapy with dicumarol has resulted in hypoglycemia by virtue of its ability to inhibit metabolism of the sulfonylureas. Adjustment in sulfonylurea dose may be necessary.

Phenytoin (Dilantin) added to therapy of the diabetic has been observed to aggravate the patient's condition. Impairment of insulin release may be responsible for the hyperglycemic response seen even at normal therapeutic doses.

Evaluation of Diabetic Therapy

How effective the therapeutic regimen for a particular diabetic patient is depends on the several factors discussed throughout this chapter. Control is reflected by objective parameters (the patient's blood glucose, the degree of glycosuria) and by subjective parameters (the absence of diabetic symptoms, freedom from hypoglycemia, and general feeling of well-being in everyday living). Some parameters are measurable, while others may not be as easily quantified. Therefore, the question of control related to future complications remains unanswered. The primary measure of success becomes the degree to which the goals of therapy are achieved.

REFERENCES

1 Raskin, P. The role of somatostatin in managing diabetes, *Drug Therapy*, March 1978, pp. 81–90.
2 McGarry, J. D., and Foster, D. W. Gluconeogenesis as a target for diabetic therapy, *Drug Therapy*, March 1978, pp. 95–103.
3 Bonar, J. R. *Diabetes—A Clinical Guide* (Flushing, N.Y.: Medical Examination Publishing Company, 1977).
4 Bressler, R., and Galloway, J. A. The insulins: pharmacology and uses, *Drug Therapy*, March 1978, pp. 43–61.
5 Ibid.
6 Bonar. Loc. cit.
7 Bressler, R. The controversy over blood glucose control, *Drug Therapy*, March 1978, pp. 24–37.
8 Lilly Research Laboratories. *Diabetes Mellitus,* 7th ed. (Indianapolis, Ind.: Eli Lilly and Company, 1973).
9 Ibid.
10 Kimble, M. A. Diabetes: current therapeutic concepts, *J. Am. Pharm. Assoc.,* NS14 (2): 80–90, 1974.

11   Bressler and Galloway. Loc. cit.
12   Lilly Research Laboratories. Loc. cit.
13   Kimble. Loc. cit.
14   Bressler and Galloway. Loc. cit.
15   Lilly Research Laboratories. Loc. cit.
16   Kimble. Loc. cit.
17   Bressler and Galloway. Loc. cit.
18   Young, L., and Kimble, M. A. *Applied Therapeutics for Clinical Pharmacists* (San Francisco: Applied Therapeutics, Inc., 1975), pp. 225–260.
19   Ibid.
20   Bressler and Galloway. Loc. cit.
21   Bressler and Galloway. Loc. cit
22   Ibid.
23   Ibid.
24   Herfindal, E. T., and Hirschman, J. L. *Clinical Pharmacy and Therapeutics* (Baltimore: Williams and Wilkins, 1975), pp. 278–298.
25   Bressler and Galloway. Loc. cit.
26   Bonar. Loc. cit.
27   Lilly Research Laboratories. Loc. cit.
28   Bonar. Loc. cit.
29   Boyden, T. W. The proper place of oral hypoglycemics in diabetes management, *Drug Therapy*, March 1978, pp. 66–77.
30   Shen, S. W., and Bressler, R. A. Clinical pharmacology of oral anti-diabetic agents, *N. Engl. J. Med.*, **296**: 493–499, 787–792, 1977.
31   Young and Kimble. Loc. cit.
32   Boyden. Loc. cit.
33   Young and Kimble. Loc. cit.
34   Boyden. Loc. cit.
35   Skillman, T. G., and Tzagournis, M. *Diabetes Mellitus* (Kalamazoo, Mich.: The Upjohn Company, 1977).
36   Shagan, B. P. Diabetes in the elderly patient. Symposium on geriatric medicine, *Med. Clin. North Am.*, **60**: 1191–1207, 1976.
37   Cutler, P., Kudzma, D. J., Schiffer, S., Seltzer, H. S., and Young, R. Managing diabetes—which way should you go? *Current Prescribing*, **2** (8), 1976.
38   Ibid.
39   Bressler. Loc. cit.
40   Cutler et al. Loc. cit.
41   Goldstein, H. A. Therapy of maturity onset diabetes—oral hypoglycemic agents and insulin. From presentation to American Diabetes Association and ADA Colorado Affiliate, Inc., Vail, Colorado, 1977.
42   Ibid.
43   Runyan, J. *The Primary Care Guide* (Univ. of Tennessee College of Medicine, 1974), pp. 62–67, 116–127.
44   Bonar. Loc. cit.
45   Lilly Research Laboratories. Loc. cit.
46   Young and Kimble. Loc. cit.
47   Lilly Research Laboratories. Loc. cit.
48   Bressler, R., and Galloway, J. A. Insulin treatment of diabetes mellitus. Symposium on diabetes mellitus, *Med. Clin. North Am.*, **55**:861–876, 1971.

49 Ibid.
50 Chase, H. P. Pediatrics—office management of diabetes mellitus in children, *Postgrad. Med.*, **59**:243–252, 1976.
51 Jackson, R. L., and Guthrie, R. A. The child with diabetes, in *Current Concepts* (Kalamazoo, Mich.: The Upjohn Company, 1975).
52 Goldstein. Loc. cit.
53 Lilly Research Laboratories. Loc. cit.
54 Gibbs, G. E. Outpatient initiation of insulin treatment in the juvenile diabetic, *Nebr. Med. J.*, August 1976, pp. 297–300.
55 Chase. Loc. cit.
56 Lilly Research Laboratories. Loc. cit.
57 Molnar, G. D., et al. Metabolic effects of exercise and of multiple dose insulin regimens in hyperlabile diabetes mellitus, *Metabolism*, **12**:157, 1963.
58 Jackson and Guthrie. Loc. cit.
59 Bressler and Galloway. Loc. cit.
60 Jackson and Guthrie. Loc. cit.
61 Herfindal and Hirschman. Loc. cit.
62 Goldstein. Loc. cit.
63 Bressler and Galloway. Loc. cit.
64 Goldstein. Loc. cit.
65 Bressler and Galloway. Loc. cit.
66 Jackson and Guthrie. Loc. cit.
67 Lock, J. P., and Sussman, K. E. Diabetes mellitus in the adult, in *Conn's Current Therapy*, (Philadelphia. Saunders, 1977) p. 427.
68 Young and Kimble. Loc. cit.
69 Ibid.
70 Ibid.
71 Bonar. Loc. cit.
72 Boyden. Loc. cit.
73 Gebhardt, M. C., Garnett, W. R., and Pulliam, C. C. Recognition and management of secondary failure to oral hypoglycemic agents, in *Clinical Pharmacy Sourcebook*, The American Society of Hospital Pharmacists (Alton, Mass.: Publishing Sciences Group, 1976).
74 Bonar. Loc. cit.
75 Ibid.
76 Lilly Research Laboratories. Loc. cit.
77 Duncan, G. G., and Gill, R. J. Clinical value of a simple qualitative test for plasma acetone in diabetic coma. *Diabetes*, **2**:353, 1953.
78 Boehm, T. M. Advantages of continuous low dose insulin infusion in diabetic ketoacidosis, *Resident and Staff Physician*, May 1975, pp. 123–128.
79 Boehm. Loc. cit.
80 Ibid.
81 Hofeldt, F. D. Diabetic ketoacidosis—1974. Unpublished material.
82 Crofford, O. B. Multiple methods of insulin therapy. From presentation to the American Diabetes Association and ADA Colorado Affiliate, Inc., Vail, Colorado, 1977.
83 Madison, L. L. Phosphate and bicarbonate therapy in the treatment of diabetic ketoacidosis, in *Diabetes in Review: Clinical Conference 1976* (American Diabetes Association and ADA New England Affiliate, Inc., Boston, Mass. 1976).

84 Young and Kimble. Loc. cit.
85 Bonar. Loc. cit.
86 Ibid.
87 Lilly Research Laboratories. Loc. cit.
88 Mattron, J. R., Patterson, R., and Roberts, M. Insulin therapy in patients with systemic insulin allergy, *Arch. Intern. Med.*, **135**:818–821, 1975.
89 Galloway, J. A. *Insulin Therapy—New Insulins, Insulin Resistance and Allergy* (Indianapolis, Ind.: Eli Lilly and Company).
90 Ibid.
91 Bonar. Loc. cit.
92 Galloway. Loc. cit.
93 Shipp, J. C., Cunningham, R. W., Russell, R. O., and Marble, A. Insulin resistance: clinical features, natural course and effects of adrenal steroid treatment, *Medicine,* **44**:165, 1965.
94 Kahn, C. R. Insulin receptors: their role in obesity and diabetes, *Drug Therapy,* March 1978, pp. 107–118.
95 Shipp et al. Loc. cit.
96 Lilly Research Laboratories. Loc. cit.
97 Galloway. Loc. cit.
98 American Medical Association. *AMA Drug Evaluations*, 3d ed. (Littleton, Mass.: Publishing Sciences Group, 1977).
99 Hayes, J. S., and Kaye, M. Inappropriate secretion of antidiuretic hormone induced by chlorpropamide, *Am. J. Med. Sci.*, **263**(3):140, 1972.
100 Moses, A. M., Howanitz, J., and Miller, M. Diuretic action of three sulfonylurea drugs, *Ann. Intern. Med.*, **78**:541–544, 1973.
101 Earley, L. E. Editorial, *N. Engl. J. Med.*, **284**:103–104, 1971.
102 Garcia, M., Miller, M., and Moses, A. M. Chlorpropamide-induced water retention in patients with diabetes mellitus, *Ann. Intern. Med.*, **75**:549–554, 1971.
103 O'Sullivan, J. B., and D'Agestino, R. B. Decisive factors in the tolbutamide controversy, *J.A.M.A.*, **232**:825–829, 1975.
104 American Medical Association. Loc. cit.
105 O'Sullivan and D'Agestino. Loc. cit.
106 American Medical Association. Loc. cit.
107 Moss, J. M. Twenty years of hypoglycemic drugs, *The Diabetes Educator*, **3**(4):10–12, 1977–1978.
108 Bonar. Loc. cit.
109 Young and Kimble. Loc. cit.
110 Bonar. Loc. cit.
111 *Evaluations of Drug Interactions*, 2d ed. (Washington, D. C.: American Pharmaceutical Association, 1976).
112 Hansten, P. D. *Drug Interactions*, 3d ed. (Philadelphia: Lea and Febiger, 1976).
113 Rosenberg, J. M. Antidiabetics—as always, the problem is maintaining control. *Current Prescribing*, **3**(3):57–60, 1977.
114 Coleman, J. H., and Evans, W. E. Drug interactions with alcohol, *Med. Times*, **103**(6):145–155, 1975.
115 Sczupak, C. A. Drugs and the diabetic: licit and illicit. Unpublished outlined summary, Buffalo, New York.
116 Halushka, P. V., Lurie, D., and Calwell, J. A. Increased synthesis of prostaglandin E-like material by platelets from patients with diabetes mellitus. *N. Engl. J. Med.* **297**:1306–1310, 1977.

Chapter 8

The Hospitalized Diabetic

Dorothy R. Blevins

In hospitals there are more contact hours between patients and nurses than in most other settings, and between patients and nurses than between patients and other health care professionals. These hours must be used effectively if patients are to achieve and maintain optimal health status during their hospital stay and after discharge. Nurses who make valid decisions about care requirements and who teach, counsel, and give care to diabetic patients can make significant contributions to their well-being.

This chapter discusses aspects of nursing care needed by adults who are hospitalized and who have diabetes mellitus; the focus of the chapter is on that care directly related to the endocrine component of diabetes mellitus. All diabetic people have the potential for acute disorders of hyperglycemia from insulin deficit; those who are treated with insulin or other hypoglycemic agents also have the potential for hypoglycemia from insulin excess. Nurses should attend to the endocrine status of all those identified as diabetics, not just those who are receiving therapeutic interventions for acute physiological crises. In addition to monitoring the endocrine status of and providing care for diabetic patients when they are acutely ill, nurses must also attend to the adequacy of patient self-care practices. Many diabetic people—regardless of the duration of the disease—have inadequate knowledge, skills, and attitudes for competent self-care and can benefit from an educational program. Diabetic people who are able to maintain optimal well-being after discharge are well served.

Current developments in the field of nursing include evolving systems of assessment, standards of care, and quality-assurance programs; these are assisting individual nurses and groups of nurses in delineating roles, functions, and activities in particular settings. Patient care outcomes, assessment guides, and audit criteria can provide guidelines for nurses as they make decisions about care requirements of diabetic individuals and plan care activities. When patients are acutely ill, one high-priority goal is restoration of physiological well-being; when patients are well enough to learn, an equally important goal is patient education. Early assessment of learning needs and potentials is necessary if early implementation of teaching plans is to occur. Throughout this chapter, examples of patient care outcomes and assessment guides are presented which can be useful to nurses who are planning and providing care for adults with diabetes mellitus.

THE DIABETIC PERSON IN ACUTE METABOLIC IMBALANCE

It is important for the reader to understand that the adult population of hospitalized diabetics includes many who are not admitted for acute disorders of insulin deficit or excess; that is, adults with diabetes mellitus who are hospitalized are not always admitted because of an endocrine problem. In fact, the majority of diabetic adults are diagnosed and their endocrine disease is managed on an ambulatory basis. Most diabetic adults found in hospitals have been previously diagnosed and are undergoing treatment for problems other than hyperglycemia; some of these people will develop more severe carbohydrate intolerance with the stress involved in the diagnosis precipitating admission and during hospitalization and therapy. Some diabetic adults in hospitals will be newly diagnosed after admission. Although screening blood glucose tests are generally used on all patients upon admission, it is a fact that hyperglycemia—and even ketosis—may first develop some time during a hospital stay. Those who are admitted as newly diagnosed diabetics may be acutely ill or may have had an unsuccessful trial of management on an ambulatory basis.

The first part of this chapter discusses nursing care requirements of the diabetic adult with acute disorders resulting from insulin deficit or excess. There are three situations in which skilled nursing care is critical; nurses must be able to respond appropriately to (1) diabetic coma, (2) hypoglycemia, and (3) disruption of day-to-day control measures. Any of the patients described previously may be in one or more of these situations.

Continuing Assessment: A Requirement

Continuing assessment of the patient's endocrine status is important for all diabetic patients admitted to hospitals. Measuring urinary glucose and acetone provides one index of the level of achieved control of hyperglycemia; measuring blood glucose level is another. Clinical observations are also important in detecting early signs of hyperglycemia (e.g., polyuria, polydipsia and polyphagia, and fatigue) and those seen when dehydration, hyperosmolarity, and acidosis develop (e.g., lethargy, coma, Kussmaul's breathing, etc.). The onset of fever or other signs of infection, abdominal pain, nausea, and vomiting may portend serious changes in the patient's endocrine status. The increasing incidence of hospital-induced infections must be remembered; often infection precipitates more severe hyperglycemia and can lead to ketoacidosis.

Regardless of the chief reason for admission—or the time of diagnosis—the identification of a patient as a diabetic requires that nurses systematically look for signs of hyperglycemia. The change in environment, the stress related to episodic illness, and the institution of various therapies (e.g., steroids, thiazides) often make the degree of hyperglycemia more severe. In addition, hypoglycemia is always a potential threat for insulin-dependent patients, and this threat becomes more likely when food intake decreases or insulin dose increases. When hyperglycemia is being treated by increasing insulin doses, or as acute illness subsides and insulin requirements decrease, close attention for early signs of an insulin reaction is important.

Corrective Measures When There Is Insulin Deficit

When patients are acutely ill with disorders of insulin deficit, the extent of physiological change is determined largely by measuring levels of blood glucose and ketones, blood gases, blood urea nitrogen, and serum potassium, as discussed in Chapter 5. Essential clinical observations relate to levels of consciousness, cardiopulmonary function, and renal output. Plans of care should include frequent observations of these parameters, as well as interventions used to correct the metabolic imbalance and support of the patient. When there is an acute disorder of insulin deficit, it is essential that care be implemented promptly and in coordination with the care plans of other health professionals and technicians. Effective communication is necessary between members of the health care team so that evaluative data about the response of patients to therapy can be used to plan appropriate measures.

Medically prescribed measures differ in kind, sequence, and frequency for individual diabetics who are in acute crisis states of insulin deficit. Priority measures are those related to insulin replacement, fluid and electrolyte replacement, and reversal of acidosis. It is difficult to predict the rapidity of an individual's response to treatment measures, and surveillance of the preceding parameters is necessary for evaluation of patient progress. A flow sheet is often used to record essential treatment information. The flow sheet in Table 8-1 shows the changes in physical status in response to therapy of one patient in ketosis. Unexpectedly rapid response to therapy should be reported to the physician, as well as specific levels of blood glucose, urinary glucose and ketones, and mental status. As blood glucose levels approach normal, insulin becomes more effective and there is an increased possibility of hypoglycemia.

Nurses should make systematic observations as they carry out therapeutic and supportive measures. A brief discussion follows of those measures and

Table 8-1 Changes That Occurred during Treatment of a Patient with Ketosis
(Corrective Measures Included Insulin and Fluid Replacement)

Time	Blood glucose (serum), mg per 100 mL	Urine			pH	Blood gases			Insulin (intravenous)	
		Volume	Percent glucose	Acetone		P_{O_2}	P_{CO_2}	HCO_3	Injection	Infusion
9 P.M.	405	300	5	moderate	7.39	98	24	21	15 U	1 U/h*
10 P.M.	335	300	5	moderate					15 U	2 U/h
12 P.M.	225	200	5	moderate	7.43	98	26	23		5 U/h†
4 A.M.	208	150	2	small	7.43	95	28	28		3 U/h
8 A.M.	165	125	1	0	7.47	96	33	23		1 U/h

* 25 U per 250 mL 5% dextrose in water begun at 9 P.M.
† 50 U per 250 mL 5% dextrose in water begun at 12 midnight.

assessments frequently used for patients in acute diabetic comas. The reader is referred to preceding chapters for further explanations.

Crystalline zinc insulin (regular) is the only insulin administered intravenously. There may be decreased absorption of insulin administered subcutaneously when the patient is severely dehydrated and circulatory inadequacy is present. Intramuscular injection and intravenous infusion of regular insulin are becoming more widely used. Maintenance of the prescribed flow of intravenous fluid is always important; the addition of regular insulin to an intravenous infusion intensifies the need for frequent and careful monitoring of flow rate. A monitoring and/or pumping device may be used to regulate flow.

The dosage of intravenous insulin by infusion is regulated by attention to the *units* per milliliter per minute and the milliliters (or drops) per minute. A change in insulin concentration or in the size of intravenous infusion sets can make significant differences in dosage. The nurse should recalculate the delivered dosage when equipment is changed or the concentration of insulin in the infusion is changed. See Table 8-2 for an example. The following formula is useful in calculating the units of insulin infused per minute:

$$\text{Units per minute} = \text{concentration} \times \text{number of drops per milliliter} \times \text{number of drops per minute}$$

An electrocardiogram is often taken to determine the effect of potassium imbalance on the heart's electrical function; in fact, continuous cardiac monitoring may be ordered so that potassium may be replaced according to the evaluation of cardiac function. Change in the configurations of the T wave, ST segment, PR interval, and QRS segment reflect the extracellular potassium levels. Figure 8-1 illustrates a large "peaked" T wave (hyperkalemia) and a

---

Table 8-2 Calculation of Delivered Dosage of Insulin

First, calculate the units and number of milliliters of fluid to be infused. If 50 U of regular insulin are added to 250 mL of fluid for a 10-h infusion, the insulin concentration is

$$\frac{50\ \text{U} + 250\ \text{mL}}{10\ \text{h}} \quad \text{or} \quad \frac{5\ \text{U} + 25\ \text{mL}}{\text{hour}} \quad \text{or} \quad \frac{0.08\ \text{U} + 0.41\ \text{mL}}{\text{minute}}$$

Second, calculate the rate of flow according to the size of the infusion set. If a minidropper set is used which has 60 drops per milliliter, the rate of flow is

$$25\ \text{mL/h} \times 60\ \text{drops} \quad \text{or} \quad 25\ \text{drops per minute}$$

If a regular infusion set with 10 drops per milliliter is used, the rate of flow is

$$25\ \text{mL/h} \times 10\ \text{drops} \quad \text{or} \quad 4\ \text{drops per minute}$$

Both of these will deliver 0.08 U/min. A change in infusion set to a different-sized dropper without changing the flow rate can result in significant error.

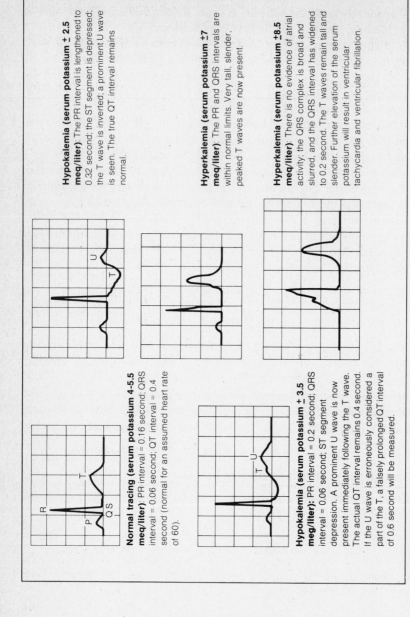

Hypokalemia (serum potassium ± 2.5 meq/liter): The PR interval is lengthened to 0.32 second; the ST segment is depressed; the T wave is inverted; a prominent U wave is seen. The true QT interval remains normal.

Hyperkalemia (serum potassium ±7 meq/liter): The PR and QRS intervals are within normal limits. Very tall, slender, peaked T waves are now present.

Hyperkalemia (serum potassium ±8.5 meq/liter): There is no evidence of atrial activity; the QRS complex is broad and slurred, and the QRS interval has widened to 0.2 second. The T waves remain tall and slender. Further elevation of the serum potassium will result in ventricular tachycardia and ventricular fibrillation.

Normal tracing (serum potassium 4-5.5 meq/liter): PR interval = 0.16 second; QRS interval = 0.06 second; QT interval = 0.4 second (normal for an assumed heart rate of 60).

Hypokalemia (serum potassium ± 3.5 meg/liter): PR interval = 0.2 second; QRS interval = 0.06 second; ST segment depression. A prominent U wave is now present immediately following the T wave. The actual QT interval remains 0.4 second. If the U wave is erroneously considered a part of the T, a falsely prolonged QT interval of 0.6 second will be measured.

Figure 8-1 Cardiac monitoring signs of hypokalemia and hyperkalemia.

216

"flattened" T wave (hypokalemia), as well as the other signs. Although additional signs of potassium imbalance may be present, the cardiac effects of either hyperkalemia or hypokalemia can lead to cardiac arrest. Table 8-3 compares the signs of hypokalemia and hyperkalemia. Frequent evaluation and reports to the physician of significant changes that affect levels of potassium are essential; these changes can be in (1) acidotic status, (2) volume of urinary excretion, and/or (3) cardiac signs. Potassium chloride is added to intravenous fluids when the physician is sure that the kidneys can excrete excess potassium and that the shift of potassium *into* the cell is under way.

Major deficits in fluids and electrolytes occur in ketoacidosis and other diabetic comas. Polyuria occurs as an early sign of hyperglycemia and glycosuria and leads to depletion of body fluids and electrolytes. In the absence of a history or signs of renal disease, oliguria or anuria is presumed to be a result of hypovolemia and a decreased glomerular filtration rate. This assumption is verified by the restoration of adequate urinary flow. Until 50 mL/h of urine are excreted, a major question exists concerning underlying renal pathology. If urine volumes do not increase after 1 to 2 h of fluid replacement, the physician should be notified. Likewise, an unanticipated increase or decrease in urine volume should be reported. This is particularly important if potassium is being infused.

In addition, evidence that fluid replacement is effective includes improvement in blood pressure, decrease in tachycardia and temperature, and improvement in mental status. Table 8-4 illustrates a typical sequence of patient response to treatment.

Table 8-3 Comparison of Signs of Hypokalemia and Hyperkalemia in Ketoacidosis

	Hypokalemia	Hyperkalemia
Serum levels	Below 3.0 meq/L (mild) Below 2.0 meq/L (severe)	Above 5.0 meq/L (mild) Above 6.0 meq/L (severe)
Most usual time of onset	After treatment restores pH balance and urinary excretion	With acidosis and/or oliguria
Shifts of K^+ and H^+	K^+ moves into cell as H^+ ion concentration decreases within the cell	K^+ moves out of cell as H^+ ion concentration increases within the cell
Cardiac	Decreased contractility, arrhythmia, cardiac arrest	Slowed conduction, arrythmia, cardiac arrest
Gastrointestinal	Decreased motility, anorexia, nausea, distention, paralytic ileus	Increased motility, colic diarrhea in mild states
Neuromuscular	Decreased irritability, flabby muscles in mild states, flaccid paralysis in severe states, loss of deep tendon reflexes	Increased irritability, twitching, hyperreflexia in mild states, paralysis in severe states

Table 8-4   Clinical Observations Correlated with the Change in Physical Status of a Patient Treated for Ketoacidosis

Time	Observations	pH	Potassium, meq/L	Blood glucose, mg per 100 mL	Insulin dosage
12:00*	Semicomatose, acetone breath, hyperpnea, rate: 34, poor skin turgor with "tenting," urine: 5% sugar, strong acetone	7.05	5.8	840	100 U
1:00		7.12			100 U
2:00	Lethargic, can be aroused by verbal stimuli, urine: 25 mL/h, 3% sugar, strong acetone				150 U
3:00		7.24		680	150 U
4:00	More alert, complains of nausea and abdominal pain	7.35	5.2	420	75 U
5:00	Skin turgor improved, taking oral fluids, respirations deep and 24, urine: 50 mL/h, 3% sugar, strong acetone				
6:00		7.42	4.0	200	

* 1000 mL .45% sodium chloride 400 mL/h began and 100 meq sodium bicarbonate given.

It is well to remember that replacement of fluids and electrolytes is based on *estimations* of the patient's needs. The ability of the patient to adapt to changes in the intravascular compartment may be impaired. Observations for circulatory overload become increasingly necessary as hydration continues. Monitoring for gains in weight, positive fluid balance, and signs of edema is essential. If sodium bicarbonate was used to treat acidosis, retention of fluid may be accelerated if the kidneys cannot excrete the sodium load. Many diabetic patients have concomitant cardiac disease and/or renal dysfunction and may not be able to manage marked increases in intravascular volume. Jugular vein distention, orthopnea in the alert patient, tachycardia, tachypnea, and cough may precede frank pulmonary edema. The use of central venous or arterial pressures may reflect more precisely the cardiac status.

Hypoglycemia

Hypoglycemia may occur when there is a rapid decrease in blood glucose concentrations. As insulin therapy reduces the acidosis and/or hyperglycemia in the acutely ill diabetic, there is an increased possibility that hypoglycemia will occur from an excess of insulin. Estimations of insulin requirement for the acutely ill patient are based on clinical observations and laboratory tests. As blood glucose levels approach normal concentrations there is more effective utilization of insulin. Frequent observations are necessary to detect the onset of hypoglycemia. Increase in restlessness, pallor, trembling, perspiration, and tachycardia are all hallmarks of an excess of regular insulin.

These clinical signs are related to excess epinephrine activity which occurs in hypoglycemia or in other states of stress. When these signs appear in the patient who is receiving treatment for ketoacidosis and whose blood glucose has approached normal concentrations, there is little doubt that hypoglycemia is the cause.

Hypoglycemia must be considered a possible cause of these clinical signs as well in other critically ill diabetics receiving insulin (e.g., patients with myocardial infarction or postsurgical patients). Hypotension, hypoxia, hypercapnia, pain, and strong emotional states can also elicit increased epinephrine activity, and the same clinical symptoms are exhibited.[1] When doubt exists as to the cause of these symptoms in the diabetic, the patient's response to glucose administration and blood glucose levels can verify whether hypoglycemia was the cause. Certainly measures to increase blood pressure, blood volume, and ventilation and to relieve pain should be instituted as needed. Evaluation of the response of the patient to these measures can be useful in planning future treatment.

A cycle of alternating hypoglycemic reactions and periods of hyperglycemia can be initiated during blood glucose regulation. Instead of achieving relatively normal blood glucose levels, sometimes repeated episodes of hypoglycemia may alternate with increasingly higher levels of hyperglycemia. One cause of this is the Somogyi reaction, in which endogenous hormonal responses to hypoglycemia raise blood glucose levels. When additional insulin is administered, even more severe hypoglycemia is provoked, thus:

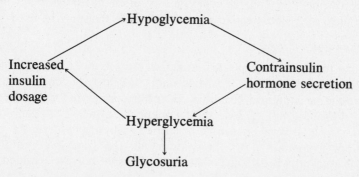

Careful documentation of insulin reactions, glucose intake, blood and urine concentrations of glucose, and insulin dosage aids the physician in planning appropriate dosages of insulin to avoid alternating hyperglycemia and hypoglycemia.

The critical actions to be instituted when hypoglycemia is suspected are

1 Obtain blood samples for testing
2 Administer glucose
3 Notify the physician

The order in which these actions are taken may vary with individual patients. Delay in providing glucose can be costly to the patient's well-being; waiting for urine excretion from an oliguric patient, or for a "second voided" specimen, is inappropriate when symptoms of hypoglycemia occur.

The choice of method of glucose administration depends on the patient's ability to swallow and retain food and liquids, the patency of the intravenous line, and the availability of a physician. The institution's medical and nursing practice guidelines should provide for a rapid treatment response for hypoglycemia. How to treat insulin reactions should be clearly defined for each patient when he or she first receives insulin. Figure 8-2 shows a flow sheet with a record of observations, actions taken, and evaluation of a patient's response to treatment.

As symptoms of hypoglycemia subside, review is made of past insulin dosages and prescribed carbohydrate intake. Additional and more slowly absorbed carbohydrate or protein may be needed to "cover" the insulin already administered. Estimations of response are used to prescribe dosage of insulin, but the actual response of the patient may necessitate changes in insulin dosage and carbohydrate intake. The patient's mental and cardiac status following a hypoglycemic episode should be assessed and documented. Did mental and cardiac function return to the prehypoglycemic state? The nurse should observe changes in behavior, rate and rhythm of pulse, and presence of angina. Failure to return to the prehypoglycemic status should be reported to the physician.

Relatively small amounts of glucose are usually adequate in treating hypoglycemia; improvement in clinical symptoms is often noted within 5 min. Refer to Chapter 6 for recommended amounts of foods that may be used.

Supportive Measures

Plans of actions to maintain respiratory function are based on assessment of ventilatory adequacy, fluid balance, cardiac status, and level of consciousness. Unless the presenting acute problem involves respiratory pathology, diabetics in metabolic acidosis are not hypoxic and do not need oxygen. The respiratory pattern of Kussmaul's breathing can be described as hyperpnea and the rate specified ("labored breathing" and "respiratory distress" are inaccurate descriptions of Kussmaul's breathing). This type of respiration is identified by

Name: Daily flow sheet

Date:							Intake					Output		Treatments
Vital signs							Intravenous			Oral				Comments
Time	Temperature	Pulse	Respiration	Blood pressure	Time up	Site	IV number, type, and amount solution	Time down	Amount absorbed	Type of fluid	Amount	Volume	Sugar acetone	
8 AM	38	84	18	120/74						SKIM MILK, JUICE, COFFEE	320		½ %	NPH 85 u
9														
10														
11		120		150/100	11:05		50 mL 50% D/W IV push 1000 mL D/5W 100 mL/h started		50	orange juice	120			Hypoglycemia; BS 42
12		84		124/70										
1 PM										SKIM MILK	100		1%	Ate all of Lunch
2										SOUP, COFFEE	290			
3														

8° Totals:

Figure 8-2 A daily flow sheet can be used to record onset of hypoglycemia and its treatment. Details can be reported on the progress notes: e.g., at 11:00 A.M.

S   Could not state place or time, or describe reaction.
O   Skin warm and dry except forehead. Facial tics on right side disappeared after glucose, and patient stated name, place, and time.
A   Hypoglycemia—patient unable to perceive signs. Mental status returned to normal.
P   Monitor frequently, maintain IV for 24 h, encourage eating. Reduce insulin to 75 U in A.M.

regularity of deep chest excursions. Suctioning may be necessary to maintain an open airway in the comatose patient. Positioning the patient on his or her side prevents aspiration of secretions and/or vomitus. Continuous evaluation of ventilatory patterns is necessary. Moist breath sounds are unusual in the dehydrated and acidotic patient. As rehydration occurs, secretions are liquefied and mobilized. Increasing moistness, change in symmetry of breath sounds, or adventitious sounds may be heard as the patient regains consciousness and Kussmaul's breathing subsides.

Frequent turning and encouragement of deep breathing and coughing are continued as long as there is evidence of retained secretions. Mists, intermittent positive pressure, and postural drainage may be used to assist in removal of secretions.

Infection may be the precipitating cause of the metabolic imbalance. It may be the reason for admission or may develop after the patient is in the hospital. The diabetic patient has depressed defenses against infection during ketoacidosis: decreased phagocytosis, circulatory stasis, and an interstitial medium of glucose. Normal flora suppression by antibiotics may result in overgrowth of secondary organisms. Chest x-ray and sputum culture and sensitivities are commonly done upon admission of the patient with diabetic coma. Antibiotic therapy is started after the sputum sample is obtained. The presence of respiratory infection increases the need for surveillance and respiratory assistance. Pulmonary infections may increase fluid losses and decrease respiratory compensation of acidosis.

When urinary tract infection is suspected, a urine sample for culture and sensitivities is collected and evaluation for signs of urinary infection is ongoing. Indwelling catheter drainage is often required in the early treatment of the comatose patient in order to titrate amounts of fluid and electrolyte replacement and to monitor the urine for glucose and acetone. Meticulous aseptic technique is necessary for the insertion and maintenance of a closed system of drainage and for collection of the specimen. The catheter should be removed as soon as possible.

As the patient regains consciousness, he or she is questioned concerning frequency of urination and symptoms of pain and burning upon urination, and he or she is instructed to report these if they develop. Often culture and sensitivity studies are done to detect subclinical infections, and observation of the clarity and color of urine is done routinely. Continued attention to fluid intake is given so that urinary stasis does not develop.

Activities to maintain the integrity of the skin as well as to prevent any other complications of bed rest are incorporated into the plan of care. If indicated, special equipment may be used. Air mattresses, flotation pads, water beds, and foot cradles can be used to decrease pressure points. These are helpful when combined with frequent changes of position, massage, cleansing, and gentle touch when moving the patient. Proper alignment and range of motion exercises promote integrity of joint function. Passive or active leg exercises are used to decrease stasis of circulation, which is aggravated by bed rest in a dehydrated patient.

Comfort measures are important as the patient regains consciousness. The patient requires orientation to time and place and explanation concerning the care underway. The noncomatose patient who is dehydrated and/or acidotic is usually uncomfortable, drowsy, and irritable. Abdominal tenderness or pain, nausea, and vomiting are not unusual. A nasogastric tube may be in place, as well as a urinary catheter. Blood and urine samples and examinations of mental and physical status are frequent. Activities are grouped to allow the patient as much rest as possible. The patient needs a quiet environment with care proceeding in an efficient manner.

Frequent mouth care and attempts to relieve immobile areas or pressure points can promote comfort. The nasogastric tube is left in place until the patient is able to retain fluid. Small sips of fluids are *gradually* increased as nausea and vomiting subside. Fluid intake and output are measured, abdominal distention and discomfort are observed, and the recurrence of pain, nausea, and/or vomiting is monitored. Evaluation of gastrointestinal status also includes assessment for return of bowel sounds, passage of flatus or stool, and decrease in abdominal tenderness or distention. Constipation is a frequent sequela of dehydration. The nurse should report to the physician if pain or distention increases.

Support to the family is an integral part of the plan of care. Families and patients vary in their understanding of the nature and treatment of hyperglycemia and related complications. They have been under stress during evaluation of the severity of illness, and while arranging transportation and admission and providing care during the preadmission period. They often fear death or disability and may be apprehensive about the kind and quality of care the patient will receive. Feelings of relief that the patient is admitted may be mixed with feelings of anxiety.

Interactions with the nursing staff can offer a family the opportunity to verify the presence of caring and competence and allow development of trust. Nurses should explain the care underway and indicate when the family may talk with the physician. Privacy and comfortable surroundings should be offered.

Before family visits, the nurse should check the appearance of the patient and remove any unnecessary intrusive equipment. Guidance can be offered the family concerning voice levels, closeness or touch, and length and frequency of visits. Support given to the family may promote their ability to console and comfort the patient. Clues about coping ability and the understanding of diabetes mellitus and its treatment can be obtained during the acute phase. These will suggest the support systems available to the patient and family during the crisis and later.

Setting the Stage for Learning

The plan of care is designed to allow increasing independence in all daily activities as the patient's status improves. Assessing acuteness of illness is basic to deciding when to increase independence or begin instruction. Alertness, comfort, and energy are necessary for learning self-care techniques. As the patient recovers, appraisal is made of his or her learning abilities: memory, anxiety, attention span, interest, and literacy. All these have bearing on the plan of approach and the methods of teaching to be discussed in Chapter 9.

Evaluation of learning needs can begin as recovery ensues. Diabetics receiving insulin or hypoglycemic agents should be able to state (1) the specific medication, dosage, and time of last dose, (2) the results of the day's urine tests by recall or by referring to flow sheets, and (3) why blood sugars are taken in relation to medication and diet. Repetition and reinforcement are used as necessary to assist the patient and significant family members in achieving these behaviors. Modeling can be used as a teaching technique as the nurse discusses and performs tasks in the presence of the patient and family. The higher the level of anxiety, the more important it is that the nurse direct discussion toward expressed concerns and interests.

It is not unusual for newly diagnosed adults or children to state that some other person will take responsibility for part or all of the therapeutic measures after discharge. The consequences of this decision should be explored with the patient, as well as with the other person. Fear of injections, low self-esteem, or a desire for the interpersonal gains achieved through dependency, may be the basis for such a decision.

If the patient experiences a hypoglycemic reaction, the nurse should help him or her recall and state the inner feelings during the reaction so that this knowledge can be used in detecting other reactions. Other glucose sources should be compared with the one the patient was given. Sometimes patients are ordered to have a glucose source at the bedside. In hospitals, usually the most convenient and easily obtained source is orange juice (refer to Chapter 6 for other foods with comparable glucose content).

Patient Outcomes

The following outline delineates the purposes of nursing care for diabetic patients in physiological crisis. These "patient outcomes" can guide assessments and interventions and serve as evaluative criteria for nursing practice.[2]

I   The patient shall have improvement of signs and symptoms:
   A   Decreased hyperglycemia
   B   Decreased ketonemia
   C   Elimination of Kussmaul's respirations
   D   Return to normal blood gases
   E   Decreased glycosuria
   F   Decreased ketonuria
   G   Elimination of nausea and vomiting
   H   Decreased pain
   I   Improved sensorium—ability to respond verbally
II   The patient shall remain free of avoidable complications:
   A   The patient shall maintain a normal blood pressure and heart rate.
   B   The patient shall maintain a patent airway and a normal respiratory rate.
   C   The patient shall be free of hyperkalemia and hypokalemia.
   D   The patient shall be free of insulin reactions.
III   The patient and/or significant others shall be able to discuss plans for nursing care:
   A   The patient can explain the reason for admission.
   B   The patient can relate that he or she is receiving insulin.
   C   The patient can relate that his or her urine is being tested.
   D   The patient can relate that blood is being drawn frequently for blood glucose readings.

Throughout hospitalization, regardless of acuteness of illness, the following nursing activities are continued:

1   Observation of signs and symptoms of hyper- and hypoglycemia
2   Monitoring of intake and output
3   Monitoring of glucose and acetone contents of urine
4   Administration of medications prescribed to control blood glucose
5   Prompt recognition and treatment of insulin reactions
6   Assisting patient to select and eat foods and to monitor food intake

SURGERY AND DIAGNOSTIC TESTS

When decrease in food intake occurs in the insulin-treated patient, increased monitoring for hypoglycemia is necessary. Sometimes this is due to anorexia; however, in the hospital this may be due to fasting requirements for surgery or diagnostic tests. Nurses are not responsible for the prescription of insulin or food intake; however they are responsible for monitoring the metabolic status of the patient and for identifying when conditions may be harmful to the patient.

Surgery and many diagnostic procedures increase the dangers of hypoglycemia for the insulin-dependent patient. Whenever fasting is required, changes in insulin management and the use of intravenous glucose infusion are often necessary. How insulin is to be managed should be clarified when surgery and diagnostic tests are scheduled. Several options are available including (1) reduction in dosage or delay of subcutaneous injection of insulin until the patient can eat (when a relatively short fasting period is anticipated); (2) inclusion of insulin in a glucose intravenous infusion; or (3) change to regular insulin at scheduled intervals during the day. The latter option may be correlated with food intake and/or the amount of glycosuria and ketonuria.

Early morning scheduling of insulin-dependent diabetics for surgery or diagnostic tests is necessary so that minimum disruption of daily control measures occurs. Personnel in other departments should be alerted when patients have had alterations in insulin and food intake that predispose them to hypoglycemia so that prompt response can be made to symptoms of hypoglycemia. Increased chance of hypoglycemia in the surgical patient is related to decreased food intake, the inability of the patient under sedation or anesthesia to detect symptoms of hypoglycemia, and, in some patients, the rapid decrease in insulin requirement as treatment corrects the precipitating infection or physiological stress.

As a general rule, patients undergoing surgery also need more insulin than when they are well. Catabolism induced by the surgical experience or the presence of infection results in contrainsulin hormonal changes that increase blood glucose levels. The use of a "sliding scale" or "rainbow schedules" to correlate additional amounts of regular insulin with glycosuria and ketonuria were discussed in Chapter 7.

The postoperative carbohydrate requirement is usually 125 to 250 g per day.[3] The presence of ketonuria in the absence of glycosuria may indicate starvation ketosis. Too slow a rate of glucose infusion may lead to hypoglycemia in the insulin-treated patient or ketosis, while too rapid a rate may increase the level of hyperglycemia and lead to caloric loss through glycosuria.

Steinke states that the risks of surgery for the diabetic patient include increased chances for hypoglycemia and hyperglycemia and the presence of cardiovascular disease in many diabetics.[4] Silent myocardial infarctions may occur in the diabetic patient during surgery, and surgical risk is increased in the presence of poor metabolic control, obesity, arteriosclerosis, and cardiovascular disease.[5]

EDUCATING THE HOSPITALIZED DIABETIC

Expertise is needed for judgment of when to begin teaching and when to begin increasing self-management. Effective use of hospitalization for teaching is mandatory if diabetic patients and families are to be competent and confident at the time of discharge.

Assessment of Learning Needs

The following outline lists the desired "patient outcomes" at the time of discharge. They guide assessments, plans, and records of patient behavior and illustrate knowledge, attitudes, and skills of self-management.[6]

I   The patient and/or significant others shall be able to discuss those changes required in life-style upon discharge:
  A   Can explain the meaning of diabetes, how treatment measures regulate blood sugar
    1   Signs and symptoms of hypoglycemia and hyperglycemia
    2   Actions to be taken during infections and other illness
    3   Actions to be taken to prevent hypoglycemia and hyperglycemia
    4   Actions to be taken to treat insulin reactions
  B   Can explain a specific health maintenance program at home:
    1   Diet prescription
    2   Foot care
    3   Medications
    4   Urine testing and recording
  C   Can state purpose and time of scheduled return visit for health supervision
II The patient and/or significant others shall be able to demonstrate those skills required for self-care:
  A   Can test urine for sugar and acetone accurately and record results in a diary
  B   Can perform proper foot care
  C   Can measure and inject insulin accurately
    1   Can use at least two body areas for injection sites
    2   Can maintain a site rotation schedule

Adult patients recovering from acute diabetic syndromes form a minority of the diabetics with whom hospital nurses work. The "patient outcomes" just listed can serve as a guide for initial assessment of baseline skills of any diabetic patient who is not acutely ill. It is important that there be a continuity of self-care practices which leads to optimal health status. Opportunity for review of knowledge and self-care practices can be incorporated into a planned educational program during hospitalization regardless of the reason for admission or the length of time the patient has had diabetes.

Guidelines for Assessment

Most hospital-based nurses practice in settings where diabetics form only a portion of the patient population. Assessment models work best when tailor-made for a particular group of patients and when they are designed to help nurses identify the problems most commonly seen. It is not feasible for nursing staffs to develop unique assessment models based on the specific requirements of the many differing diseases their patient populations manifest. Assessment models used by nursing should be complementary to those used by the other disciplines in a particular setting. Certainly, effort must be made to prevent inundation of the patient with data gatherers of various and sundry disciplines, all asking the same questions. Nor should the patient be repeatedly assessed by several nurses. Nursing assessment models should reflect teaching, counseling, and care giving in the selection of information categories. Plans of care communicate those approaches, methods, and sequences of events that seem most appropriate for the particular patient. Written care plans as well as verbal shift reports can be used to inform all nurses involved in a patient's care of particular needs and the interventions to be used.

A general assessment of nursing needs precedes the use of a specialized diabetic-focused assessment. To focus too soon on diabetes and related activities may result in an overlooking of the concerns most pressing to the patient. Patients in pain or other discomfort, those undergoing frightening diagnostic or therapeutic procedures, or those awaiting conclusion of ambiguous diagnostic processes may be quite uninterested in discussing the aspects of their diabetic state, much less in learning more about self-care practices. In contrast, patients who find the hospital dull may welcome a diabetic care assessment and educational program as distracting and "time filling."

1   Why have you come to the hospital?
2   What does the doctor plan for you while you are here?
3   Have you been in the hospital before? Why?
4   What good things do you remember about your stay?
5   What was upsetting to you during your stay?

Simply phrased questions such as these have been used as part of the standard assessment for all patients admitted to wards of one medical-surgical department.[7] They are asked first and convey to the patient interest in and concern for his or her perceptions and expectations. They elicit from the patient important information that can be used to judge his or her understanding of the present circumstances. In addition, they can be used to identify fears and concerns about the hospital stay. (Whether the diabetic patient identifies himself or herself as a diabetic and discusses the control measures is most useful to observe.) Often the nurse can detect evidence of trust or mistrust as the patient and nurse engage in mutual planning of how these measures will be continued in the hospital. The patient's use of terminology to describe his or her diabetic status can provide some indication of the level of understanding of the disease. Certainly, specific follow-up questions should be asked of the insulin-dependent patient regarding the last dose of insulin taken, recent food intake, presence of vomiting, and the last urine-test results.

When the patient is admitted for one of the diabetic vascular complications, the nurse can listen for expression of beliefs about the complication and diabetes. Some patients will reveal quite sophisticated knowledge about diabetes and its relationship to their present state. It is not unusual for patients to reveal some feelings about their past levels of compliance and to relate concern about their effects. Expressions of guilt or anger or of fatalistic attitudes by the patient or family may be apparent. Chapter 10 discusses the specific needs of patients with diabetic complications.

The initiation of assessment should be combined with the introduction to the patient of the roles of the nurse as care giver, counselor, or teacher, depending on the content of the initial interview. Simply stating "We like to use the hospital stay for review of learning needs" can present to the patient the nurse's expectations. Initial plans for continuity of care and methods to be used to alleviate pressing concerns should be shared before leaving the patient.

The daily activities of living should be reviewed as early after admission as possible in order to determine the kinds of assistance needed and whether special equipment should be ordered. Again, the following questions can be used with all patients, not just with diabetics. However, the high incidence of vascular and neurological complications in the adult and elderly diabetic make these questions particularly applicable to those patients.

1 Do you have any difficulty walking or getting into or out of a chair?
2 Will you need assistance with your bath? With meals?
3 Do you sleep through the night at home?
4 What helps you get to sleep at home?
5 Do you have any difficulty with urination?
6 What are your usual bowel habits?
7 How often do you use enemas or laxatives?
8 Are you receiving any special treatments or doing special exercises?

These questions often elicit information about the patient's basic nursing care requirements. When combined with careful inspection of the patient's gait, transfer techniques, and walking ability, these questions can help the nurse determine the level of assistance needed for mobility. The condition of the skin surfaces of the legs and feet should be inspected in all adult diabetics. Appropriate measures to ensure safety of the patient should be instituted, and foot cradles, air mattresses, or an overhead trapeze should be obtained if necessary. Close attention to the condition of shoes and stockings, as well as the feet, gives clues as to whether foot-care practices are adequate.

Nurses should listen particularly to diabetic patients as they describe any problems with urination. Polyuria and nocturia may interfere with sleep.

Dysuria may indicate bladder infection, and incontinence may be present in the patient with neuropathy.

Life-style Questions about available help at home and the kind of environment from which the patient comes are helpful in identifying particular resources or factors to be considered in making realistic plans.

1 With whom do you live?
2 Upon whom do you rely when you need help?
3 Do you live in an apartment? House? Other?
4 Do you have to climb stairs?
5 What kinds of activities do you usually do during the day?
6 What do you do at work?

Certain life-styles make it more difficult to adequately control the blood glucose level in insulin-dependent diabetics. Rotating schedules of work, inconsistency in the amounts and kinds of food intake and energy expenditures from day to day, traveling, meals away from home, and lack of privacy for urine testing or insulin administration are factors which require problem solving. Sometimes these can be modified. One diabetic nurse chose to work as a permanent night nurse rather than rotate on three shifts. Rotating shifts requires frequent manipulation of insulin dosages and food intake to match the inconsistency in activity and sleep patterns. Many people do not have the option to change work hours and thus need considerable assistance in regulating insulin and diet.

When patients report fear of hypoglycemia and restrict their activities on this basis, the nurse can ascertain whether they have sufficient information to make valid decisions. There is some trial and error involved in learning to regulate food, exercise, and insulin, and this lack of preciseness about "how much" to increase food intake (or to decrease insulin) on days of planned exercise contributes to the lack of confidence in the new diabetic. Sims and Ethan suggest that some new diabetics may need to decrease insulin dosage by 20 percent and increase food intake by an equal amount.[8] Certainly, food sources should be readily available and the diabetic person should be able to recognize and treat hypoglycemia. In addition, as the patient records particular responses to exercise, food intake, and insulin dosages, he or she can learn to predict more precisely the modifications needed prior to and during activity. Supportive counseling can be useful to the diabetic in reviewing plans for activities perceived as necessary to a full life (see Chapter 3).

Asking the patient to describe a typical day is useful; attention to description of work and home can reveal problem areas. Sometimes the work environment is potentially hazardous. For example, a car wash attendant or mail carrier may require problem-solving assistance in terms of how to maintain dry and warm feet. The home environment may be quite limited in material resources. For example, an aged pensioner may be cooking on a hot plate in his or her one-room "apartment" and sharing a bathroom with eight other people; an

alcoholic diabetic on insulin may live in a halfway house where the only carbohydrate available is in a vending machine; or an elderly diabetic in a wheel-
chair may report that a neighboring drug addict steals her syringes and needles.

A number of elderly widows have reacted to the diagnosis of diabetes by
initiating more contacts with others in the community. These women reported
fatalistic resignation about aging and approaching death prior to the diagnosis,
but after diagnosis voiced fears of "dying alone" where "no one would know."
Although they understood the relative slowness of symptoms of diabetic coma
in the insulin-independent patient, they viewed the diagnosis of diabetes as an
"acceptable" reason to ask for more regular contacts from neighbors and
members of church groups.

Early assessment of home and work environments makes teaching plans
more realistic and enables the patient to move from hospital to home more
easily. If social services need to be contacted, early referral is possible when
thorough assessments have been made soon after admission.

Alcoholism   Alcoholism is a critical consideration in assessing life-style.
Large numbers of people in the United States have alcohol addiction or excessive
drinking patterns. These are often not revealed by patients seeking health care.
Hidden information about the extent of drinking can mislead diagnosis and
treatment and make self-care plans unrealistic for diabetic people. When diabetes and alcoholism coexist, change in self-care behavior must occur if optimal
health is to be achieved. (See Chapter 6 for incorporation of occasional drinking
into the diet.)

There are many relationships between alcoholism and diabetes. Diabetes
may be caused by alcoholic destruction of pancreatic tissue. The severity of
insulin deficit can be magnified by further drinking, and alcoholic disease states
can mimic or magnify such complications of diabetes as neuropathy, cardiac
myopathy, optic atrophy, and organic brain disease. The many diseases caused
by alcohol and the crisis states of acute alcoholism and withdrawal can alter
metabolic control of diabetes as well as be life-threatening in themselves. Alcoholic ketosis can precipitate coma and metabolic acidosis; and hypoglycemic
coma (in the diabetic treated with insulin or sulfonylureas) potentiated by alcohol is particularly hazardous. Well known are the symptoms of cerebral and
cerebellar dysfunction that occur in both drunkenness and hypoglycemia. Jail
confinement has precluded prompt treatment by glucose administration of hypoglycemia in both drinking and nondrinking diabetics.

All diabetics should be encouraged to carry diabetic identification. They
also need to eat when drinking because drinking without eating can lead to
hypoglycemia in both nondiabetics and diabetics. In addition, alcoholic intake
decreases the rate of recovery from insulin-induced hypoglycemia, and glucagon is ineffective in restoring an adequate level of blood glucose.[9]

When the alcoholic diabetic is undergoing detoxification or convalescing
from acute illness, frequent evaluations of his or her learning potential should
be made. Increased concentration and improvement in thought processes

should be matched with gradual assumption of diabetic self-care activities. A forthright and nonjudgmental manner is necessary to involve the patient in discussions of drinking patterns and the effects of alcoholic behavior on diabetic control.

Varying patterns of behavior are presented by those who are labeled alcoholics. To assist in altering these patterns, stages have been devised to aid in treatment, prevention, and rehabilitation. Basic to alcoholism is the tension-reducing effect, which inhibits growth and the development of more adaptive coping mechanisms. Whether the alcoholic can relate information about alcohol to his or her life depends on the amount of denial he or she uses. As alcoholism progresses, there is increasing preoccupation with drinking and, at the same time, discomfort about drinking. This leads to the use of rationalization, increased isolation, and sporadic attempts to stop drinking. These behavior patterns and blackouts occur before true addiction, according to Jellinek.[10] Life becomes increasingly alcohol oriented, and choices about drinking are restricted. Loss of control is a central feature of chronic addiction. At this stage, the person no longer has freedom of choice, except the choice of taking the first drink.

A major contribution of nurses can be the exploration with the alcoholic of his or her willingness to use supportive services to modify the drinking pattern. The first step is to determine whether alcohol is perceived as a problem that affects well-being. Giving advice is rarely useful; however, focusing on current life experiences can help the alcoholic confront the problems caused by drinking and the choices available. Certainly the alcoholic should be informed of the dangers of the combination of alcoholism and diabetes. The occurrence of blackouts and loss of recent memory make the use of insulin and hypoglycemic agents extremely hazardous.

The choice of life without alcohol may be untenable to the addicted alcoholic, but choices within smaller time frames can be more reality focused. Whether to take a drink is a choice the patient can review within a day's activities related to the diabetic regimen. A counseling approach is useful in exploring those situational factors which trigger drinking and in reinforcing both the choices available to the patient and the consequences of the decisions.

At some point, the chronic alcoholic may be unable to continue independent living, and a supervised living situation may be the best course of action. Alienation from family members and social groups often narrows the options available to the patient. Self-help groups have been useful to many. Moreover, increasing kinds and numbers of services are developing in the field of alcoholism rehabilitation. Early referral of the diabetic who has a problem with alcohol is recommended.

Specific Diabetic Assessment

The diabetic assessment guide illustrated in Fig. 8-3 was designed and tested by nurses. Like the questions discussed earlier, these are simply phrased. They elicit information useful in providing continuity of care and in judging the level

Diabetic control	*Prior to admission*	*Since admission*

Insulin type and amount

Oral agent

Diet

Has been a diabetic for _____years

Insulin

Administered by _____

Drawn by _____

Time taken _____

Condition of injection sites _____

Equipment used _____

Vision _____

Urine testing

Frequency at home_____

How much do you spill?_____

Method used _____

Test for acetone?_____

Where equipment kept?_____

What do you do if spilling? _____

Foot care

Condition of feet and toenails _____

_____

Who cuts toenails?_____

Special care at home?_____

Diet

Who prepares and shops for food?_____

When do you eat?_____

Snacks?_____

Do you use exchange list?_____

Drink alcoholic beverages?_____

How much?_____

General knowledge and attitude

How do you feel when your sugar is high?_____

How do you feel when your sugar is low?_____

Do you carry candy?_____

Have you known anyone in the past with diabetes? _____

How did this person get along? _____

Employment _____

Do people at work know you are a diabetic?_____

Do you carry diabetic identification?_____

When do you retire?_____   Clinic you attend _____

Arise? _____   How do you get to clinic?_____

Figure 8-3 Diabetic admission information guide used at University Hospitals, Cleveland.

of education about diabetes. The timing of a specific diabetic assessment depends on the nurse's judgment of the acuteness of the illness and the ability of the patient to focus on diabetic care activities. Sometimes, particularly for the insulin-dependent diabetic, certain aspects of the information will have been obtained in the initial interview, as discussed earlier.

Hypoglycemic Reactions Patterns of hypoglycemic reactions must be discovered as soon after admission as possible so that monitoring and treatment can be more effective. Some patients can describe symptoms quite easily, while others report that they have never experienced an insulin reaction. Although avoidance of hypoglycemia is a generally accepted goal of treatment, if the patient has not experienced hypoglycemia after several years of insulin therapy, one can wonder about the adequacy of control. With institution of a calorie-controlled environment for this patient, the chances of hypoglycemia may be greater. It is true that some diabetic patients cannot perceive the symptoms of insulin reaction and must rely on others to detect them. Family members can give very helpful hints. "When he starts arguing, I know I should give him sugar," said one wife of a usually easygoing man. "When she talks crazy and her skin is cold," said a sister of an elderly woman.

It is essential that the entire nursing staff be notified of the particular signs and symptoms the patient exhibits. In addition, the plans to treat the insulin reaction should be clear to all.

Weight and Diet Refer to Fig. 8-3 for specific questions about weight control and dietary managment. If the diabetic person fails to mention a special diet for diabetes, follow-up questions are in order. What past instructions have been given for dietary management? Does the patient expect the physician to order a special diet? The "fit" of the hospital routine of times of meals can be estimated by finding out the patient's usual pattern. Whether regularity of eating is a habit is as important to report as the quantity of food intake. How the patient describes food intake, whether he or she anticipates a change while in the hospital, and his or her interest in and willingness to learn more about diet management are all useful to observe. Communication to other nurses and to the dietitian should include the patient's specific motivating factors about diet as well as any lacks in education or compliance.

Recording of admission weight is routine for all patients; for the diabetic patient it is an essential base line against which change will be gauged. The patient in acute metabolic disorder from insulin deficit may have weight loss from dehydration and catabolism; as treatment becomes effective, this will be reversed. For the diabetic with edema, institution of diuretics, sodium, and/or water restriction is evaluated by the amount of weight loss. For the obese diabetic who is in the hospital, where food intake is relatively more controlled than at home, weight loss may occur on a diet that seems to have a "normal" caloric value. How patients perceive their weight status, and their ability to manipulate it are important indications of the amount of motivation or concern they have for dietary management. Refer to Chapter 6 for ways in which to facilitate dietary management.

Medication History A survey of medication usage is important for all patients admitted to a hospital. Diabetic patients should be able to name their insulin or hypoglycemic agent, the dosage, frequency, the last dosage taken, and the reason for taking it. On admission, policies are clarified regarding self-medication in the hospital, and medications brought by the patient are identified. Medications bought over-the-counter as well as prescription drugs may have significant amounts of glucose (or alcohol, e.g., Geritol); and some interfere with urine tests. Others may alter carbohydrate tolerance (see Table 7-6). Refer to Chapter 7 for drug-disease and drug-drug interactions.

Plans should be shared with the patient regarding the physician's orders for insulin or hypoglycemic agents, and the patient should be told the approximate time to expect the medication. Initial discussion should determine whether the patient will self-administer insulin on a routine basis or whether nurses will give the injection. Sometimes the adult is glad of a "rest" or asks that nurses use the sites that are difficult for the patient to reach.

Diabetic Self-Care Activities

In addition to the interview, observation of the patient's abilities in performing the skills of diabetic care is essential. Accurate assessment of patient learning needs can only be based on direct observation. Early in the hospital stay, the nurse should ascertain the accuracy and skill with which the patient administers insulin, tests urine, chooses diet, and practices foot care. Plans for teaching can be implemented in accordance with this assessment. (Principles of teaching are explored in Chapter 9.)

An essential component of diabetic self-care is the patient's ability to *monitor* and *evaluate* the extent of metabolic imbalance. The diabetic monitors the level of glycosuria and ketonuria rather than the more direct blood glucose. Attention to the presence or absence of symptoms that indicate metabolic imbalance is just as important as urine testing. Refer to Fig. 8-3 for questions that are helpful in initially determining adequacy of self-care practice.

Urine-Testing Accuracy Several studies have demonstrated serious inaccuracies in patient urine testing. There is little doubt that patients—and nurses—need to read directions for urine tests carefully and at periodic intervals. In one study, 86 percent of diabetics timed the test inaccurately, 19 percent used outdated materials, and 67 percent stored the test materials improperly.[11] Other problems in testing relate to incorrectly obtained urine, inadequate mental or physical ability, and incorrect test procedures.

A study by Derr indicated that bias of the tester influenced the accuracy of tests for acetone. Errors increased when nurses knew prior test results for glucose and acetone and when they knew glucose concentrations were high. The more frequently urine tests were performed by an individual, the more bias appeared.[12] Another study found high numbers of inaccuracies by nurses testing for glucose and suggested that errors are increased when testing becomes routine.[13] These reports indicate a need for periodic review of urine-testing directions and for evaluation of technique by another person.

Urine-Testing Materials Two kinds of test materials are available for determining the presence and amount of glycosuria. Clinitest tablets (and Benedict's solution, which is rarely used) are based on copper reduction of sugars. They detect the presence of other sugars as well as glucose. Three dilutions of urine are used—the 1-drop, 2-drop, and 5-drop methods; all three require 10 drops of water and one tablet, and are read 15 s after boiling has stopped. The 1-drop method is rarely used. It and the 2-drop method can differentiate concentration levels of glucose above 2 percent. In the past, most patients were taught the 5-drop method; now many are being taught the 2-drop method. The 5-drop test is limited in determining percentages above 2 percent; one does not know whether the urine contains 2 percent or a higher glucose concentration. Those patients with unstable diabetes are advised to use only the Clinitest 2-drop method or to retest urine with this method if other tests show 1 or 2 percent glucose concentration. Shaking the tube during reaction, slanting the dropper, or using a different-sized dropper from the one that comes with Clinitest can change the dilution of urine to water and affect the accuracy of the test. Caution must be taken to use the color-coded test chart that corresponds with the test being used—the 2-drop or the 5-drop method; there are significant differences in the charts. Watching the urine *during* the 15-s waiting period is essential in the 2-drop test, for sometimes a "pass-through" reaction occurs when a large sugar content is present. Failure to watch can result in the inaccurate reading of 1 or 2 percent, when in fact 5 to 10 percent glucose may be present. If clean test tubes and medicine droppers are not used, residues of glucose can change the test results.

There are some potential hazards in the use of Clinitest tablets. Caustic burns can occur from ingestion of the tablets, and handling of the test tube during the boiling phase may result in burns on the hands or fingers—so can handling the tablets with moist fingers. Moisture added to a sealed bottle of Clinitest can result in an explosion. For these reasons, if children are in the home, the patient may choose to purchase individually wrapped tablets or tablets packaged with a childproof cap. All urine-testing materials will deteriorate if moisture is added to them. Clinitest tablets are packaged with a dessicant which should be kept in the container. Patients—and nurses—should keep containers tightly sealed and in an area free of excessive moisture. (At home, the kitchen or bathroom is not the best place to store urine-testing materials.)

Clinitest tablets can deteriorate and lose their ability to detect glucose accurately. These tablets should be off-white, with only a few light blue specks, and whole, not chipped or broken. They should completely dissolve after boiling. If any of the preceding characteristics are absent, the tablets may no longer be of use in accurately determining the level of glucosuria.

Clinistix, Diastix, and Tes-Tape measurements of glycosuria are based on reactions of an enzyme, glucose oxidase, with glucose; thus they are specific tests for glucose in contrast to Clinitest. They too are read by comparison to color charts. Patients often value their convenience. Diastix and Keto-Diastix are paper-impregnated plastic strips which are dipped *quickly* in urine (2 s) and read *while held in air* after a specified time period (30 s). Clinistix is read in 10 s and has only three color gradations. One inch and a half of paper tape from the Tes-Tape roll is partially dipped in urine and read *while held in air* at either 1 or

2 min. With the combination Keto-Diastix, it is important that the glucose be read at 30 s and the ketones be read at 15 s.

With Tes-Tape, a yellow-to-green color change at 1 min indicates 1¼ percent (2+); a change to dark green at 2 min indicates a glucose content of ½ percent (3+) or more; and a darker greenish black color indicates 2 percent or more (4+). Selzer recommends that all 3+ reactions of Tes-Tape be read as 4+, since the difference in 3+ and 4+ is difficult to detect and sometimes full color development does not occur.[14]

These products can be tested for deterioration by using a solution of 1 tsp of freshly opened Coca-Cola or 7-Up mixed with ⅓ cup of water (instead of urine and water). When this solution is tested by Diastix or Keto-Diastix, the result should be ¼ to ½ percent if the product is performing accurately.[15] Moisture can cause these products to deteriorate, so patients should be taught to keep the containers tightly capped. Expiration dates should be checked on all test materials.

Choice of Urine Test   Two factors influence patient choice of test materials: cost and convenience. The tape and dip sticks require little equipment beyond the test material and a watch. Many patients learn simply to dip the stick or tape into the stream of urine rather than to collect a specimen. The importance of careful timing should be emphasized when this method is used. Clinitest tablets in bulk (100 tablets per bottle) and Tes-Tape (100 tests per spool) are the least expensive to purchase, while Diastix and individually wrapped Clinitest tablets are more expensive.

The choice of urine test is sometimes determined by drug interactions. False-positive Clinitests can result when large amounts of vitamin C are taken, when more than six tablets of aspirin are used daily, and with the use of such other drugs as Gantrisin, injected tetracycline, levodopa, Benemid, isoniazid, NeGram, and p-aminosalicyclic acid (PASA). Selzer states that no false-negatives occur with Clinitest; however, glucose may not be detected accurately when certain drugs are used with Tes-Tape or Diastix, e.g., ascorbic acid, salicylates, levodopa, and Pyridium. No false-positives occur with Tes-Tape or Diastix according to Selzer.[16] Cephalosporins (e.g., Keflex) often cause color reactions with Clinitest that are difficult to read.

The ability to perform urine tests often influences the choice of test. Particular assessment is made of visual ability: Can the patient see individual drops fall for the Clinitest method? Can he or she identify color changes? One patient who labeled himself color-blind was able to differentiate the extreme color changes of negative and 5 to 10 percent with Clinitest. Color changes seem easiest to read with Clinitest. However, the Ames Company has recently announced a new product that is designed for the visually handicapped person. Mega-Diastix has a bigger test area (¾ in²) and larger color blocks for easier reading. Instruction sheets are also printed in large type. Changes in visual ability occur during periods of excessive hyperglycemia. For the diabetic being regulated, therefore, another person may be needed to carry out the testing.

Because of the transient nature of these visual changes, however, the diabetic may be able to test his or her urine after control is established.

Besides lack of visual ability, certain mental deficits, such as memory loss for recent events, inability to incorporate a time schedule into daily living, or inability to concentrate on completion of a task, may be present. Diabetics with these deficits should be helped with testing and evaluation of the results, as well as with supervision of other self-care activities.

The diabetic with a hand dysfunction because of weakness or tremors may need special adaptations to manipulate equipment. If he or she is independent in toileting, hygiene, and eating, he or she can usually learn to test urine. Increasing the stability of the urine container and the hand can facilitate independence and accuracy in the number of drops of urine and water. Placing the test tube in a heavier container such as a water glass or a test tube rack adds stability, as does resting the forearm on a firm surface. Tes-Tape or a dipstick may be easier for this person. Clinitest tablets can be purchased in a bottle with a regular cap if Clinitest is required by a patient with a disabled hand.

Frequency   The minimal frequency with which a diabetic must test urine and the kind of test depend on the judgment of the primary care provider. Considered are: renal threshold, stability of blood glucose, resistance or "proneness" to ketoacidosis and/or hypoglycemia, and the appraisal of the diabetic's ability and/or willingness to comply with the proposed schedule. The period of regulating blood glucose levels in the new diabetic serves to establish a habit of testing at specified times. A testing schedule may increase the ability of the asymptomatic diabetic who feels well to incorporate regularity of food and activity into his or her life-style. By repeated attention to urine testing, the patient has repetitive reminders that his or her diabetic status now requires surveillance. Since most asymptomatic diabetics are obese and should lose weight, frequent testing for glycosuria may be useful in their perception of the need to change behavior. Once satisfied that a diabetic has relatively stable blood glucose, that he or she is not prone to ketoacidosis and/or hypoglycemia, and that he or she is reasonably compliant with diet, the physician may decrease the frequency of testing to once or twice daily.

Initially, testing four times a day is prescribed (before breakfast, lunch, dinner, and bedtime snack). This is true for the newly diagnosed diabetic whether hospitalized or not. Frequent daily testing is necessary for the diabetic with unstable blood sugar.

Testing for Acetone   This should be a skill available to all diabetics. Usually new diabetics are taught to test for ketonuria as well as glycosuria. Those diabetics who have stable blood sugars, are nonketotic, and are resistant to hypoglycemia may test for acetone only when the level of glycosuria is increased over the usual pattern or when they feel ill.

Testing for ketonuria can be done by Acetest tablets or the more convenient Ketostix or Keto-Diastix dipsticks. Color changes indicate relative presence of ketones: "trace," "small," "moderate," or "large." No percentages are used in either of these tests. One particular disadvantage of Keto-Diastix is that moderate or large amounts of ketones may interfere with the reaction for glucose, thus low readings may result. Rechecking the urine by Clinitest is advised when the Keto-Diastix indicates ketonuria. The glucose test is read in 30 s, while the ketone test is read in 15 s.

The Acetest tablet is placed on a piece of white paper, one drop of urine is added directly to the tablet, and in 30 s the color change of the tablet is compared to the Acetest color chart. Acetest tablets should be white and completely absorb one drop of urine.

Moisture can affect the performance of these test materials also, and patients should therefore store them properly. To test Diastix for product performance, Ames Company recommends testing a strip in a solution of ¼ tsp of freshly opened Cutex or Revlon nail polish mixed with ⅔ cup water. A reading less than "small" or a color development quite different from that on the color chart indicates that the test strips should be replaced.[17]

Most often the patient tests a *single specimen* of urine. A first morning specimen, prior to breakfast, is tested to measure the level of nocturnal, or fasting, glycosuria, while other specimens are tested to measure amounts of postprandial glycosuria. Both fasting and postprandial results are useful in determining whether treatment measures are adequate. The pattern of glycosuria is used to determine modifications of insulin type and dosage and distribution of food. When second-voided specimens are tested, they indicate the amount of glycosuria at a specified time; patients are taught to void 30 to 60 min prior to testing, drink a glass of water, and then collect the specimen at the specified time. Less precise information is gained from testing urine that has collected in the bladder over a period of hours and would be tested if a first-voided specimen were collected.

Sometimes patients will be asked to collect all urine voided during certain hours (or for 24 h). They then test a sample(s) or take the sample(s) to the physician. *Fractional* urines might be collected between 7:30 and 11:30 A.M., 11:30 A.M. and 4 P.M., 4 and 9 P.M., 9 P.M. and 6 A.M., and 6 and 7:30 A.M. Testing these five samples can give information about the pattern of glycosuria and ketonuria. In addition, quantitative measurement can be made of the amount of glucose and ketones lost in the urine when fractional or 24-h urine collections are used. (Refer to pages 183 and 188.)

Record Keeping   Urine testing results are recorded on a sheet that relates time and test results sequentially. Most urine-testing diaries have spaces for recording insulin or hypoglycemic medication, food intake, and special comments about occurrence of symptoms of hyperglycemia or hypoglycemia. Many primary care providers, hospitals, diabetes clinics, and other health care agencies design and duplicate their own forms. Commercially prepared forms are also available.

Regardless of the particular form of recording, the information should be such that a retrospective review is possible. Both the health care provider and the diabetic use this information to decide whether changes are necessary in the therapeutic measures. The diabetic is advised to present the urine-test record to any health care provider he or she contacts. Problems in recording urine tests most often result from a lack of understanding of the purpose of the information or a lack of commitment. Reinforcement of both testing and recording can be given by a show of approval, discussion of the test record, and use of the information in planning.

Seeking Consultation The diabetic should know which actions to take when glycosuria is above a specified level and acetone is present. Several actions are possible when the patient is well educated:

1 Test more frequently
2 Increase dosage of regular insulin
3 Note whether there is polyuria, thirst, hunger, and drowsiness
4 Note whether there are other changes in health status
5 Call the health care provider

The newly diagnosed diabetic is often told to call the physician if the urine test is "orange" and acetone is present. This may be the only realistic direction to the new diabetic in ambulatory care because of the complexity of other alternatives. Directions can then be given for self-care or arrangement can be made for a visit for further evaluation and treatment.

Ideally patients are taught to read and record urine tests in percentage rather than by color or plus signs. Variations among the tests can be misleading (see Table 8-5). For example, ½% glucose concentration is 1+ by the Clinitest 5-drop method, 2+ by the Diastix, and 3+ by Tes-Tape (plus signs are not available for the Clinitest 2-drop method). It should be noted that Clinistix is less precise than others because it does not determine percentage but only the relative presence of glucose. Test results of 4+ on the Clinitest 5-drop method, Diastix, and Tes-Tape all indicate 2 percent or more glucose concentrations. (Of these, only the 2-drop Clinitest method can differentiate above 2 percent).

Table 8-5 Comparison of Readings with Various Urine-Sugar (Glucose) Tests

Product	Glucose concentration							
	1/10%	1/4%	1/2%	3/4%	1%	2%	3%	5%
Clinitest, 5-drop		Tr	+	++	+++	++++		
Clinitest, 2-drop*			‡		‡	‡	‡	‡
Diastix	Tr	+	++		+++	++++		
Clinistix†	Light (+)		Medium (++)		Dark (+++)			
Tes-Tape	+	++	+++			++++		

* The 2-drop chart provides a "trace" color block without a percent value; a trace result only indicates less than ½%.
† Estimates relative presence of glucose, but cannot show percent amount.
‡ Measures percent at these levels, but equivalent + signs not available.
Note: Blank spaces mean color blocks are absent for those concentrations.
Source: Ames Company, Division of Miles Laboratories, Home Urine Testing for the Diabetic, p. 7, 1976.

The more knowledgeable the diabetic is about symptoms of hyperglycemia and the warning signs of ketoacidosis, the more able he or she is to make valid decisions about the need for consultation with the physician. The diabetic and the members of the family who have learned to *evaluate* the diabetic's health status and *respond appropriately* to increased glycosuria and/or ketonuria are able to use all the preceding options. When signs of ketosis appear, they may increase the insulin dosage within the limits set by the physician and call the physician when signs of ketosis persist. Figure 8-4 illustrates directions for the handling of minor illness. (Refer to Chapter 6 for modifications in food.)

In the adult, changes from ketosis to ketoacidosis may occur over hours to days. This change contrasts with the rapidity of an insulin reaction. The insulin-treated patient and key members of his or her family must know the required response to an insulin reaction, i.e., the administration of glucose. There are no options for delay, except to obtain glucose if it is not readily available. Glucagon may be prescribed for home emergency use also.

Figures 8-5 and 8-6 illustrate types of identification items that are used by diabetics to alert others to their need for special attention. Carrying identification information is an essential part of self-care practice.

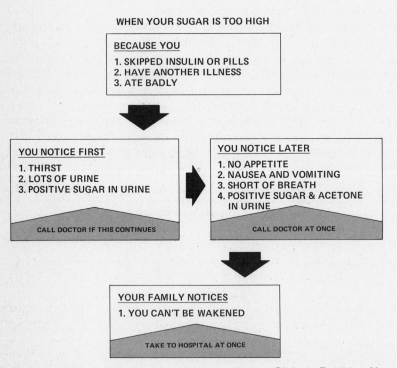

WHEN YOUR SUGAR IS TOO HIGH

BECAUSE YOU

1. SKIPPED INSULIN OR PILLS
2. HAVE ANOTHER ILLNESS
3. ATE BADLY

YOU NOTICE FIRST

1. THIRST
2. LOTS OF URINE
3. POSITIVE SUGAR IN URINE

CALL DOCTOR IF THIS CONTINUES

YOU NOTICE LATER

1. NO APPETITE
2. NAUSEA AND VOMITING
3. SHORT OF BREATH
4. POSITIVE SUGAR & ACETONE
   IN URINE

CALL DOCTOR AT ONCE

YOUR FAMILY NOTICES

1. YOU CAN'T BE WAKENED

TAKE TO HOSPITAL AT ONCE

Figure 8-4 Instructions for handling minor illness. *(Diabetic Teaching Manual, Mt. Sinai Hospital, Cleveland, Ohio.)*

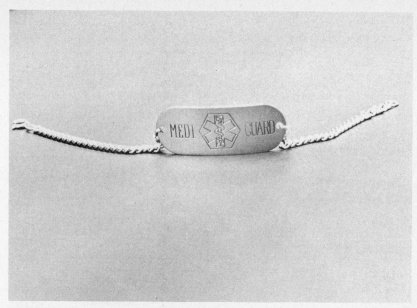

Figure 8-5 This identification bracelet is available from the New York Diabetes Association, 104 East 40th Street, New York, N.Y. 10016. On the reverse side, the tag bears the following information: name, emergency phone number, and the word *diabetic*. Additional wording can be added at extra cost over the base cost of $7.24.

Hygiene

The diabetic person can ill afford to omit hygienic practices that are considered healthful for all people. There are few hygienic "rules" that are special for the diabetic person. However, more severe complications may occur from injury and infection in the diabetic person, hence attention to self-care hygienic practices is an important consideration in assessment of teaching needs.

Skin that is supple, clean, and free from lesions is a barrier to bacterial invasion. In the elderly diabetic with dry skin, daily washing may be as deleterious as infrequent washing in the younger diabetic who actively perspires and receives more frequent "minor" skin wounds.

Areas of intertrigo or chafing may occur when there is rubbing of moist skin surfaces; this develops more frequently in those who are obese. Two areas of intertrigo are more frequent in women: perineum and thighs and the chest wall under pendulous breasts. Intertrigo is not only a source of discomfort but predisposes the diabetic patient to more serious infection of fungi or bacteria. The obese patient may be unable to cleanse or inspect areas easily, and may therefore benefit from suggestions about "airing," types of clothing, and cleansing and drying measures. For example, the patient with perineal inflammation can be taught to flush with tap water after each voiding, gently dry the area, and position so that air can reach all surfaces. The best rule for intertrigo is to avoid home remedies other than cleansing, drying, and airing. Certainly,

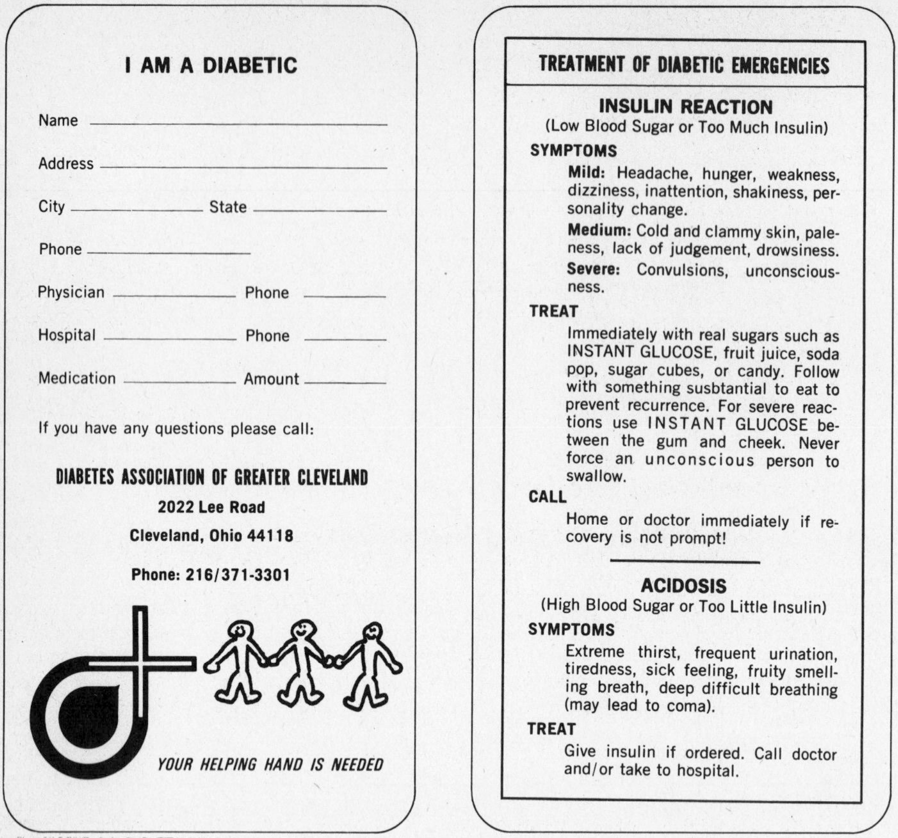

I AM A DIABETIC

Name _____

Address _____

City _____ State _____

Phone _____

Physician _____ Phone _____

Hospital _____ Phone _____

Medication _____ Amount _____

If you have any questions please call:

DIABETES ASSOCIATION OF GREATER CLEVELAND

2022 Lee Road

Cleveland, Ohio 44118

Phone: 216/371-3301

YOUR HELPING HAND IS NEEDED

TREATMENT OF DIABETIC EMERGENCIES

INSULIN REACTION
(Low Blood Sugar or Too Much Insulin)

SYMPTOMS

Mild: Headache, hunger, weakness, dizziness, inattention, shakiness, personality change.

Medium: Cold and clammy skin, paleness, lack of judgement, drowsiness.

Severe: Convulsions, unconsciousness.

TREAT

Immediately with real sugars such as INSTANT GLUCOSE, fruit juice, soda pop, sugar cubes, or candy. Follow with something susbtantial to eat to prevent recurrence. For severe reactions use INSTANT GLUCOSE between the gum and cheek. Never force an unconscious person to swallow.

CALL

Home or doctor immediately if recovery is not prompt!

ACIDOSIS
(High Blood Sugar or Too Little Insulin)

SYMPTOMS

Extreme thirst, frequent urination, tiredness, sick feeling, fruity smelling breath, deep difficult breathing (may lead to coma).

TREAT

Give insulin if ordered. Call doctor and/or take to hospital.

Figure 8-6 Wallet cards for identification are furnished by many diabetes associations and pharmaceutical companies. This card, produced by the Diabetes Association of Greater Cleveland, also provides directions for treatment of diabetic emergencies. (Instant Glucose is available from this agency.)

diabetics with persistent or increasing signs of inflammation should report them to their physician.

Foot Care   Health care professionals and many lay people can give vivid examples of amputation following minor injury in diabetic individuals. Inadequate or dangerous home remedies often precede physician visits and delay treatment. The establishment of *daily* inspection and *daily* care of the feet is a major goal in educating the diabetic. Keeping feet clean, dry, and free from lesions and keeping the skin supple are a good practice for all people. The diabetic individual may have vascularly deprived tissue that is less resistant to infection, and many have diminished ability to perceive injury or infection (see Chapter 10). Foot care should be taught early to all diabetics so that it becomes routine. Protocols for teaching of foot care principles and methods are readily available (see Chapter 9). Most lists of dos and don'ts are similar to those of Dr. Joslin reported in 1929 in the *American Journal of Nursing:*

Hygiene of the Feet

1 Wash feet daily with soap and water. Dry thoroughly, especially between toes, using pressure rather than vigorous rubbing.

2 When thoroughly dry, rub well with hydrous lanolin as often as necessary to keep skin soft, supple, and free from scales and dryness, but never render the feet tender.

3 If the feet become too soft, rub once a day with alcohol.

4 If nails are brittle and dry, soften by soaking in warm water, one-half hour each night; apply lanolin generously under and about nails and bandage loosely. Clean nails with orange wood sticks. Cut the nails only when very clean. Cut the nails straight across to avoid injury to the toes. If you go to a chiropodist, tell him you have diabetes.

5 Wear shoes of soft leather which fit and are not tight (neither narrow nor short). Wear new shoes one-half hour only on the first day and increase one hour daily.

Treatment of Corns and Callosities

1 Wear shoes which fit and cause no pressure.

2 Soak foot in warm, not hot, soapy water. Rub off with gauze . . . dead , skin on or about callus or corn. Do not tear it off.

3 Do not cut corns or callosities.

4 Prevent calluses under ball of foot:
   a By exercises such as curling and stretching toes 20 times a day
   b By finishing each step on the toes and not on the ball of the foot

Aids in Treatment of Imperfect Circulation

Cold Feet:

1 Exercises. Bend the foot down and up as far as it will go six times. Describe a circle to the left with the foot six times, and then to the right. Repeat morning, noon, and night.

2 Massage with lanolin or cocoa butter.

3 Do not wear circular garters. Do not sit with knees crossed.

Treatment of Abrasions of the Skin

1 Proper first-aid treatment is of the utmost importance even in apparently minor injuries. Consult your physician immediately.

2 Avoid strong irritating antiseptics. . . .

3 Elevate and, as much as possible until recovery, avoid using the foot.

4 Consult your doctor for any redness, pain, swelling, or other evidence of inflammation.[18]

Education about foot care should focus on particular hazards in the daily life of the individual and provide guidance for incorporating foot care in the home, work, and play environment. More frequent inspection, change of socks and shoes, and use of protective foot gear may be indicated when patients report that (1) their feet are often cold and wet, or moist and warm, (2) they go barefoot, (3) they frequently receive "minor" injuries. Some patients may have to revamp priorities about use of money to purchase shoes that give support, fit well, and allow for a change of shoes.

Yearly consultation with a podiatrist is recommended. This may be done by referral by the private physician or clinic or by seeking the services of podiatrists in private or group practice in the community. As vascular and neuropathic complications develop, the use of podiatry services are often effective in minimizing and delaying disability.

Dental Hygiene* It is advisable for the diabetic patient to have regular oral and dental examinations and prophylaxes so that good oral health, once established, can be maintained. The tissues of the oral cavity can be sensitive indicators of the general health status. Certainly, the oral mucous membranes are affected by pathologic processes which affect other body systems.

The oral symptom complex which can be associated with diabetes is a reflection of the metabolic, nutritional, and vascular problems the diabetic patient presents. These symptoms include xerostomia, loss of lingual filiform papillae, gingival swelling and hyperemia, and oral and perioral burning sensations. Also, periodontitis seems to be more severe in the diabetic and its onset is earlier, with alveolar bone loss as one of the first signs. This accounts for the complaint of loose teeth with which the diabetic patient may present. Generally, diabetics do not show an unusually high dental caries incidence.

Dental consultation should be a basic, routine part of the diabetic's treatment program. A specific system of home oral hygiene practices (brushing, flossing, and gingival massage) should be outlined so as to eliminate all local irritants from the teeth and soft tissues.

Since proper nutrition is such a vital part of the treatment program for diabetics, oral and dental abnormalities should be corrected so that the foods in the prescribed diet can be properly chewed as an aid to normal digestion, absorption, and utilization.

Insulin Administration

Chapter 9 discusses the development of teaching programs, including insulin administration. It is assumed that the reader is skilled in the technique of subcutaneous injections to another person. Special considerations are necessary when self-injections are done daily or more frequently. Both knowledge and skill are necessary if the patient is to use insulin safely. Early identification of those patients requiring initial instruction or reeducation is necessary so that the patient can be both skilled and knowledgeable by discharge. Assisting the patient in giving his or her first injection requires skill in support as well as technique. Fear and hesitancy must be overcome before the patient can focus on manipulative skills. For adults, assistance with self-injection is the first step before details of syringe preparation are given and practice with it is started. Once adults have injected themselves they can proceed with the acquisition of other necessary skills.

---

* This section was written by Theodore A. DiSantis, D.D.S., Staff, Euclid Clinic Foundation, Assistant Clinical Professor, Case Western Reserve University School of Dentistry, Cleveland, Ohio.

The questions in the assessment model in Fig. 8-6 are helpful in determining the need for instruction in patients not new to insulin therapy. These questions are not sufficient, however; actual demonstration by the patient of his or her practice with insulin injection is essential.

Errors   Errors in administration of insulin are more likely to occur than errors with other medications because of the multiple kinds and strengths of insulin and the differing scales on various syringes. Until U-100 insulin concentrations and U-100 syringes (100 U/mL and 50 U per 0.5 mL) become standard and U-80 and U-40 products are phased out, errors from mismatching syringe and insulin concentration can continue to occur. It is necessary to ask patients what kind of syringe they use; some are still using glass dual-scaled syringes (U-40 and U-80), and some will report using syringes which do not correspond to the strength of insulin they are now using.

The patient should be able to check that the purchased insulin is the same as that prescribed—both by type and concentration—and that it matches the unit dosage on the syringes. The patient must know that errors in dosage can result either in insulin reaction or in increased hyperglycemia—even ketoacidosis. Although patients need not know all the details of other insulin preparations, it is essential that they understand that others exist and differ in strength and length of action. In addition, they must know to check expiration dates.

Other errors can occur if the technique of preparing the syringe is faulty or inconsistent. While an air bubble is commonly used to clear the needle after injecting an intramuscular medication, this is not done with a subcutaneous injection which contains a small amount of liquid. In this injection, the use of an air bubble results in a significant change of dosage if the syringe and needle contain much dead space.* For example, if the syringe and needle contain 0.1 mL dead space, an increase of 10 U of insulin would be injected (if U-100 insulin was the prescribed strength) if an air bubble were used to clear the syringe and needle. Patients need supervised practice to learn how to expel all air prior to measuring the insulin in the syringe.

When mixtures of short-acting and longer-acting insulins are prescribed, another problem involving dead space can develop. Whichever insulin is withdrawn into the syringe first, an amount of that insulin equal to the dead space of the syringe is also withdrawn as the second insulin is pulled into the syringe. (After the plunger is pushed in all the way, a mixture of the two insulins remains in the dead space.) If the sequence of withdrawing insulin is changed, changes occur in the amounts of both the insulins. Consistency in the daily dose can be achieved only if the same sequence is followed. Because syringes and needles differ in the amount of dead space they contain, changing to another type of syringe can result in an inadvertent change of dosage. For this reason, patients

---

* *Dead space* refers to that area of the syringe tip and bore of the needle which contain insulin after the plunger is pushed all the way in.

are advised to use only the type prescribed. Refer to Chapter 9 for further details of teaching insulin administration.

Rotation of Needle Insertion Sites   Because daily injections are usually continued for life, it is very important that the patient use as many injection sites as possible in order to avoid frequent reuse of the same site, which can lead to decreased absorption and cosmetic disfigurement. An informed patient understands that reuse can cause changes in blood glucose control and that tissue in the area may become enlarged and hardened (lipohypertrophy) or may become hollowed out (lipoatrophy). Some patients incorrectly continue to use a site that has had tissue hypertrophy or atrophy because they discover they experience less pain in these sites.

The nurse can assist the patient in developing a workable plan for remembering past injection sites in the selection of the current site. A stick figure is useful in quickly determining not only the general areas used but also whether there is a planned sequence for using the areas (see Fig. 8-7). Many patients can report no plan other than alternating thighs from day to day, as illustrated in Fig. 8-7. Inspection and palpation of those areas used can also indicate whether tissue changes are occurring and reinforce in the patient the need to avoid the same site. (In some instances, the physician may prescribe trial injections of U-100 insulin into areas of atrophy. This practice is based on findings that in some patients, growth of atrophied tissue can be stimulated.[19])

First, the patient must grasp the idea that each of the areas shown in Fig. 8-8 can yield 10 to 20 *needle insertion sites* and that these are the sites to be

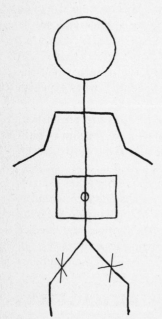

Figure 8-7   A stick figure for quickly assessing those sites generally used by diabetics for injecting insulin. This patient could indicate no other sites than thighs and could not indicate any sequence.

rotated. Moving a 1-in-diameter paper circle over the arm, leg, abdomen, etc., is useful in teaching this concept. Also, an insertion guide is available that illustrates eight insertion points for each area in a similar manner. This guide also includes a log for recording insertion sites.[20] Patients can record the site used on the urine-testing record or on a calendar for easy reference. Some patients may mark the skin or use a small adhesive strip to identify the next injection site.

Second, the nurse can assist the patient in determining the number of insertion points that can be used and the sequence to follow in each area. Sufficient sites should be used so that at least 1 to 2 months elapse before that site is reused. Patients differ in size of available areas and in dexterity. For example, a right-handed person often is unable to inject the right arm and must stabilize the tissue of the left arm on a chair back, table, or wall in order to inject it. Many patients need to use the abdomen in order to have sufficient numbers of insertion sites, or they need to have another person give injections in the posterior sites.

A recent study suggests that athletes engaging in vigorous exercise which uses leg muscles might have less chance of incurring hypoglycemia if they use the abdomen or arm for injection rather than the legs. Seven of eight insulin-

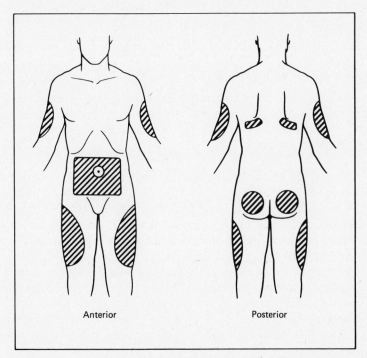

Anterior   Posterior

Figure 8-8 Commonly used sites for insulin injection. *(Adapted from D. A. Jones, C. F. Dunbar, and N. M. Jirovec, "Medical-Surgical Nursing: A Conceptual Approach," New York, McGraw-Hill, 1978, p. 685.)* Authorities differ on whether upper or lower abdomen is preferable. The belt area is avoided since skin there may be thickened.

dependent diabetics who injected insulin in the legs had marked increase in insulin absorption while using a cycle ergometer.[21]

Angle and Depth of Insertion   The end of the needle should neither be in muscle nor close to the skin; it should be closer to muscle than to the skin. The angle of insertion depends on the depth of the fatty tissue in the chosen site: when little fat is present, a short needle (⅜ or ½ in) is inserted at an angle near 45° and the site pinched or folded. Using a longer needle (⅝ or ⅞ in), an angle of 90°, and stretching the skin allow deeper deposition when more fat is present.

Burke has described a different method, in which insulin is injected under the fat pad in the "space" or "pocket" between fat layer and muscle, and reports that fewer localized reactions or atrophy occur when this method is used.[22] The depth of insertion and needle length are determined by measuring the distance of the base of folded tissue, and an angle of 25° is routinely used. For example, a 1½-in needle is used if the width of the fat fold is 1½ in, and the needle is inserted through the base of the fold.

One should be careful that the patient is not confused by the unnecessary introduction of different techniques. The patient needs a safe way of injecting insulin. Simple cleansing of the skin and top of the vial, handling the syringe and needle so that sterility is maintained, and drawing up the accurate dosage are important in meeting this goal. Many descriptions of procedures are available that differ only in small details; it is usually wise, therefore, if one standard procedure is agreed on by nurses who work together in teaching a patient or groups of patients.

New patients on insulin therapy commonly use disposable syringes and needles; these are more convenient yet more costly over a period of time. Cotton in bulk or balls and a bottle of 70% alcohol are less expensive than individually wrapped alcohol swabs.

Sterilization   If the patient chooses a reusable glass syringe, he or she may use disposable or reusable needles. Some patients reuse disposable syringes and needles to save money; this practice can result in the distortion of syringe markings if the syringes are boiled or kept in alcohol and in dull or breaking needles. When reusable products are chosen, the patient should learn a sterilization technique. Boiling the syringe and needle for 10 min can be done daily prior to injection or at weekly intervals if the syringe and needle are kept immersed in 70% alcohol between injections. (A small covered jar is filled with alcohol, cotton is placed in the bottom so that the needle point is protected, and a string is wrapped around the syringe so that it can be pulled out. Air drying is accomplished by pulling the piston back and forth several times prior to drawing up the insulin.)

Prior to boiling, the syringe and needle are washed with soap and water. If cloudy deposits appear, soaking in vinegar can restore clarity of the syringe or a tablespoon of baking soda or vinegar can be added to the water used to cover the syringe and needle. If reusable needles are chosen, the patient can check their sharpness at this time. A strainer that can fit in a saucepan is useful for boiling a syringe and needle. The needle is inserted through the mesh of the strainer with the piston and barrel separated and laid in the strainer. After boiling for 10 min, the strainer is removed, the water emptied, and the strainer replaced in the pan until the equipment is cool. No forceps is necessary to place the barrel into the hub of the needle and then to insert the piston—only the ends of the piston and barrel need be touched. The syringe and needle are then ready for use or for immersion into the cleaned, boiled, and refilled alcohol container.

SUMMARY

This chapter has presented the nursing care requirements of diabetic patients who are hospitalized. While a minority will be admitted for acute disorders of insulin deficit or insulin excess, the potential for metabolic imbalance is a concern of all hospitalized diabetics. Skilled nursing care includes expertise in corrective and supportive measures for the patient in physiological crisis.

Hospitalized diabetics also benefit when nurses use time of recuperation to assist them to review and learn how to improve their diabetic management after discharge. Patient care outcome and assessment models provide a basis for determining the needs for education, counseling, referral, and interdisciplinary consultation.

The extent to which a patient has achieved desired patient outcomes is documented in the patient's record. Supportive interventions are also documented when patients are unable to achieve the desired goals. Not all patients have the capacity for achieving self-confidence and competence in the management of diabetes. Some may never achieve safe self-care; some need continual assistance by family members or other caretakers. Communication with those responsible after discharge may be by written referrals or phone consultation.

Chapter 9 explores the development of educational programs for the hospitalized diabetic. Education can be provided during hospitalization of the diabetic if assessment of learning needs is systematic and nurses are committed to the teaching role. Beginning the teaching early in hospitalization is necessary, and as the day of discharge approaches, the energy of the patient and family should be directed toward resumption of an interrupted life and the specific matters of discharge. It is generally ineffective to use that day for introduction of new knowledge or skills; however, review of plans for the next 24 h is often helpful to both patient and family.

REFERENCES

1 Vander, A., Sherman, J., and Luciano, D. *Human Physiology: Mechanisms of Body Functions* (New York: McGraw-Hill, 1975), pp. 166, 270, and 271.

2 *Standards of Nursing Care for Patients with Diabetes Mellitus.* Department of Medical-Surgical Nursing, University Hospitals of Cleveland, Ohio, 1976.

3 Beaser, S. B. Surgical management, in M. Ellenberg and H. Rifkin (eds.), *Diabetes Mellitus: Theory and Practice* (New York: McGraw-Hill, 1970), p. 749.

4 Steinke, J. Management of diabetes mellitus and surgery, *N. Engl. J. Med.,* **282:**1472, 1970.

5 Steinke, J., and Soeldner, J. S. Diabetes mellitus, in Thorn et al. (eds.), *Harrison's Principles of Internal Medicine* (New York, McGraw-Hill, 1977), pp. 563–583.

6 *Standards of Nursing Care.* Loc. cit.

7 Admission Information. Department of Medical-Surgical Nursing, University Hospitals of Cleveland, Ohio, 1976.

8 Sims, D., and Sims, E. H. Exercise and diet = good health, *Diabetes Forecast,* **29:** 24, 1976.

9 Berger, H. Hypoglycemia: a perspective, *Postgrad. Med.,* **57:**83, 1975.

10 Jellinek, O. M. Phases of alcohol addiction, *Q. J. Stud. Alcohol,* **13:**673–684, 1952.

11 Leifson, J. Glycosuria tests performed by diabetics at home, *Pub. Health,* **84:**28–32, 1969.

12 Derr, S. Testing for glycosuria, *Am. J. Nurs.,* **70:**1513, 1970.

13 Dobson, H. L., et al. Accuracy of urine testing for sugar and acetone by hospital ward personnel, *Diabetes,* **17:**281–285, 1968.

14 Selzer, H. S. Urinary glucose tests: a consumer's guide, *Diabetes Forecast,* **30:**25–27, 1977.

15 Ames Company, Division of Miles Laboratories, Inc. *Home Urine Testing for the Diabetic, Instructional Aid for Diabetes Educators,* 1976, p. 12.

16 Selzer. Loc. cit.

17 Ames Company. Op. cit., p. 7.

18 Moores, W. The care of the diabetic, *Am. J. Nurs.,* **29:**499–503, 1929.

19 Galloway, J. A. Insulin therapy, in *Diabetes in Review: Clinical Conference, 1976.* American Diabetes Association and the American Diabetes Association, New England Affiliate, Inc., p. 42.

20 Becton, Dickinson and Company. An illustrated step-by-step introduction to proper site selection and preparation for insulin injections.

21 Koivisto, V. A., and Felig, P. Effects of leg exercise on insulin absorption in diabetic patients. *N. Engl. J. Med.,* **298:**79–83, 1978.

22 Burke, E. L. Insulin injection—the site and the technique, *Am. J. Nurs.,* **72:**2194, 1972.

BIBLIOGRAPHY

American Nurses' Association. *1973 Standards of Nursing Practice.* American Nurses' Association, Kansas City, 1973.

Beland, I., and J. Passos. *Clinical Nursing: Pathophysiology and Psychosocial Approaches.* New York, Macmillan, 1975.

Danowski, T. J. Diabetic acidosis and coma, in M. Ellenberg and H. Rifkin (eds.), *Diabetes Mellitus: Theory and Practice.* New York, McGraw-Hill, 1970, pp. 674–681.

Fajans, S. S. (ed.). *Diabetes Mellitus,* Fogarty International Center Series on Preventive Medicine, vol. 4. DHEW Publication No. (NIH) 76-854, 1976.

Guthrie, D. W., and R. T. Guthrie. *Nursing Management of Diabetes Mellitus*. St. Louis, Mosby, 1977.

Haunz, E. A. Diabetes mellitus in adults, in H. F. Conn (ed.), *Current Therapy, 1973*. Philadelphia, Saunders, 1973, pp. 365–385.

Hornback, M. Diabetes mellitus—the nurse's role, *Nurs. Clin. North Am.,* **55**:3–12, 1970.

Haung, S. Nursing assessment in planning care for a diabetic patient, *Nurs. Clin. North Am.,* **6**:135–142, 1971.

Jones, D. A., C. F. Dunbar, and M. M. Jirovec. *Medical-Surgical Nursing: A Conceptual Approach*. New York, McGraw-Hill, 1978.

Lawrence, P., and M. Gebhardt. Is dead space really dead? *Diabetes Forecast*, **30**:12–14, 1977.

Martin, M. M. Insulin reactions, *Am. J. Nurs.,* **67**:328–331, 1967.

Matz, R. Coma in the nonketotic diabetic, in M. Ellenberg and H. Rifkin (eds.), *Diabetes Mellitus: Theory and Practice*. New York, McGraw-Hill, 1970, pp. 684–690.

Meltzer, L., et al. *Intensive Coronary Care: A Manual for Nurses*. Philadelphia, Charles Press, 1975, pp. 106–115.

Nursing 77 Books. *Managing Diabetics Properly*. Intermed Communications, Horsham, Pa., 1977.

Shafer, K. N., et al. *Medical-Surgical Nursing,* 6th ed. St. Louis, Mosby, 1975, pp. 745–769.

Simon, J. and M. Stewart. Assessing patient knowledge about diabetes, *Mt. Sinai J. of Med.,* **43**:189–202, 1976.

Snyder, V. Cognitive approaches in the treatment of alcoholism, *Social Casework,* **56**:480–485, 1975.

Stuart, S. Day to day living with diabetes, *Am. J. Nurs.,* **71**(8):1548–1549, 1971.

Sussman, K. E., and R. J. S. Metz (eds.). *Diabetes Mellitus,* 4th ed. New York, American Diabetes Association, Inc., 1975.

Watkins, J. D., and F. I. Moss. Confusion in the management of diabetes, *Am. J. Nurs.,* **69**(3):521–524, 1969.

Williams, R. *Textbook of Endocrinology,* 5th ed. Philadelphia, Saunders, 1974.

Chapter 9

Elements of the Teaching Program

Carol E. Hartman

Since the management of the diabetic requires daily self-care, the importance of education for the diabetic patient has long been recognized. However, added emphasis for considering diabetic education as an *integral* part of treatment has come from the National Commission on Diabetes.[1] They found inadequacies in diabetic education resulting in poor management. Among their recommendations is one that health professionals in every patient care setting use a planned approach to meet patients' educational needs. It is critical for people with a lifelong disease such as diabetes to understand their disease and their special health care needs. When the well-educated diabetic applies knowledge and understanding of the disease in everyday self-care, the effects of diabetes can usually be regulated well enough for the person to lead an active, satisfying life. The incidence of hospitalizations for diabetic complications also decreases. Lack of proper management on a day-to-day basis, however, can result in repeated crises, a higher risk of death and chronic complications, restricted activities, and damaging psychosocial effects.

Adequate education is necessary to control the disease and to avoid such acute metabolic crises as hypoglycemia, hyperglycemia, and ketoacidosis. Education to decrease the risk factors of atherosclerosis and to delay complications is also important. For the optimal well-being of people with diabetes, their everyday habits should contribute positively to their health.

Inadequate teaching programs resulting from poor planning and/or inadequate information account for some of the gaps in knowledge and self-care practices of diabetic people. Inconsistencies by health professionals certainly explain some of the confusion and poor management practices of patients and their families. Other problems of patient education for diabetic management relate to physical changes such as decreased visual acuity, poor memory, and diminished touch sensation. Further problems result from failures in educational evaluation and follow-up of initial diabetic education, often leaving many of the learning needs unidentified and uncorrected.

Many different approaches to diabetic education have been tried. Because the self-care of diabetes involves many fields of expertise, the use of teaching teams benefits the patient. Good planning and communication among the team members is essential. Lack of consistency in expectations can lead to confusion, frustration, and apathy on the part of the patient. Some programs focus on individualized teaching; others use group teaching. Audiovisual aids have been used in both the group and individual approaches. Some programs have a purely educational function, with no provision for ongoing diabetic management, while others incorporate both the medical management and the educational aspects of diabetic control. The settings and length of time of educational offerings also are varied. In the Grady Memorial Hospital program, diabetics are brought into the Diabetes Day Care Center for a full day of education and medical evaluation. Some hospitals offer group classes for inpatients 4 or 5 days a week. These classes are usually about 1 h in length and the series is repeated weekly. It is not uncommon for families to be included, and sometimes after discharge from the hospital, the patient returns for the classes again. Often clinics will have group classes that are spaced 3 or 4 weeks apart to correspond with the patients' return visits. In many communities, several hospitals concentrate their educational efforts in one central place and patients and their families are referred from the cooperating hospitals. Local diabetes associations frequently sponsor ongoing education through seminars, workshops, and discussion groups. These associations are good resources for the diabetic and his or her family as well as for the health team members who are working with diabetics. Diabetes information and tapes on diabetic care are available through dial-access systems in some areas. Educational television has also been used for diabetes education.

INVOLVEMENT OF THE DIABETIC PERSON

Some of the problems of diabetic education relate to failure to gain active involvement of the diabetic in self-care. The purpose of a diabetic education program is to improve self-care practices, and thus it is necessary for the person to be involved in the learning process. One way of promoting involvement is for the diabetic person to contribute to the development of the goals and the means of achieving them. This mutual give-and-take of teacher and learner in deciding what learning is to be accomplished and how it will take place is a form of contract. What the health professionals think the person ought to know is shared and identified, as well as what the patient thinks she or he needs to know. The approach focuses first on those particular aspects of care which are of greatest concern for the patient.

One should remember that just giving information is not teaching, and that the learning process, or changing behavior, is usually slow. The speed of learning depends on content, the learner's ability, and the degree of motivation. A brief review of the components of the learning process provides a framework for a more specific discussion of diabetic learning. Woodruff lists the common sequential steps in the learning process as follows:[2]

1 Motivation from within makes the learner receptive to stimulation.
2 A goal becomes related to the motivation.
3 Tension arises and the learner is ready to act.
4 The learner seeks an appropriate line of action to reach the goal.
5 The learner fixes the appropriate line of action.
6 Inappropriate behaviors are dropped.

The steps are often not as clear-cut as the list implies, but they operate to some extent in any learning situation. One learns through meeting situations, trying out responses, and discovering the consequences of each response.

In making plans for a diabetic education program, the planner will find it useful to focus on important aspects of the teaching/learning process. In addition to content, one must consider the learner, the teacher, the teaching/learning climate, the learning objectives, the methods and learning materials, and the evaluation of the learning.

THE LEARNER

The learner should be the prime focus of an educational plan that is based on a realistic appraisal of the learner.* This means that one needs to identify the strengths of the person which can facilitate learning as well as the weaknesses which may be barriers to the learning process. In some situations it may be necessary to call on a family member or a friend to supplement self-care. These significant people then become the learners along with the patient.

ASSESSING THE LEARNER

The nurse uses all kinds of assessments and knowledge about diabetes and its control to identify the learning needs. Information about the patient, his or her customs, beliefs, interests, social groups, and past experiences with formal and informal learning as well as physical and mental capabilities gives clues for planning an effective learning program. To tailor a program for the learner

---

* Although the individual is the focus of the following discussion about the learner, the concepts can be applied to aggregates and groups.

requires that one take into consideration such things as age, living situation, and occupation. One often finds age-related differences that are important in planning and carrying out a teaching plan. In adults between the ages of 30 and 50 there is a slight decrease in the sensory, motor, and intellectual functions, with more pronounced changes apparent after age 60. With increasing age there is a loss of speed.

Individual variations also occur because of pathological changes and metabolic imbalances. Diminished visual acuity and changes in tactile sense in the diabetic patient can affect perceptions, and therefore, one may find it necessary to rely more heavily on hearing and movement as part of the teaching strategy. Decreased dexterity and a lower level of confidence may be found in the older diabetic. Motor skills are learned and performed slowly. In contrast, the young adult often has confidence and much dexterity. Motor skills are performed quickly by the younger adult. One must remember that there will be individual differences, and it is necessary to determine each person's capabilities.

One should find out what knowledge and skills the patient already has and what his or her current practices are. Using an interview guide will help ensure that information is collected about areas important for diabetic self-care. The use of open-ended questions allows the patient to expand on the information given. Actual practice of the diabetic may not be what is described verbally. Therefore, a part of the assessment of the diabetic should include direct observation of the self-care. To observe the person's everyday situation would be best; this is often impractical, however. Observation of such skills as foot care, urine testing, and insulin preparation and injection in the hospital or ambulatory setting can give the nurse valuable information.

Knowledge and skills of the patient are usually easier to determine than are values and attitudes, although these are major factors in effecting lasting behavior changes. How one spends time reflects tastes and values as well as lifestyle. "Tell me about a typical day" or "How do you spend your time?" often give valuable clues for learning needs as well as pointing up positive habits which should be reinforced. Possible barriers to diabetic self-care may be identified by obtaining information about the person's life-style. Asking which activities give the greatest satisfaction and which give the least may further elicit values and attitudes.

In working with a new diabetic, it is especially important to determine the person's perception of the disease. Such questions as, "Do you know anyone who has diabetes?" "How does that person get along?" and "How do you think diabetes will affect your life?" may help determine the present attitude toward diabetes. A need for reshaping perceptions or positive attitudes on which to build may become evident. It is useful also to identify how oriented the person is to health and how past illnesses have been handled.

For the patient with diabetes who presents for reevaluation, the interview can serve to identify knowledge gaps and compliance problems. Such questions as, "How do you feel when your sugar is high?" and "What do you do when this happens?'' can reveal many misconceptions regarding diabetic management. One should not assume that just because a patient has been a known diabetic for a long time, his or her knowledge and practices are satisfactory. Follow-up studies of people who have long-standing diabetes describe many faulty practices and gaps in knowledge.[3-5]

It is easier to help people change when they are dissatisfied with their own behavior. Wanting to learn involves knowing what is to be learned and understanding why it is important. The key to successful learning is to start with what the learner sees as important, that is, what the learner perceives as learning needs. As the patient gains more knowledge and recognizes the importance of other aspects of care, his or her perception of learning needs will change.

THE TEACHER

The teacher's tasks are to identify learning needs, stimulate learner interest, serve as an expert resource person, and facilitate learning. An effective teacher is able to listen, question, give criticism, and offer encouragement. Patient education requires adequate education of the patient educator. The knowledge, skills, and experience of the teacher are important in the teaching/learning process. Those who hope to support a diabetic through a teaching program must feel comfortable with their own knowledge and attitudes concerning diabetes. It is important that nurses have accurate and up-to-date knowledge about diabetic management. Feustel's study of nursing students' knowledge about diabetes mellitus points up the need for nurses to upgrade their knowledge of diabetes and its management if they are to be effective teachers of the diabetic.[6]

The teacher should be able to explain facts in a clear, concise manner and in terms and language the patient can understand. Professionals often have difficulty reorganizing their own knowledge so that they can relay knowledge to the diabetic in a simple, concise form. Many of the terms used by professionals in diabetic teaching are not understood by the patients. Reading literature prepared for diabetics and reviewing health education materials prepared for the public can be helpful in learning simple terms. Listening to and noting the terms that patients use in talking about diabetes are also useful.

In order to support a patient with a new diagnosis of diabetes and to help him or her deal with the anxieties, the professional must exhibit a positive attitude concerning diabetes and its management. The new diabetic needs factual information and his or her questions answered accurately. Hedging replies and nonverbal behavior that hints of mystery will increase the patient's anxiety. The patient watches carefully how the nurse answers the questions. Admitting lack of knowledge is far better than giving a vague or inaccurate reply.

An important principle of learning is to gain the person's attention before presenting new material. Reducing distractions in the environment sometimes calls for imagination, but often such simple things as turning off a radio or television set helps reduce distractions. One nurse and patient from a busy medical ward found a quiet place on the fire escape to go over a picture presentation of diabetic care. The patient was a longshoreman used to being outdoors. He had not had much formal education but was interested in learning to do what was needed. He remembered and was practicing what was taught when he returned for clinic follow-up. Timing also plays a part in gaining attention. Giving a lot of information and instruction the day of discharge from the hospital violates these principles of learning. There should be an opportunity for review, questions, and reinforcement of learning. To assimilate new learning and incorporate it into one's life-style takes time.

THE LEARNING CLIMATE

One of the tasks of the teacher is to create a climate that affords the patient a comfortable feeling—a feeling that the teacher understands what he or she might be experiencing and will help in the adaptation to this new "condition." The climate should be such that the person is willing to be exposed to new experiences. The learner must feel safe in expressing feelings and in trying new behaviors. Patients are entitled to courtesy and respect. As one patient so ably expressed it, "I don't have much schoolin' but I've got feelings." When working with clients from a specific cultural background, understanding how this may influence their ability to follow a prescribed program is essential. Interest and enthusiasm on the part of the teacher along with genuine learning expectations generally contribute favorably to the learning climate.

LEARNING GOALS AND OBJECTIVES

Behavioral objectives form the backbone of the plan for learning. They clearly define for the teacher the goals toward which the teaching activities are directed and provide for an evaluation of the learning. For the patient, objectives make clear what behavior is expected. The conditions under which the behavior is to be performed and the measures of satisfactory performance further provide the patient with a standard for self-monitoring progress.

The direction of plan implementation flows from the objectives. The more specifically the large goal of learning self-care is broken down, the more precise can be the teaching, the evaluation of the amount of learning, and the assessment of the need for reinforcement or reteaching. Behavioral objectives described by Mager and others include (1) an action verb, that is, what the learner will do; (2) the criterion, or the measure of acceptable performance; and (3) the "givens," or the conditions under which the action is carried out.[7,8] Such specificity also provides for consistency and continuity if more than one person is involved in the teaching program.

To foster learning, one should set realistic goals. As discussed previously, it is desirable to develop the objectives in collaboration with the patient. Sometimes the desired outcomes and necessary learning activities need to be negotiated in terms of what the patient feels can reasonably be accomplished.

The nurse may set objectives for the teaching program but find that the patient is not making progress. The difficulty may lie in the fact that the patient was not consulted concerning what he or she felt could be achieved. The patient needs to express what he or she feels can be accomplished and together with the nurse reach a compromise. Your priorities may not be the same as those of the patient in his or her unique situation.

One 50-year-old woman hospitalized for a serious blood condition was also newly diagnosed with diabetes mellitus. Even though she was quite intelligent, the daily instruction regarding insulin administration was not progressing satisfactorily. She could not remember much information from day to day. When the patient was consulted regarding her overall management problems and the skills she would need to acquire for her diabetic management, she was able to plan realistically with the nurse. Together they agreed on the skills which the patient could learn and carry out independently and those skills which a family member could provide. From that point on, the teaching program progressed rapidly.

The value of the patient's involvement in all aspects of the learning process is emphasized. For changes in behavior to be long-lasting and practiced regularly, they need to be self-imposed. Helping the patient set goals fosters the development of self-confidence, personal responsibility, and competence in self-care practices.

PRIORITIES AND SEQUENCE OF LEARNING

There is a limit to the amount of new information that can be handled, especially when the patient is trying to deal with the emotional aspects of a new diagnosis as well as trying to learn the essential skills. In presenting new information it is necessary to be selective and to set priorities for immediate learning. For the patient directed to take insulin on an ambulatory basis, there is no question that the first priority is assistance with safe dosage, sterile technique, and correct injection sites. With this priority in mind, the nurse will also assist the patient in giving the injection before the patient leaves the health care setting. It is helpful for the patient to experience self-injection while receiving the support of another person.

In addition, the patient, or someone in the family, must know the signs and symptoms of too much or too little insulin, as well as the actions to take in hypoglycemia, and be able to test urine and interpret the results. Supervision and assistance should be provided enough times that the patient can prepare the syringe and needle in a sterile manner, draw up and administer the correct dosage of insulin, and select the right site for injection. This initial instruction in insulin administration may take several hours. If this is done in an ambulatory setting, the patient is given choices of support for the following days. Clinic return visits, a referral to a visiting-nurse association, or a telephone call while preparing the injection are all possible avenues of support. If the patient is not able to learn within one clinic day, return visits for repeated instruction are scheduled.

Hospitalizing the patient for teaching is a last resort used only if other avenues of teaching are not suitable for the particular patient. If the person is hospitalized, he or she is expected to learn and practice the daily injections under supervision, not to mention the other aspects of self-care.

It is better to have the patient learn a few skills well than to deluge him or her with facts. One should limit new material and the time of the teaching sessions according to what the person can take in. Years after the initial diagnosis of diabetes, one young woman tearfully described her feelings at that time with great intensity: "I just felt awful. All I wanted to do was cry. I didn't understand what was happening, and when they gave me all those books to read, I couldn't concentrate on them and I felt like I'd never be able to manage. I was so overwhelmed I didn't even feel like trying." This patient's experience points up that patients need to have opportunities to express their feelings and cope with the impact of the disease. They need time to assimilate new information. The timing of learning activities and the methods used should be based on the learner's current needs.

Once the nurse and the patient have agreed on objectives and learning activities, the level of difficulty and the steps in the learning process should enable the person to cope and to succeed. Content too easy or a pace too slow is likely to result in boredom. However, if the content is too hard or the pace too fast, the patient is apt to become discouraged. The learning tasks should be just challenging enough for the person to have a sense of accomplishment.

DIFFERENT KINDS OF LEARNING

Learning involves changes in what people know and understand (cognitive behavior), what people want to do (affective behavior), and/or what people actually do (action or psychomotor behavior). Learning objectives can be classified according to these three areas of behavior. Appropriate learning materials and activities, depending on the area in which change is desired, are then selected. Facts, information, and concepts needed for cognitive learning can be gained from lectures, discussions, reading materials, and audiovisual aids such as films and tapes. Effective learning usually occurs slowly as a result of experiences; facts alone are not enough. Discussions, encouraging expression of feelings, role play, and games are methods that can be used to help the person gain insight into feelings and attitudes. Enacting desired behavior and publicly stating an attitude play a part in changing attitudes.

Psychomotor skills are learned through observing a demonstration and then having an opportunity to practice. The speed of acquiring a skill can be hastened if attention is directed to the manner of performing the action. Guided participation is also useful in the acquisition of skills, since the actual motor response influences perception. A sense of accomplishment serves to reinforce the behavior. In adults there is usually a quicker response if verbal explanations are included with the demonstration. Performance of skills improves with practice, provided there is feedback on how the skill is being performed. Generally short periods of practice with rest periods in between are the most effective for learning psychomotor skills.

CHOICE OF METHOD

The choice of method is dependent on the learner, the desired objectives, and the teacher's capability in using the particular method. Cost and availability of materials and technology are also factors in the selection of methods to be used for particular content.

Lecture

The lecture method is useful for giving factual information to a group of people. It must be remembered that the learner may be quite passive in a lecture situation and often only a portion of the content is retained. Answering questions and providing for some active involvement of learners enhances the use of the lecture. (For one-to-one teaching, the lecture is inappropriate.) Some ways to make the most of lectures include getting the learners' attention and interest, asking questions to provoke thought, using examples to illustrate key points, varying the lecture pace, rewarding participation, and summarizing key points. The content should be organized logically, and the presentation should be paced for the learners.

Group Discussion

A small group discussion with 6 to 10 members provides for more active involvement of learners. The group members can learn from one another. The discussion leader must keep the group discussion flowing and be prepared to be a resource person for the group. As with the lecture method, the group discussion should be summarized. Group discussions which include some decision making and publicly stated commitments have a positive influence on behavior change. In a group of peers there is value in the interchange of ideas, and sometimes the experiences of another diabetic lends credibility for the learner. One problem with open discussion is how to handle the "expert" who is giving wrong advice. Tact on the part of the leader in correcting unsafe practices is necessary for the maintenance of a productive learning climate. The group discussion method can help newly diagnosed diabetics express their feelings and recognize that others with diabetes are living active lives. Discussion groups can also provide help for family members and friends. Some diabetes associations sponsor regular discussion groups and provide resource people and discussion leaders.

Audiovisual Materials

Materials for diabetic teaching are available in the form of booklets, pamphlets, charts, slides, tapes, films, filmstrips, and videotapes. Learning is usually speeded or reinforced by the use of materials and methods that stimulate several senses. Knowing what methods have been successful in the past for a particular patient helps the nurse make more rational selections. Many materials for diabetic teaching can often be obtained from diabetes associations and pharmaceutical companies. It is important to select materials wisely, keeping in mind the learner and the objectives. Many times a specific teaching aid needs to be altered for an individual prior to use. It is important to avoid inconsistencies in directions and materials given to the patient.

For some content and for some learners, written materials in the form of books and pamphlets may be used. One must be certain that the language is understandable and that the reading level is not above that of the learner. A well-chosen booklet in print large enough to be seen and in language appropriate for the learner can emphasize important points and serve as a memory aid. One should choose the size of print and the format the person can best use. Much of the material available contains too many concepts and variations, which may lead to confusion on the part of the patient. Items that do not pertain to the patient are best eliminated before the materials are given to the patient. One advantage of written materials is that the learner may proceed at his or her own pace. However, the use of books and pamphlets should not be a substitute for personalized instruction. Too often one finds the diabetic inundated with books and pamphlets without an opportunity to discuss feelings and perceptions.

One also should not assume the person can read unless this has been assessed. In one situation, a hospitalized patient was given a book as part of the diabetic teaching program. It was not until weeks later that the family mentioned to the visiting nurse, "John never learned to read." No matter how excellent resource material may be, it must be in a form that the person can use in order to be of benefit in learning self-care. Tape cassettes accompanied by illustrated booklets can be very helpful in the preceding situation. Audio materials also are useful when visual problems accompany diabetes.

Space limits a review of the many materials that are available. However, a few examples will be given as a guide for the beginning teacher. The series of five booklets for diabetes teaching developed and published by the Diabetes Association of Cleveland (DAC) has proven quite useful.[9] Each small booklet is devoted to one topic. The content is concisely and attractively presented. The print is large and the line drawings are clear enough to accommodate diminished vision. The colorful illustrations are especially good in the sections on foot care and high and low blood sugar. This booklet also provides a diabetic identification card and a chart for recording urine test results. *You and Diabetes* also gives a brief overview of diabetes and its control; however, the print is smaller.[10] *Feet First,* a booklet published by the Department of Health, Education and Welfare, contains good information for people with decreased peripheral circulation and sensation and therefore is suited for use by the diabetic.[11] At first glance this booklet may seem too simple, but many patients like the presentation. The cartoon-like illustrations are eye-catching and, even if the patient has limited reading skills, serve to get across the important points of foot care. *Que es diabetes* presents a general overview of diabetes in Spanish.[12]

Diabetes Forecast, a bimonthly publication of the American Diabetes Association, helps diabetics keep posted on what is new in patient self-care and education. It also regularly carries a section in Spanish.[12a] Manufacturers of urine-testing supplies often furnish brochures describing the test procedure. One company sends a newsletter to patients on request.[13] *Getting Started* is an example of a general overview of diabetes that is presented by audiotape and flip chart.[14] It is possible also to obtain a booklet of the material covered for the patient to keep for future reference. *Exchange Lists for Meal Planning* with color-coded lists and attractive illustrations is a useful tool for the dietitian to use in helping the patient translate the diet prescription into actual foods.[15] In lieu of supervised cafeteria selection for practicing meal planning and the use of diabetic exchanges, food models may be used to assist the learner in the selection of foods. Pictures of foods from magazines and advertisements may also be adapted. Leapley describes the use of nutrition cubes for teaching patients diabetic exchanges and nutritive values.[16] The *DAC Index* is a listing of teaching materials currently available for health care personnel; it is available from the Cleveland Diabetes Association, Lee Road, Cleveland, Ohio, for $10.00.

Local videotape productions or slides with familiar faces and surroundings are an effective way of reaching patients if the equipment and technical services are available. Following the use of community-based videotapes in a clinic serving a bilingual population, the number of people participating in health education programs increased from 26 to 1260.[17] Television and dial-access systems can also be used for giving information about diabetes and diabetic care.

Programmed Instruction

Programmed instruction is another method used to present knowledge. The content is presented in small steps which are followed by testing and feedback. Programmed learning provides for a consistent presentation. The learner proceeds at his or her own pace. With this method the learner is required to be more active. Again with this method one must take care that the content and format are not overwhelming to the patient. Different types of programming and different levels of complexity are used. If the person has not used programmed instruction previously, some assistance at the beginning of the program will be required to make certain the learner knows how to use the program. After becoming familiar with the use of the program, the learner proceeds independently of the teacher.

Demonstration and Practice

Demonstration and practice are useful for learning the skills of insulin administration, urine testing, and foot care. In demonstrations it is important that the learner can see the demonstration clearly. Placement alongside the teacher is helpful if both the learner and the teacher are same-handed; if, however, the learner and the teacher are opposite-handed, the demonstration will usually be more effective if the participants are facing each other. A verbal description of the steps as they are being demonstrated improves the learning of motor skills in adults. After a demonstration, the learner needs an opportunity to try the new skill immediately and to receive feedback on his or her efforts. From the very beginning it is helpful to establish good habits. In teaching new skills, one should use the kind of equipment that the person will be using at home, since this makes the transfer of learning from the practice situation to daily management easier. Short practice periods interspersed with rest periods pay off in teaching skills.

Guided Performance

High levels of anxiety interfere with concentration and memory, both of which are essential for diabetic self-care. Being told that daily insulin injections will be required is often quite anxiety provoking. It is more difficult to deny the existence of diabetes when insulin is required. Getting over the hurdle of the first self-administered insulin injection usually helps allay much of the anxiety related to one's ability to give the needed injection. For this reason, the patient is encouraged to give his or her own injection before being exposed to all the details of insulin administration.

Guided performance of a new behavior may be used before the person understands all the intricacies of an action. The motor response uses kinesthetic sense, and the response itself affects perceptions of the skill. Handling and manipulating the equipment facilitates skill learning. Guided performance is particularly effective in coaching the person through a first insulin injection. The successful performance of the injection gives the person confidence in his or her ability to do a difficult task. It is not uncommon for the person to heave a sigh of relief or beam a smile after doing this. Discussion of the performance and the patient's feelings about it contributes positively to the learning experience. The learner is then able to concentrate better on some of the other necessary learning.

Role Play

Role play in which two or more people are assigned roles in a hypothetical situation can be used to increase the individuals' awareness of feelings and ability to anticipate and rehearse some of the situations that may be problematic. In role play, the players are given character descriptions and the context of the situation, but the drama itself is played out spontaneously. An essential aspect of this method is the careful analysis of what occurred in the role play. What and how to tell peers and coworkers about diabetes is one situation that can be explored through role play. With role play there is active participation of the learner, and this enhances learning.

Instructional Games

Games are another approach to learning. They, too, actively involve the learner and can be developed with different levels of complexity and sophistication. Instructional games can present new information and provide practice in a simulated situation. Games, as a teaching strategy, fall about midway between a lecture and a real-life situation. They have the advantage of condensing a real-life situation into a short span of time so that one can see the consequences of trying a course of action in a nonthreatening situation. The game chosen should be neither too easy nor too difficult for the learner. Some of the commercially available games pertain to nutrition and meal planning. Others deal with general health practices. A card game using nutritive values and exchange lists is available from the British Diabetes Association.[18] The written portion of the cards is done in French and German as well as in English. One can also use some of the principles of bingo to provide repetition and reinforce learning in a manner that will sustain interest. Hayman points out that games for instructional purposes should be carefully planned and presents a model for the design of games.[19]

Example or Modeling

Teaching by example or through modeling is important for nurses to keep in mind when they are caring for diabetics. Sometimes the unintentional examples of professionals lead to undesirable or unnecessary behavior. One patient changed his syringe storage container to be more like that in the physician's office—a large, flat, uncovered pan into which he reached to remove the syringe. Unable to grasp the differences in sterilization techniques between office and home, he made the following modifications. He did not boil the pan because it was too large. He never emptied it, but simply kept adding alcohol so that the level was over the syringe. This practice was unsafe from the standpoint of sterility and also was costly in terms of the amount of alcohol used. Although this patient reported no history of infection, the potential for infection was increased. More important, however, this example illustrates that unintentional modeling may occur and that assessment of our own professional practices is necessary.

An example of appropriate modeling that may be missed is that regarding foot care. Carrying out foot care in the manner verbally described while the patient is in an acute or chronic care facility takes advantage of the principles of reinforcement through practice. However, when the patient is only told about good foot care but never receives such special foot care, he or she is likely to pick up the disparity between words and actions. This reinforces the status quo and results in no behavioral change. Another example of appropriate use of modeling is the nurse's rotation of the sites used for insulin injection. Making a conscious effort to point this rotation out to the patient as one is doing it reinforces the importance of this practice. For positive results one should use learning by example or modeling purposefully. A "share-your-skills" program for teaching principles and skills of diabetic care is based on modeling. In this program, lay diabetic volunteers are used to teach new diabetics, but only after the volunteers are carefully screened and certified.[20] It is important that the helpers understand the principles of care and that they themselves have good, safe practices.

BEGINNING TO TEACH

The behavioral objectives listed in Table 9-1 can be used as an assessment model for "what diabetics should know and be able to do" for competent self-care. If the person is not able to perform the behavior, the objective can be used as a teaching goal (or defined learning outcome) with that individual. The emphasis in this particular list is performance of specified behaviors. If the person can perform these "tasks," he or she can manage safely until more complex concepts about the condition itself can be learned. After the learning activities have taken place, these same objectives are a guide for evaluation of learning.

Some simple tasks accomplished early in the educational program give the patient a feeling of confidence that is helpful when more complex learning is needed. Since techniques of foot care and urine testing are usually easily learned, these should be incorporated early and reinforced as needed until the patient is independent in their use. Teaching centered around these two techniques can easily flow into basic concepts about blood glucose, glycosuria, and diabetes itself. Furthermore, the teacher who evaluates the teaching/learning process can gain clues about the learner's ability and the effectiveness of the teaching approach. Before proceeding further, it is useful to draw conclusions about further plans, specifically,

1 Length and frequency of instruction periods
2 Amount and kind of reinforcement
3 Sequence of new learning tasks
4 Teaching strategy

It is helpful to outline the teaching plan with the patient. Reviewing the results of an assessment of self-care along with the objectives helps the patient see what it is he or she should know and should be able to do. Patients themselves are the best resources regarding their strengths and should play a part in determining the order and manner in which things are presented and learned.

When group classes for diabetes education are used, there needs to be planned follow-up to evaluate the learning and to answer special questions. In hospital settings, education programs either in groups or for the individual have been offered for the newly diagnosed diabetic. Much less attention has generally been given to "refresher courses" for the person who is a known diabetic of several years. Keeping in mind the rate of forgetting over time, one should not be surprised at the poor practice and high error rate in day-to-day management by known diabetics. Initial instruction may have been satisfactory, but often there has not been reinforcement of good practice. It would be beneficial to reevaluate the total management program at intervals and make revisions if necessary.

It is important to document what the person is able to do and what he or she knows rather than just noting what he or she has been exposed to. Much of the evaluation of diabetic education programs to date has focused on an in-

Table 9-1 Behavioral Objectives for Competent Diabetic Self-Care

Foot care

1 During daily care, the patient:
  a Washes feet in warm water
  b Inspects feet carefully
  c Uses lubricating substance if skin is dry; uses powder if skin is moist
  d Wears clean stockings or socks each day
  e Wears appropriate slippers or shoes when out of bed
  f Asks for medical attention for any new lesion
  g Asks for podiatry service if needed
2 During interview, the patient is able to:
  a Explain the need for extra attention to feet
  b Describe adequate foot care at home

Urine testing

1 At specified times, the patient collects a specimen of urine for testing—first or second as directed
2 During urine testing, the patient:
  a Manipulates dropper, test tube, tablets, or other materials according to the test used
  b Measures correct number of drops if test requires
  c Times test accurately
  d Interprets color charts correctly
  e Records results accurately
3 During interview, the patient is able to:
  a Relate time of urine testing to meals and/or insulin
  b Relate effects of insulin to test results
  c Name the test used and describe it accurately
  d State reason for collecting a second voided specimen
  e Explain meaning of test results
  f Describe actions to take based on results
  g Describe safe storage of materials

Insulin administration

1 During insulin administration, the patient:
  a Uses a syringe that corresponds to strength of insulin
  b Handles syringe and needle with sterile technique
  c Rotates bottle if long-acting insulin
  d Inverts bottle and looks for suspension of insulin
  e Inserts required amount of air
  f Withdraws accurate amount of insulin
  g If regular insulin is to be mixed with long-acting insulin, inserts air into both bottles, withdraws the regular insulin first, and then adds the long-acting insulin to the syringe.
  h Cleanses skin adequately
  i Injects insulin into appropriate site
  j Uses planned sequence of sites for injection
2 During interview, the patient is able to:
  a State insulin dosage(s) taken that day
  b State insulin type(s) taken that day
  c State insulin dosage and type used at home
  d Explain an effective method of sterilization
  e If disposable syringes and needles are used, describe a safe method of disposal
  f Explain an effective method of rotating sites

Table 9-1   Behavioral Objectives for Competent Diabetic Self-Care (Continued)

 g   Relate the time of insulin to food intake
 h   Relate the time of insulin to urine testing
 i   Relate the effects of insulin to urine test results
 j   Relate the effects of insulin to symptoms
 k   Relate the effects of insulin and exercise
 l   State symptoms of a past insulin reaction or state probable symptoms
 m   State actions to be taken to prevent or treat an insulin reaction
3   The patient has ready access to a source of glucose

Meal planning (refer to Chapter 6)

1   The patient is able to:
 a   Plan meals according to diet prescription using exchange lists (or other system)
 b   With the assistance of a dietitian, adjust meal plan to accommodate ethnic and religious restrictions and personal preferences
 c   Select food according to diet prescription when eating away from home

Identification

1   The patient carries a diabetic identification card or wears a diabetic identification tag

Ability to assume self-care at home: summary

1   The patient is able to:
 a   State prescribed insulin: kind, strength, dosage
 b   State times urine testing is to be done
 c   State symptoms of high blood sugar, ketoacidosis, and low blood sugar (insulin reaction)
 d   State actions to be taken for ketoacidosis and insulin reaction
 e   State plans for diabetic follow-up, including place and time of next appointment
 f   Plan for obtaining needed equipment and supplies
 g   Plan daily schedule of insulin, diet, and urine testing in relation to home and work/school activities
 h   Administer insulin safely
 i   Test urine accurately
 j   Care for feet properly
 k   Plan, shop, prepare, and eat prescribed diet
2   The patient has:
 a   Diabetic identification card
 b   Necessary equipment and supplies
 c   Written instructions
 d   Phone number(s) of resource people

crease in knowledge and facts. It should be remembered that having knowledge about something does not necessarily mean that that knowledge is what is practiced. Graber et al. state that diabetic patient care and education are inseparable.[21] They propose that performance at home, day-to-day control states, school and work absenteeism, hospital use, frequency of acute complications, and total health care costs be used as measures in evaluating diabetic patient education programs. If diabetic patients are to achieve optimal health control, their self-care practices must be evaluated no matter how long they have been known and they must participate in ongoing learning opportunities, which ultimately will benefit them.

REFERENCES

1 *Report of the National Commission on Diabetes to the Congress of the United States,* vol. I, The Long Range Plan to Combat Diabetes, NIH-76-1018; vol. III, part V, Diabetes Education for Health Professionals, Patients and the Public, NIH-76-1031, Washington, D.C., U.S. Department of Health, Education and Welfare, 1975.

2 Woodruff, A. D. The learning process, in T. L. Harris and W. E. Schwann (eds.), *The Learning Process* (New York: Oxford Univ. Press, 1961), pp. 10–19.

3 Stafford, R. A study of patients with recently diagnosed diabetes to ascertain the extent of utilization of instruction, unpublished master's thesis, Loma Linda University, 1963.

4 Watkins, J. D., et al. A study of diabetic patients at home, *Am. J. Public Health,* 57:452–459, March 1967.

5 Montgomery, L. H. A study to ascertain the effectiveness of the teaching team in the preparation of the newly diagnosed diabetic, unpublished master's thesis, Loma Linda University, 1967.

6 Feustel, D. E. Nursing student's knowledge about diabetes mellitus, *Nurs. Res.,* 25(1):4–8, 1967.

7 Mager, R. *Preparing Instructional Objectives* (Palo Alto, Calif.: Fearon, 1962).

8 Jones, P., and Ortel, W. Developing patient teaching objectives and techniques: a self-instructional program, *Nurse Educator,* 2:3–18, 1977.

9 *DAC Kit,* Diabetes Association of Greater Cleveland, 2022 Lee Road, Cleveland, Ohio 44118.

10 *You and Diabetes,* G-5712-6, Upjohn Company, January 1977.

11 *Feet First, A Booklet about Foot Care,* U.S. Department of Health, Education and Welfare, 1970.

12 Covarrubias, A. P. *Que es diabetes,* División Nutrición, Departamento de Investigación Científica, Centro Médico Nacional, Instituto Mexicano del Seguro Social.

12a. *Diabetes Forecast,* American Diabetes Association, 600 Fifth Avenue, New York, New York 10020.

13 Ames Company, Elkhart, Indiana.

14 *Getting Started,* Becton, Dickinson & Co., Rutherford, New Jersey.

15 American Diabetes Association, Inc., and American Dietetic Association. *Exchange Lists for Meal Planning, 1976* (Chicago: American Dietetic Association, 1976).

16 Leapley, P. Nutrition cubes—a tool for teaching individuals the new ADA exchange lists, *Diabetes,* 26:343, October 1977.

17 Lazes, P. M., and Snyder, D. Community oriented videotapes—a low cost effective teaching tool, *Int. J. Health Ed.,* 20(1):68–70, 1977.

18 Food Exchange Playing Cards (1975), British Diabetes Association, 3/6 Aflred Place, London WC1E7EE, England. In Sleet, D. A., and Stadsklev, R. Annotated bibliography of simulations and games in health education, *Health Ed. Monogr.,* 5(Suppl. 1):74–90, 1977.

19 Hayman, J. Games—a teaching strategy, *Nurs. Outlook,* 25:302, May 1977.

20 Austin, D., et al. Share-your-skill program in diabetes, *Diabetes,* 26(Suppl. 1):363, 1977.

21 Graber, A. L., et al. Evaluation of diabetes patient-education programs, *Diabetes,* 26:61–64, January 1977.

BIBLIOGRAPHY

Bachscheider, J. E. Self-care requirements, self-care capabilities, and nursing systems in the diabetic nurse management clinic, *Am. J. Public Health,* **64**:1138–1148, December 1974.

Bernheimer, E., and L. H. Clever, *The Team Approach to Patient Education: One Hospital's Experience in Diabetes,* U.S. Department of Health, Education and Welfare, Public Health Service, Center for Disease Control, Bureau of Health Education, Atlanta, Georgia, 1977.

Bilodeau, E. A. (ed.). *Principles of Skill Acquisition.* New York: Academic, 1969.

Blair, G. M., et al. *Educational Psychology.* New York: Macmillan, 1967.

Bloom, A. *Diabetes Explained.* Baltimore: University Park Press, 1971.

Bohdan, S. T., and K. Jans, A new diabetic with complications, *Nurs. Clin. North Am.,* **12**(3):393–406.

Brown, G. I. *Human Teaching for Human Learning.* New York: Viking, 1971.

Clarke, W. D., et al. Health education in the doctor's waiting room—an experiment, *Health Educ. J.,* **35**(1):135–141, 1976.

Cosper, B. How well do patients understand hospital jargon? *Am. J. Nurs.,* **77**:1932–1934, December, 1977.

Garber, R. The use of a standardized teaching program in diabetes education, *Nurs. Clin. North Am.,* **12**(3):375–391, 1977.

Greenblat, C. S., and H. Owen (eds.). Gaming-simulation and health education, *Health Ed. Monogr.,* vol. 5 (Suppl. 1), 1977.

Guthrie, D. W. and R. A. Guthrie, *Nursing Management of Diabetes mellitus.* St. Louis: Mosby, 1977.

Haggerty, R. J. Changing life styles to improve health, *Prev. Med.,* **6**(2):276–289, 1977.

Hebron, M. *Motivated Learning.* London: Methuen, 1966.

Huang, P., and R. W. Alexander, A model for a diabetic outpatient teaching program, *Diabetes,* **26**(Suppl. 1):402, 1977.

Laugharne, E., and G. Steiner, Tri-hospital diabetes education centre—a cost effective, cooperative venture, *Can. Nurse,* **73**(9):14–19, 1977.

Meyers, S. A. Diabetes management by the patient and a nurse practitioner, *Nurs. Clin. North Am.,* **12**(3):415–426, 1977.

——— *Patient Education Workshop: Summary Report.* U.S. Department of Health, Education and Welfare, Public Health Service, Center for Disease Control, Atlanta, Georgia, 1976.

Plant, J. Educating the elderly in safe medication use, *Hospitals,* **51**(8):97–8, 100–102, 1977.

Pohl, M. L. *The Teaching Function of the Nursing Practitioner.* Dubuque, Iowa: Brown, 1968.

Porter, A. L. Student participation in diabetic education, *Nurs. Clin. North Am.,* **12**(3):407–414, 1977.

——— (ed.). Symposium on diabetes education and care, *Nurs. Clin. North Am.,* **12**(3):361–445, 1977.

Redman, B. *The Process of Patient Teaching in Nursing.* St. Louis: Mosby, 1976.

Rosenthal, H., and J. Rosenthal, *Diabetic Care in Pictures.* Philadelphia: Lippincott, 1960.

Stevens, B. J. The teaching-learning process, *Nurse Educator,* May-June 1976:9–20.

Sturdevant, B. Why don't adult patients learn? *Sup. Nurse,* May 1977, pp. 44, 46.

Suren, J. V. Education of the culturally and educationally deprived diabetic, *Nurs. Clin. North Am.,* **12**(3):427–437, 1977.

Chapter 10

The Diabetic with Vascular Complications

Dorothy R. Blevins

Violet A. Breckbill

The diabetic is more likely to develop cardiovascular-renal disease earlier or more rapidly than is the nondiabetic. A 16-year follow-up study of the Framingham population revealed that more people with diabetes mellitus developed cerebral vascular accidents, cardiac disease, and peripheral occlusive disease than did those without diabetes. Insulin-treated women had the highest mortality rate.[1] In the course of 10 to 15 years of having diabetes, most people have developed significant vascular abnormalities.

Indeed, about 80 percent of diabetic patients die of some form of cardiovascular disease, including renovascular disease, compared to 40 to 50 percent of nondiabetic patients. Diabetes now ranks as the fifth leading underlying cause of death by disease in the United States. The current system of codifying and reporting deaths does not reflect the contribution of diabetes mellitus to cardiovascular-renal deaths. The National Commission on Diabetes suggests that diabetes probably ranks as the third cause of death if its contribution to underlying causes is considered.[2]

ATHEROSCLEROSIS

Vessels of all sizes are affected, from the aorta down to the smallest arterioles and capillaries.[3] The aorta and large- and medium-sized arteries are affected by accelerated, severe atherosclerosis.

It is generally believed that the predisposition to vascular disease in diabetes stems from some genetic trait separate from but in some way related to the metabolic derangement. In support of this belief, reports cite patients with strong hereditary backgrounds for diabetes who suffer from accelerated atherosclerosis but who have no demonstrable carbohydrate or lipid abnormalities. The advance of atherosclerosis correlates better with the duration of the disease than with its severity. Any patient with a 10-year history of diabetes is almost certain to have at least moderate, and more often severe, atherosclerosis. Development of vascular disease may well be promoted by the hyperlipidemia and hypercholesterolemia so characteristic of diabetes. In addition, diabetics have an increased incidence of hypertension, which is known to accelerate the development of atherosclerosis.

Biochemical Changes

The basic process of the formation of atheromatous lesions is still a controversial issue. They occur in areas where there are high flow rates and turbulence; their correlation with hypertension also supports a mechanical component. Factors in the blood, such as platelets, also play an important role. It has been suggested that the initial lesion is the loss of the lining of endothelial cells, perhaps due to trauma from the turbulent flow, or stress, and this is followed by a patch of platelets which cluster over the site of injury. Then there is some proliferation of smooth muscle cells which are in the tunica media of the artery, and these move into the area of injury. Proliferation of the smooth muscle cells into the site of injury is likened to a neoplastic but benign growth. If there are elevated levels of cholesterol and other lipoprotein materials, they can accumulate in the lesion. The lesion increases in size rather than regressing. Other people suggest that the lesion itself may be due to a primary lesion in the endothelial cells leading to a tumorlike growth. The accelerated atherosclerosis noted in diabetic patients may have something to do with the fact that the metabolism of the smooth muscle wall itself is different in normal and diabetic tissues.[4]

Hyaline arteriolosclerosis, the vascular lesion associated with hypertension, is both more prevalent and more severe in diabetics than in nondiabetics. However, it is not specific for diabetics because it is seen in elderly nondiabetics even without hypertension. It is an amorphous, hyaline thickening of the wall of the arteriola which causes narrowing of the lumen. Recently it has been proposed that the hyaline material is comprised of deposits of plasma proteins. Presumably these penetrate into the abnormally permeable walls of the arterioles by a process called *insudation.*[5] This concept relates the arteriolosclerosis to the exudative lesions of the glomeruli described later.

HYPERTENSION

Diabetes is considered a contributing factor to the development of hypertension and its related diseases (renal failure, hypertensive heart disease, coronary heart disease, and stroke), which account for approximately 70 percent of all deaths among the middle-aged population in the United States.[6] About 15 percent of the adult population has high blood pressure.[7] Adult-onset diabetes is associated with hypertension in 28 to 45 percent of the populations reviewed in studies on hypertension.[8] Twenty percent of juvenile diabetics develop high blood pressure within 10 years. The incidence of hypertension increases as age and duration of diabetes increases. Hypertension has been called the silent killer because of its quiescent nature for many years before stroke, heart disease, or renal failure becomes evident. Hypertension is often accompanied by nephropathy and retinopathy.

Reduction of elevated levels of blood pressure are followed by decreased risk of cardiovascular disease. The Veterans Administration Hypertension Cooperative Study gave increased impetus to the reduction of mild elevations of blood pressure as well as higher elevations. One report demonstrated a decreased risk of morbid events in people treated with antihypertensive agents with elevations of diastolic pressure of 90 to 114 mmHg.[9]

Attention is directed toward modifying other risk factors in the treatment approach to the hypertensive: weight reduction and control, reduction of sodium intake, avoidance of smoking, and decreased stress. Several studies have shown a distressing lack of compliance with self-medication of antihypertensive agents.[10] Some of the factors that patients report as reasons for noncompliance are the long-term therapy in the absence of symptoms, the inconvenience and cost, lack of access to health care facilities, inadequate instruction, and side effects.

These factors can be explored for relevance to the diabetic who also has a chronic disease, which, in the obese adult, is often asymptomatic. Anticipatory guidance can be used to assist the patient in identifying barriers to compliance.

Of importance in the hypertensive diabetic are iatrogenic effects that may alter diabetic status. Thiazide preparations are commonly used as the first antihypertensive medication; these are hyperglycemic in action, as is Aldomet, which may be used alone or with a thiazide drug. Symptoms of diabetic neuropathy may be mimicked or enhanced by several drugs; for example, guanethidine may cause orthostatic hypertension and/or impotence. Sometimes changes in drugs or dosages may be possible if the patient reports side effects he or she considers untenable. (See Chapter 7 for further discussion of drug therapy.)

HYPERLIPOPROTEINEMIAS: TRIGLYCERIDE, CHOLESTEROL, AND PHOSPHOLIPIDS

Although many diabetics have normal levels of serum lipids, about one-third have alterations in fat transport and circulating lipid levels.[11] Most commonly, a mild elevation of lipids is seen in obese diabetics with mild glucose intolerance. In these patients, the hyperlipidemia is more a function of the excessive adipose tissue than of the excessive blood glucose. Correction of the hyperlipidemia depends primarily on weight reduction in the obese adult-onset diabetic. In contrast, there is usually a marked elevation of serum triglycerides and cholesterol in ketoacidosis; with institution of adequate insulin therapy, these elevations subside. Rarely, a severe hyperlipidemia is associated with uncontrolled diabetes mellitus that is manifested by visible signs: milky plasma, eruptive xanthoma, and lipemia retinalis.

In addition to the increased free fatty acids (FFA) in the blood, all the other lipid components of the plasma also greatly increase in the absence of insulin. The excess FFA in the blood move into the liver and are used to synthesize triglycerides, cholesterol, and phospholipids which are released into the blood as lipoproteins. (The blood lipids may increase as much as 5 times.) Diabetes mellitus is one of several diseases that produces a *secondary hyperlipoproteinemia*. Hyperlipoproteinemia is any condition in which, after a 12-h fast, the plasma triglyceride concentration is greater than 150 mg/dL, the plasma cholesterol concentration is greater than 240 mg/dL, or both. The hyperlipoproteinemia in diabetes is usually identified as type IV or V, and is often due to an excess of very low density lipoproteins (VLDL) in the plasma. VLDL are the triglyceride-rich lipoproteins synthesized in the liver, not in fat cells. Much of the fatty acids used by the liver for the synthesis of triglycerides is derived from dietary carbohydrate. Differentiation of the type of hyperlipidemia allows the physician to determine the amount and type of fat restriction and carbohydrate in the diet and whether antilipid compounds will be helpful. Recent work suggests that fructose may be more involved in hypertriglyceridemia than glucose. This has led to the view that sucrose, the disaccharide that contains fructose and glucose ("table sugar"), should be reduced in the diet of diabetic patients and a fructose-free sweetener used instead. (Review the interconversion scheme for glucose, fructose, and sorbitol depicted in Fig. 4-13.)

The high lipid concentration in the blood, especially that of cholesterol, has been implicated in leading to the rapid development of atherosclerosis in people with severe diabetes (see previous discussion).

OBESITY

Obesity has long been considered a diabetogenic factor; the degree and duration of adiposity are associated with increased prevalence of adult-onset diabetes. Prevention and control of obesity are considered major thrusts of treatment for adult-onset diabetics who are prone to atherosclerosis and hypertension. Krall stated,

> It is the large population of so-called mild, often obese, diabetics without dietary regulation or adequate insulin treatments that provide the great majority of diabetics who, in later years, develop coronary artery disease, gangrene, retinopathy, and/or nephropathy.[12]

Various estimations of the degree of adiposity are used: comparisons of weight to norms of age, height and body frames, waist girths, and skin-fold thicknesses. About 80 to 90 percent of the diabetic population is above ideal weight at the time of diagnosis. Weight loss in the adult diabetic can often decrease symptoms of hyperglycemia and may reduce the necessity for insulin or other hypoglycemic agents. Weight reduction can lower blood pressure, and hyperlipidemia; it is believed that these factors may influence the progression of atherosclerosis.

An individual approach in planning for weight control, extensive education, and long-term follow-up are key factors in assisting diabetics to reduce and *maintain* weight loss.

Biochemical Factors

The relationship between diabetes mellitus and obesity is clinically recognized, but the common biochemical factors are poorly understood. The handling of dietary glucose by the obese person is abnormal and improves after the excess adipose mass has been reduced. Similarly, the obese are more resistant to the action of insulin, which is needed for the metabolism of glucose and is in reduced supply in the diabetic. An elevation of circulating plasma insulin is characteristic of the obese person.[13]

Mild diabetes often occurs in older people, and especially in older people who are overweight. As long as a person eats excessively, the blood glucose level is elevated; as soon as the dietary intake is reduced, the glucose level in the blood often reverts to normal. This diabetic effect of obesity is caused mainly by the depression of glucose metabolism in the presence of excess fatty acids in the blood.[14]

Experimental evidence suggests that obesity increases the demands on the pancreas to produce insulin. When the pancreas is unable to meet the demands because it is injured by chemical, viral, or genetic factors, then the demands of obesity may lead to failure of the pancreas. Experiments with animals would implicate obesity as a source of the "environmental stress" that can precipitate failure of the pancreas or diabetes if the pancreas is already diseased. However, an entirely normal pancreas can apparently meet the demands for extra insulin production imposed by obesity.[15]

The islets of the pancreas are enlarged in about 65 percent of obese patients. It has also been found that obese patients have increased levels of insulin, with the elevation of insulin correlated with the degree of obesity.[16,17] The data imply that the effects of obesity are manifested largely through the increased basal levels of insulin.

The factors which modulate insulin secretion are nutrients, hormones, and neural factors. Increased glucose concentration might be an important factor in enhancing the secretion of insulin in obesity. The fasting levels are higher in many obese individuals than in normal individuals.[18] The small increase in glucose observed in obese individuals might be a reflection of their state of *overnutrition* and, in turn, might signal the pancreas to secrete more insulin. Increased concentrations of amino acids may also account in part for basal hyperinsulinemia in obesity.[19] It was found that arginine, leucine, tyrosine, phenylalanine, and valine increased insulin secretion, and arginine and leucine are potent stimulators.

Rabinowitz concluded that both muscle and adipose tissue of obese subjects were less responsive (i.e., were resistant) to the actions of insulin.[20,21] Enlarged adipocytes may be the basic mechanism for resistance to insulin.

The magnitude of the response to insulin in small and large adipocytes is a function of carbohydrate intake.[22,23] Adipose tissue obtained from rats fed a high-carbohydrate diet oxidizes more glucose in the presence of insulin in vitro than adipose tissue obtained from rats on a low-carbohydrate diet. A similar effect occurs in humans. It would appear that there are the same number of insulin receptors in the membranes of the large adipocytes, but because of the increased area, they act "diluted," with a resultant decreased response to insulin.[24]

The weight loss that often accompanies the clinical onset of diabetes results from protein loss due to gluconeogenesis, which has been discussed before, and stored-fat loss due to the ineffectual stimulus of insulin on the adipocytes.

THE DIABETIC WITH MYOCARDIAL INFARCTION

Myocardial infarction is the most common cause of death in older diabetics. It is as common in the diabetic female as it is in the diabetic male; in contrast, myocardial infarction is uncommon in nondiabetic women of reproductive age.

In the diabetic, coronary artery disease often occurs after the diagnosis of diabetes mellitus is made; however, diabetes may be diagnosed at the same time or later. (Not all people with myocardial infarction are diabetic, nor do all diabetics develop coronary artery disease.) However, a transient hyperglycemia is often seen during acute myocardial infarction. One study found an incidence of 65 percent of glucose intolerance in acute myocardial infarction; this incidence had decreased to 29 percent at the end of 1 month.[25]

Priorities of care during acute myocardial infarction are those related to cardiogenic shock, arrhythmias, and other cardiac complications. Life-support measures assume more importance than short-term elevations in the level of blood glucose. Higher blood glucose levels may be permitted or desired for the insulin-dependent diabetic to avoid hypoglycemia, in which an increased work load is placed on the myocardium by tachycardia, increased contractility, and vasoconstriction of the peripheral vessels.

Occasionally, adult diabetics with delayed insulin secretion may have hypoglycemic episodes, even though they are not on exogenous insulin or oral agents. For the insulin-dependent diabetic, the similarities of symptoms of hypoglycemic reaction to those of hypotension, cardiogenic shock, and the severe pain of myocardial infarction should be remembered. Information should be obtained from the patient or significant others on admission concerning the time of the last insulin (or hypoglycemic agent), the dosage, and subsequent food intake and vomiting. Provision of adequate glucose to "cover" insulin dosage is essential. Administration of narcotics may decrease the patient's perception of inner sensations that have, in the past, assisted him or her in detecting hypoglycemia or hyperglycemia.

The responses of individuals to the life-threatening aspects of myocardial infarction and its impact on life-style are well known. Although little teaching is recommended during the acute stage, the known diabetic needs assurance that his or her diabetes is not being overlooked in the attention to cardiac treatments. High levels of anxiety are expected during the acute stage of myocardial infarction. If the nurse can explain the plan for diabetic management, the patient may be reassured and will more easily allow others to manage those activities which have become second nature to him or her. Explanations should be brief, but withholding information about results of urine tests or dosages of insulin is not reassuring to the diabetic.

The diabetic usually knows that insulin requirements increase with illness. Insulin may be necessary for the first time in the adult-onset diabetic during a myocardial episode. If polarization therapy is used to "drive" potassium into cells, this purpose of insulin should be explained as different from control of blood glucose level. Monitoring for hypoglycemia is essential regardless of the purpose of insulin administration.

Small, frequent servings of food are often recommended for the first few days after myocardial infarction. This change in distribution of foods and the differences from home cooking may be upsetting to the insulin-dependent patient. Recording and assessment of the caloric and nutrient intake are part of the care. Some patients in crisis will express motivation for weight control, which should be supported.

Other treatments used for the patient with myocardial infarction can affect blood glucose levels. Monamine oxidase inhibitors may be prescribed as tranquilizers; these have a hypoglycemic effect. Niacin, or nicotinic acid, is a vasodilator with a hyperglycemic effect. Of special consideration is the interference with sympathetic responses by propanolal (Inderal), which may potentiate hypoglycemia and prevent the insulin-dependent patient from perceiving early signs of insulin reaction.[26]

As the acute stage of myocardial infarction subsides, a teaching program should be planned based on the individual's needs and concerns. The patient should understand medication programs, dietary prescriptions, and activity restrictions and be able to implement these after discharge. It is necessary to incorporate modifications of diet, activity, and medication into a feasible life pattern that will allow management of both diabetes and coronary artery disease. Coping patterns and learning ability influence the amount and kind of instruction and the patient's ability to modify risk factors. Major patient concerns may include those changes in daily living that the patient perceives as threatening. These may be in any sphere of life, e.g., economic problems, role relations, sexual functioning, and fear of a second myocardial infarction.

The teaching plan must be coordinated and integrate the prescriptions of the cardiologist, the endocrinologist, and others for diet and other treatments.

If there are conflicts in these, recognition and resolution should be achieved before approaching the patient. Often the diabetic perceives differences between the prior food patterns and the postcoronary diet prescription. Exploration may lead to discovery that the patient was not fully compliant with the former prescription; in fact, it may reveal that the patient does not know the components of a diabetic diet, or that she or he is not aware of changes in therapy for diabetes over the years since she or he was first given a dietary prescription. Assessment of usual food intake will identify whether or not there are patterns to be modified in total caloric intake and fat or carbohydrate intake and distribution. For the obese adult-onset diabetic, priority is on weight control.

THE DIABETIC WITH CONGESTIVE HEART FAILURE

Ventricular hypertrophy followed by decompensation leads to diminished work efficiency and contractile strength of the myocardium. When compensatory enlargement of the myocardium no longer provides sufficient cardiac output for the body, congestive heart failure develops. Decreased organ perfusion and increased fluid volume of venous and interstitial spaces are central features of the syndrome of congestive heart failure. The reader is referred to specialized texts for more definitive explanations of diagnosis and treatment. Treatment is not different for the diabetic; however, consideration must be given to the maintenance of metabolic control. Suspicion should exist about the status of renal function in the diabetic.

The patient admitted with congestive heart failure may have decreased renal function because of decreased circulation or underlying diabetic nephropathy. As treatment progresses, changes in proteinuria and nitrogenous products in the blood help identify components of circulatory dysfunction (prerenal azotemia) and renal disease (renal azotemia). The presence of hypoalbuminemia indicates more severe glomerular disease, contributes to the edema, and makes diuresis more difficult. With hypoalbuminemia, a contracted intravascular compartment may preclude rapid diuresis. Postural hypotension (defined as a 10-mmHg decrease in blood pressure from lying to standing position) is often used to gauge the effect of diuresis on blood volume.

As with most other drugs, *estimation* of the effects of diuretic treatment form the basis of dosage prescription in any one patient. How much is enough? can only be answered by accurate observations of the patient and accurate measurements of weight loss, intake, and output. If volume loss through diuresis decreases renal perfusion, prerenal azotemia and oliguria may result. Decreased perfusion increases the danger of nephron damage in a kidney already at risk because of diabetes. Early detection of oliguria and postural hypotension are necessary for prompt restoration of adequate renal perfusion.

Diuretics usually cause potassium loss; two exceptions are the drugs triamterine (Dyrenium) and sprironolactone (Aldactone). For the diabetic, losses of potassium and other electrolytes may occur from glycosuria and/or diuretic therapy. Hyperglycemia is a side effect of several diuretics, including the thiazides, furosemide (Lasix), and ethocrynic acid (Edecrin). Hypokalemia retards the transport of glucose into the cell, thus increasing hyperglycemia. Hypokalemia enhances the toxicity of digitalis and its derivatives. Careful monitoring of blood and urine levels of glucose, of volumes of urine, and for signs of digitalis toxicity are aspects of care for the diabetic with congestive heart failure.

Potassium replacements may be given along with diuretic therapy by medication or in food. The carbohydrate and caloric content of potassium-rich foods should be calculated within the daily diet. If the potassium medication is mixed with a fruit juice, the amount of juice should be recorded on the dietary record.

Diabetic patients receiving diuretic therapy may believe their diabetes is worsening because of polyuria and nocturia. Knowing the results of glucose testing and the expected results of the diuretic may decrease anxiety. However, a source of confusion for insulin-dependent patients is weight loss, a criterion they may have used to estimate their control of diabetes. For adult-onset diabetics who are obese, listening to their perceptions of change in body weight may provide clues about their motivation for weight loss. One patient told these writers that she was "wasting away" after she lost 20 lb of fluid. She perceived herself as weak and sick, even though she no longer had dyspnea or orthopnea and had more energy and mobility than before. She was 5 ft 3 in tall and weighed 180 lb.

Patients recovering from episodes of congestive heart failure require a teaching program designed to assist them in carrying out prescribed medication, sodium restriction, rest, and/or exercise; identifying early signs of recurrent congestive heart failure; and modifying those factors which endanger their well-being. Integration of new treatments into daily plans must take into account established patterns of diabetic self-care. (Refer to Chapter 7 for further discussion of drug therapy in congestive failure.)

OTHER CARDIOVASCULAR CRISES

The diabetic may suffer other cardiovascular events such as stroke, aortic aneurysm, and hypertensive crisis. As in myocardial infarction and congestive heart failure, priority measures are those directed toward life support and often involve modification of diabetic control measures. Basic considerations include monitoring of diabetic status and integration of previous patterns of therapeutic self-care into new regimens. Although late, increased motivation for reduction of risk factors should be encouraged.

THE DIABETIC WITH RENAL DISEASE

Diabetic nephropathy may occur alone or with other complications of diabetes; the term *diabetic triopathy* is used when neuropathy, retinopathy, and nephropathy occur together. Hypertension is often a component of diabetic nephropathy, and renal disease aggravates the severity and consequences of hypertension. Renal disease severely limits the patient's ability to respond to treatments for congestive heart failure, hypertension, and other circulatory disorders. Diabetic nephropathy results from a combination of vascular changes within the kidney and infection.

The importance of diabetic nephropathy is indicated by the fact that renal disease is the leading cause of death among juvenile diabetics; nearly one-half die of complications of nephropathy.[27] Between ages 20 and 39, two-thirds of the deaths of people with proliferative retinopathy result from renal failure. The average life expectancy of juvenile diabetics is approximately 25 years after the onset of diabetes.

Chronic Processes

Diabetic nephropathy is often suspected when there are symptoms and laboratory evidence of renal insufficiency in a patient previously diagnosed as diabetic. It is not always possible to perform a renal biopsy to confirm the nature of the renal lesions; there are many contraindications to this examination. When chronic renal failure occurs, the confirmation of the specific etiology makes little difference in treatment, which is supportive rather than corrective.

The kidney is responsible for filtering the wastes from the blood, and this filtration occurs in thousands of little clusters of capillaries called glomeruli (see Fig. 10-1). In diabetic patients with renal failure, the basement membrane of the capillaries of the glomeruli is thickened just as in the eye. This thickening leads to plugging and leaking of the glomerular capillaries. The kidney is a prime target of diabetes; renal failure is second only to myocardial infarction as a cause of death from the disease.

Four types of lesions are seen: (1) glomerular, (2) renovascular, principally arteriolosclerosis, (3) pyelonephritis, including necrotizing papillitis, and (4) glycogen and fatty changes in the tubular epithelium.

Diffuse Glomerulosclerosis   This condition is found in at least 90 percent of patients who have had diabetes for more than 10 years. The basement membranes of the glomerular capillaries are thickened throughout; biochemical analysis of these altered membranes discloses an increase in the hydroxylysine content and in the number of glucosyl-galactose disaccharide units. These changes are definitely related to the disturbed carbohydrate metabolism.[28] These lesions almost always begin in the vascular stalk and sometimes appear to be continuous with the hyaline arteriolosclerosis in the afferent and efferent arterioles. When the diffuse glomerulosclerosis is advanced, these patients manifest severe proteinuria and the glomerular cells exhibit loss of their "foot" processes. The glomerulosclerosis leads to narrowing of the capillaries and eventually total sclerosis of the glomerular vascular tufts. Since the glomerular involvement is usually diffuse and invariably bilateral, the lesions lead to renal failure.[29]

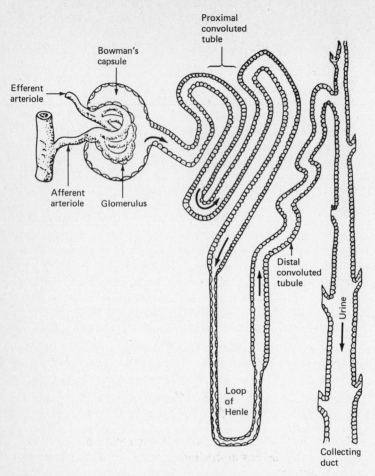

Figure 10-1 The functional unit of the kidney is the nephron, made up of a glomerulus, Bowman's capsule, and tubular system, as illustrated and identified here. The various mechanisms of filtration, reabsorption, secretion, and excretion take place at specific areas in the nephron. (*Adapted from M. J. Kluger and L. G. D'Alecy, "Workbook to Accompany Vander Human Physiology," New York, McGraw-Hill, 1976.*)

Nodular Glomerulosclerosis or Kimmelstiel-Wilson Lesions   These are distinctive because of the spherical deposits of a laminated matrix within the core of the lobule. These nodules tend to develop in the periphery of the glomeruli, pushing the peripheral capillary loops ahead of them. Often these patent loops create halos about the nodule. These lesions also have been referred to as "intercapillary glomeruloscleroses" by Kimmelstiel and Wilson in 1936; they occur randomly throughout the kidney. In advanced disease, many nodules are present within a single glomerulus, and most glomeruli are involved. The deposits are PAS-positive and contain mucopolysaccharides, lipids, and fibrils, as well as collagen fibers, and have the same composition as the matrix deposits of diffuse glomerulosclerosis. Nodular glomerulosclerosis is also related to the duration of diabetes. The nodular form is specific for diabetes; it is seen in 10 to 35 percent of diabetic patients.

These two lesions, nodular and diffuse glomerulosclerosis, along with arteriolosclerosis, usually lead to obliteration of the vascular channels and the glomeruli, and to serious, usually fatal, impairment of renal function. In late stages, adhesions appear between the visceral and parietal layers of Bowman's capsule (see Fig. 10-1), sometimes with considerable proliferation of the glomerular epithelial cells. Interstitial fibrosis and tubular atrophy become marked; ischemia is induced and causes fine scarring of the kidneys, as seen by a finely granular cortical surface.

Exudative lesions take two forms. The first are glassy, homogeneous, strongly eosinophilic deposits in the parietal layer of Bowman's capsule called "capsular drops." They may hang in the uriniferous spaces. Similar-appearing deposits, called "fibrin caps," may develop over the outer surface of glomerular capillary loops, between the visceral epithelium of Bowman's capsule and the basement membrane. These two lesions are probably the result of leakage of plasma proteins due to diffuse and/or nodular glomerulosclerosis. The capsular drop is virtually diagnostic of diabetes; the fibrin cap is nonspecific and may be seen in other glomerular diseases.[30]

Renal Atherosclerosis and Arteriolosclerosis These constitute only one part of the systemic involvement of vessels in diabetes. The kidney, unfortunately, is one of the most frequently and severely affected organs. The hyaline arteriolosclerosis affects not only the afferent but also the efferent arterioles. Such efferent arteriolosclerosis is rarely if ever encountered in nondiabetic people and is said to be also virtually diagnostic of the diabetes.

Pyelonephritis This is an acute or chronic inflammation of the kidneys due to bacteria, which usually begins in the interstitial tissue and then spreads to affect the tubules and possibly, ultimately, the glomeruli. One special pattern of acute pyelonephritis, necrotizing papillitis, also called "renal medullary necrosis," is definitely more prevalent in diabetics than nondiabetics; about 60 percent of the patients with necrotizing papillitis have diabetes, although it is seen with obstructions of the urinary tract as well as with analgesic abuse. Necrotizing papillitis is an acute necrosis of the renal papillae. In diabetes, bilateral necrosis of all papillae is not uncommon and frequently leads to acute, irreversible renal failure.

Tubular Lesions Several tubular lesions are also encountered in diabetes mellitus. Perhaps the most striking is deposition of glycogen within the epithelial cells of the distal tubules and sometimes in the descending loop of Henle. Various names are given to the lesions—glycogen infiltration, glycogen nephrosis, or Armanni-Ebstein cells.[31] Glycogen creates a clearing of the cytoplasm of the affected cells; only a distinct cell membrane with a squashed, basally displaced nucleus persists. This condition is thought to be due to severe hyperglycemia and glycosuria for a period of days or weeks. The lesion is reversible; no malfunction of the tubules is associated with the glycogen deposits. Tubular basement membrane thickening may be found along with the membrane changes described in the glomeruli. A patient who dies in diabetic acidosis may *rarely* exhibit fatty changes in the proximal convoluted tubules.

While individuals vary in their rates of progression of renal disease, the sequence of development is often similar. Symptoms of renal disease may occur under stressful states, and further damage may result from ischemic or infectious injury. Laboratory evidence of renal insufficiency usually exists prior to the appearance of symptoms.

The early sign of a glomerular lesion is proteinuria. A diminished renal reserve is evidenced by the presence of nitrogenous products above the normal concentrations in the blood (azotemia). Decreased renal clearance tests give further evidence of glomerular disease. Evaluation of the kidney's various functions and the degree of each dysfunction provides the physician with direction for treatment. A major part of the treatment is a careful matching of the patient's intake of food, fluid, and electrolytes with the kidney's ability to excrete various components. Nocturia and polyuria may occur early with proteinuria; a salt-wasting phase may occur, with the patient needing unusual amounts of sodium replacement daily. More frequently, oliguria and sodium and fluid retention occur as end-stage renal failure develops. Dialysis becomes necessary to maintain life and to remove the excess accumulations of fluid, electrolytes, and metabolic wastes. Marked restrictions in intake of fluid, protein, sodium, and potassium become necessary.

Acute Processes

Infection and circulatory inadequacy cause renal disease, unmask underlying renal pathology, and severely stress homeostatic processes. *Prerenal azotemia* is the term used for azotemia that is precipitated by inadequate perfusion of the kidney; hyperglycemia and other states that involve dehydration, hypovolemia, and hypotension may provoke signs of renal failure. Congestive heart failure and hypertension are two conditions that can decrease renal perfusion, as can antihypertensive and diuretic agents. Early detection and treatment are necessary to restore the prior renal status; observation of urinary volumes and examination of constituents of the blood and urine are necessary whenever alterations in renal perfusion are suspected.

When restoration of fluid volume and/or blood pressure does not restore urinary excretion, acute tubular necrosis is suspected. If signs of acute renal failure persist, restrictions of fluid, protein, sodium, and potassium are begun. Dialysis and other symptomatic treatments are used to support the patient until renal function is restored. The regeneration of the epithelial lining of the tubule may take 2 to 6 weeks. If the kidney does not regain function, these treatments are continued for life. In acute renal failure, hyperkalemia and circulatory overload are frequent complications. The reader is referred to specialized texts for the management of acute renal failure.

Risk Factors

Pyelonephritis is considered a major contributing factor in the development of diabetic nephropathy. The effects of asymptomatic bacteriuria on the progress of diabetic nephropathy is unclear; however, many physicians believe that bacteria should be eradicated with long-term treatment by a specific antibiotic agent. Infections of the urethra, bladder, and ureter may ascend and cause either acute or chronic pyelonephritis. Indwelling catheterization and instrumentation of the urethra can induce urinary tract infections. The kidney is also vulnerable to infection carried to it by blood from another site.

Recent studies have raised questions about the best procedures for meatal care for the patient with an indwelling catheter. One study showed a greater incidence of infections of the urinary tract when a povidone-iodine cleansing agent was applied to the meatal-catheter junction on a regular basis.[32] Cleaning with soap and water with no manipulation of the catheter at the meatus is recommended. The use of asepsis and a closed drainage system positioned below the level of the bladder are essential parts of care. Specimen collections of urine are obtained through the use of a sterile syringe and needle rather than disrupting the drainage system.

Diabetic patients may have an atonic bladder from neuropathic lesions of the autonomic nervous system. Subsequent retention of urine and inability to completely empty the bladder may be factors in the increased incidence of bladder infections. If there are no restrictions of fluid intake, encouragement to drink is recommended. States of fluid retention as in renal failure and congestive heart failure may limit the amount of fluid the patient can drink. Further restriction than that ordered by the physician should not be encouraged.

Changes in Diabetic Status

As renal disease progresses there are many changes that affect glucose and increase the amount and kind of self-care activities a patient can use to maintain optimum function. Changes in metabolic processes affect diabetic self-care activities and change the methods of control of blood glucose. Oliguria makes urine testing infrequent, but more important, a rising renal threshold for glucose often makes testing valueless. Insulin requirements often decrease over a period of months; increased frequency of hypoglycemic episodes in the insulin-dependent patient may occur.

Anorexia and subsequent reduction of caloric intake become common. The diet is restricted in the amounts of sodium, potassium, protein, and water; this is a change from the diet previously used to control blood glucose. Now the patient is encouraged to eat fat and carbohydrate to minimize catabolism of body stores of protein. Changes in physiological status may cause changes in either carbohydrate or protein metabolism. Infection increases the amount of catabolism and the endogenous production of protein acid. With cell destruction, potassium is released. Infection can increase the degree of hyperglycemia, azotemia, acidosis, and hyperkalemia. Respiratory infection is additionally dangerous because of the decreased ability to excrete carbon dioxide, a compensatory response to the metabolic acidosis that accompanies renal failure and that of ketoacidosis.

An example of the rapid change that can occur in a diabetic with renal failure follows. A woman came for a regularly scheduled dialysis treatment. She had a weight gain of 9 lb in 4 days in contrast to her usual gain of 5 lb. She complained of three-pillow orthopnea and she had slight pedal edema. She reported increased hunger and food intake with no increase in oral fluids. Her urinary daily output had decreased from 375 mL per day to less than 150 mL. Blood glucose concentration was 1000 mg/dL; she was not in ketoacidosis. Treatment included dialysis and additional insulin.

Self-Care Activities

Self-care activities for the patient with chronic renal failure include adherence to diet, monitoring of fluid and electrolytic balance, and the use of medications. Diuretics and aluminum hydroxide gels are commonly used. Sodium bicarbonate may be taken to control the degree of acidosis; cation-exchange resins may be used for the excretion of potassium. Hypocalcemia is common and is a manifestation of decreased urinary excretion of phosphates.

Aluminum hydroxide gels are used to increase the excretion of phosphate through the stool; they bind phosphate within the intestinal lumen. Since calcium and phosphorous serum levels are inversely controlled, if phosphate serum levels are decreased, calcium levels will rise. (Hypocalcemia can lead to tetany and is responsible for osteoporosis, which occurs in end-stage renal failure.) These gels can also decrease the mucosal irritation common to azotemia. They differ in the amounts and kinds of electrolytes they contain, and the desire to avoid sodium and magnesium intake often determines the particular gel chosen in renal failure.

Cation-exchange resins are used to treat hyperkalemia; they can be used in acute crises as well as in maintenance therapy. The resin can be taken orally or may be administered rectally or through a Levin tube. The resin is in the form of a powder and must be mixed with fluid; water or low-potassium fluids should be used. If the exchange agent is sodium, additional fluid retention can result.

Dialysis

The patient's program of diet, medications, and frequency of dialysis is individually planned. For the diabetic, frequent testing of blood glucose is done as well as tests for creatinine, electrolytes, and hematocrit. Directions from the dialysis center for the diabetic patient specify whether the timing of insulin and food should be changed in relation to the dialysis treatment. In addition, the center will specify whether other medications that can pass through the semipermeable membrane of the dialysis machine should be delayed. Dialysis goals are set individually for each patient based on symptoms, laboratory tests, and physical findings.

Patients with limited cardiac reserve or a contracted intravascular volume may respond with symptoms of tachycardia, hypotension, and/or arrhythmias when sudden changes in fluid balance occur. For the patient with diabetic nephropathy, nephrosis and the resulting hypoalbuminemia are common. This may limit the rapidity of dialysis or the amount of fluid that can be withdrawn. If possible, dialysis is performed until a slightly dehydrated state exists.

Certain precautions must be taken to protect the integrity of the shunt or fistula that provides access to the patient's blood for dialysis. A Scribner shunt consists of a permanent implantation of two plastic cannulas, one into a vein and one into an artery. A plastic tube connects these cannulas (when dialysis is not being performed) and allows continuous blood flow. If clotting occurs in this connection the patient must report to a physician. Clotting can be detected by inspection and palpation. A thrill in the connecting tube can be felt if blood is flowing. The patient cleanses the skin insertion sites daily and wears a protective dressing over the shunt.

An arteriovenous anastomosis (AV fistula) diverts arterial blood into a vein by a surgical anastomosis. After healing, a small scar overlays a distended and pulsating vein. The part distal to the fistula may be cooler because of the decreased arterial flow. Usually an arm is used for these procedures and requires protection from injury. The arm should not be used for injections, blood pressures, or blood samples when either a shunt or fistula is present.

The patient previously discussed reported, "On the day of dialysis, all I can do is take the treatment. I have the most energy the day after dialysis; I plan most activities for this day; I get increasingly tired until the day of dialysis. After the treatment, I have leg cramps and am irritable for several hours. If I had known how bad it was, I would not have started on dialysis."

Although diabetic patients have had experience in coping with chronic illness, stress placed by dialysis and renal failure is often overwhelming. However, options are limited: continue with dialysis until a transplantable kidney is available, or refuse to continue with the life-supporting dialysis regimen. Blindness is frequent in patients with diabetic nephropathy who require dialysis. Life increasingly revolves around the dialysis treatments; major changes in life-style become necessary. The patient must learn new self-care activities at the same time he or she is confronted with severe illness, a more difficult life-style, and evidence of a decreased life span. An unhurried approach and a supportive environment often allow the patient to internalize and adapt to this major crisis with inherent resources and strengths. The dialysis staff will have long-term and frequent contact with the patient and family, and often assume a coordinating role with all others providing health care.

THE DIABETIC WITH MOBILITY AT RISK

Neuropathy, peripheral vascular disease, and microvascular changes in the lower extremities can alter the diabetic's life and mobility. In a postmortem study of diabetics in 1952, peripheral vascular disease accounted for 12.7 percent of deaths.[33] Diabetics are 5 times more prone to gangrene than are nondiabetics. Anesthesia from neuropathy often contributes to the incidence of infection and minor trauma that lead to gangrene. (Refer to Chapter 4 for discussion of neuropathy.) Gangrene increases the severity of ketoacidosis and is often accompanied with septicemic shock. Peripheral vascular disease or neuropathy of the lower extremities may occur singly or in combination with other complications of diabetes. Those risk factors discussed under atherosclerosis apply to peripheral vascular disease.

Because of the seriousness of these conditions, all diabetics are encouraged to practice good foot care. In this section, care of the diabetic with pathology of the legs and feet will be discussed.

Infection and Trauma

Infection may begin in cracks in hypertrophied skin, neurotrophic ulcers, ingrown toenails, and under corns and calluses, as well as from traumatic injuries (abrasions, incisions, burns, and puncture wounds). Fungal infections such as athlete's foot (epidermophytosis) may precede more pathogenic invasion of the skin. The diabetic with loss of sensation from neuropathy may be unable to detect lesions until infection and significant extension of tissue damage have occurred. Visual impairment, obesity, and lack of agility may interfere with ability to monitor the integrity of skin and to provide care.

Because of the decreased circulation from both supply by large arteries and capillary perfusion from microvascular changes, healing is retarded. Foot lesions in the diabetic may be deceptive on appearance; the depth and extension to subcutaneous tissue, muscle, and even bone may be quite large and masked by the appearance of a relatively small surface lesion.

Neurotrophic Ulcers

Neurotrophic ulcers may occur in the presence or absence of vascular insufficiency and are the result of pressure atrophy. Ill-fitting shoes can provide the initial stimulus to corn and callus formation. The neurotrophic ulcer can develop under the hardened skin and not be visible until the corn or callus is removed. The lack of pain perception is a significant factor that often results in delayed detection or treatment. (Fig. 10-3 shows neuropathic lesions.)

Walking can initiate pressure atrophy and ulcer formation in the patient with muscle loss and resulting bone shifting from neuropathy (Charcot's foot). These changes cause a shift in weight bearing to those areas of the foot with little protection of soft tissues; the result is ulcer formation. Limited mobility and bed rest until healing occurs are often necessary; the use of assistive devices to avoid weight bearing is frequently needed. Specially adapted shoes, foam-rubber boots, or molded sandals can be helpful in avoiding future injury.

Arterial Occlusive Disease

Signs of arterial vascular compromise range from mild and chronic changes (loss of hair, cool temperature, thin skin, diminished pulses, thick toenails) to signs of severe and acute occlusion (cyanosis, coldness, and gangrene). Inflammatory signs may be present in acute lesions and extend upward.

The patient may report claudication or pain which limits motility. Popliteal pulses are often present, but pedal and posterior tibial pulses are diminished or absent. Occlusive disease most often affects peroneal and tibial arteries in the diabetic patient.

Dry Gangrene It is possible for tissue death to occur with minimal inflammation; this is termed "dry gangrene." Figure 10-2 shows the marked differentiation of anoxic tissue. Autoamputation of toes is possible for such areas and is often the treatment of choice. Exposure to air and a drying environment is used during the time of autoamputation. The adjacent tissues are subject to trauma and infection; gentleness is necessary in touching. The surgeon may debride some of the dead tissue. There should be close monitoring for extension of gangrene or the onset of infection.

Moisture increases the chance of infection and maceration of skin. Soaking of the foot, emollients, creams, and lotions are not used on these lesions unless ordered by the physician. Care should be used in applying any substance to the skin surrounding the lesion so that it does not get onto the lesion. (An exception may be when Dakin's solution is applied for debridement and petroleum jelly mesh gauze is ordered to cover the adjoining healthy skin.) Often dressings are not used to cover the wound, and occlusive dressings are contraindicated. If cleansing must be done, alcohol has the most drying effect; in fact, it may be regularly ordered to promote drying.

The amount of pain varies; as the area becomes gangrenous, pain slowly subsides as a result of nerve destruction. Other areas of the foot and leg may be more painful than the gangrenous ones. With advanced neuropathy, pain may be completely absent, even with inflammation, infection, and gangrene.

The patient's response to death of a part of his or her body can be assessed by the nurse working with the patient. Whether the patient looks at, touches, or talks about the part can give clues as to his or her perception and acceptance of

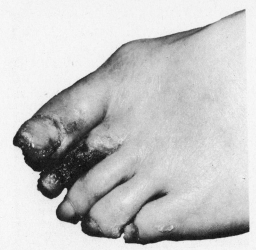

Figure 10-2 Dry gangrene of several toes of an adult-onset diabetic woman with arteriosclerosis obliterans. (*Photograph courtesy of Henry Haimovici, from Jones, Dunbar, and Jirovec, "Medical-Surgical Nursing: A Conceptual Approach," New York: McGraw-Hill, 1978, p. 669.*)

the tissue death. Although airing of the part is essential, it is not necessary that it be on view to the patient or others.

Wet Gangrene   Gangrene coupled with inflammation is termed "wet gangrene." In contrast to previously discussed dry gangrene, extension of tissue destruction is greater. Septicemia, septic shock, increased hyperglycemia, and ketoacidosis increase the threat of life. Figure 10-3 shows a toe with develop-

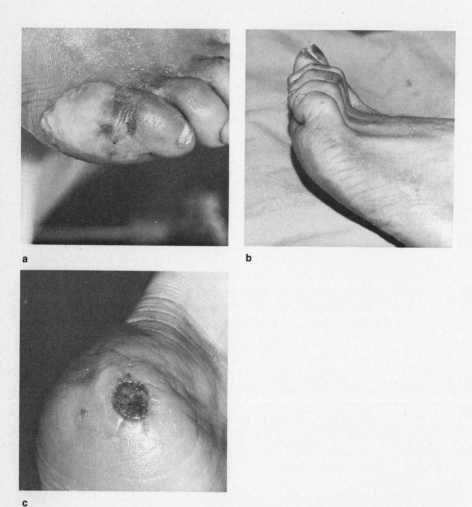

Figure 10-3   Wet gangrene in an adult man with growth-onset diabetes and neuropathy. (a) The small toe on the right foot was the source of cellulitis on admission. Line of demarcation can be seen. (b) "Cock-up toes" are one sign of advanced diabetic neuropathy. Extension of the metatarsal-phalangeal joints and flexion at the proximal interphalangeal joints are shown. Pressure areas are apparent. (c) A neuropathic ulcer on the heel is surrounded by indurated and inflamed tissue. The patient attributed this lesion to a crack in the hardened skin that was caused by pressure from shoes.

ment of wet gangrene, characteristic signs of edema, and line of demarcation. Above the toe, cellulitis with redness, edema, and increased skin temperature were observed. Amputation of this toe was performed 4 h later, followed in a week by further amputation because healing was inadequate.

Radiation diagnostic procedures are used to determine the extent and nature of lesions; radioisotope scans reveal the status of microvasculature, while peripheral arteriograms show both defects in large arteries and the extent of collateral circulation.[34] X-rays and bone scans can assist the physician in determining whether osteomyelitis and infection with aneorobic bacteria are present.

Bed rest, antibiotic therapy, supportive measures, and often amputation are methods of treatment. The reader is referred to specialized texts for the management and care of the patient with amputation and reconstructive vascular surgery. After healing of the stump, hygienic skin measures similar to those used in foot care should be used with the stump.

Bed Rest

The diabetic with problems of the feet often has extended periods of bed rest. If conservative measures are used, bed rest will be much longer than if amputation is done. All those who provide direct care to the patient should employ measures that prevent some of the complications of bed rest. Careful assessment is needed to plan activities appropriate for the individual. The patient can exercise some muscles and move some joints while eating, bathing, and performing other activities in bed. However, it is rare that the bed patient will exercise sufficiently to maintain extensors of the arm and leg for transfer, weight bearing, and ambulation. Flexion contractures do occur with bed rest and are increased with pain when positions of comfort are assumed. A program that ensures a full range of motion with active muscle exercises should be started when the patient is first ordered on bed rest, to prevent muscle atrophy and maintain joint motion.

When the diabetic has an acute foot lesion, attention should not be diverted from maintenance of the integrity of other skin areas. Because bed rest is often required for healing, pressure areas may develop. The patient with sensory loss no longer perceives the sensations of tingling ("pins and needles") that stimulate others to make small, unnoticed changes in position. Heels and bony prominences are subject to pressure areas, as are the toes from bed clothes. A foot cradle is a most important device to obtain for the diabetic with a foot lesion. When drying is ordered by the physician, one 25-W light bulb is used with the foot cradle. Heat is contraindicated.

There should be frequent changes of position and continuous monitoring of the effectiveness of devices used to decrease pressure (foam- or gel-filled pads, contoured heel protectors, and pillows). Sharp edges of foot cradle frames should be padded.

Measures designed to prevent problems of bed rest including decubitus should be planned on an individual basis. Consideration of other complications and restrictions form the medical framework within which measures are designed to prevent problems of bed rest. For example, carbohydrate restriction may limit the amount of fruits and vegetables used to prevent constipation; sodium restriction affects the choice of laxatives. Restrictions of fluid intake because of renal or cardiac disease preclude increased fluids to prevent urinary stasis.

When the patient is allowed more mobility, attention to the feet should not decrease. In fact, inspection and care of the feet should increase as the patient resumes weight bearing and ambulation. A safe environment is free of sharp objects and clutter around which the patient has to maneuver. Adequate supporting shoes should be available. The sequential steps of mobility training by physical therapists should be followed and reinforced during nursing care. If new pressure areas develop, walking is stopped until adaptations are made to decrease the irritant, if possible. Resumption of usual foot care of the involved foot should occur if it has been interrupted. Throughout the bed-rest experience, the patient should be learning more appropriate foot care.

Exercise to the Foot and Extremity

The physician should clarify the amount of exercise appropriate for the individual with a diabetic foot lesion. However, rarely will dorsiflexion, plantar flexion, and rotation of the ankle be contraindicated (or quadriceps setting and straight leg raising). These are exercises that promote muscle and joint function. Vascular exercises may be ordered to stimulate the development of collateral circulation. These are used several times a day for a set number of timed movements. See Fig. 10-4 for a description of Buerger-Allen exercises. The patient can learn to do these exercises without supervision. Frequently, however, the patient needs guidance on equipment to use at home. Evaluation of the effects of these exercises should focus on the extent of changes in color, temperature, and pain.

The use of a foot board for exercise or positioning is often ill-advised in the diabetic with neuropathic or plantar lesions for the same reasons that walking is avoided. Frequent dorsiflexion is an alternative measure to prevent foot drop. If the patient has a tightened Achilles tendon, extension of the ankle is equally important.

THE DIABETIC AT RISK FOR VISUAL IMPAIRMENT

Diabetes is the leading cause of blindness in people between the ages of 20 and 64 each year in the United States.[35] Sixty-two percent of the juvenile diabetic population will develop some retinopathy after a disease duration of 10 years, and 7.5 percent of patients with good vision and nonproliferative retinopathy will develop visual impairment annually. Of these, 50 percent will ultimately be blind. If the duration of disease extends over 30 years, 18 percent will develop proliferative retinopathy.[36] Although proliferative retinopathy is considered an

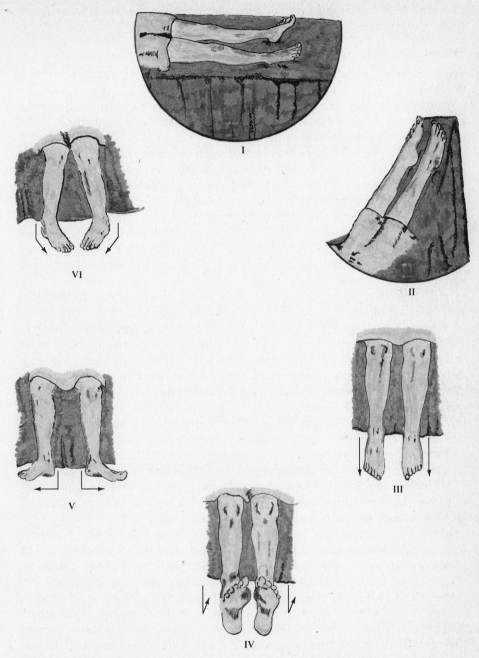

Figure 10-4 Buerger-Allen exercises are prescribed in different positions and follow this sequence: (I) starting position; (II) elevating the legs for 2 min (pain or blanching on elevation may necessitate a decreased time); (III) lowering the legs for 3 min; (IV, V, VI) moving the feet through full range of motion (in addition, the toes are spread); and, resting for 5 min (I). (*Drawn by Martha Allen.*)

advanced stage of the same process, macular edema in the earlier stage is the single greatest cause of blindness from retinopathy in the diabetic.

Retinopathy

The basic lesion of retinopathy is the outpocketings of "microaneurysms" in the retinal capillaries, which is followed by intraretinal hemorrhages, changes in blood flow through the retina due to vascular shunts between small arteries and veins, and new formation of vessels with scar tissue and hemorrhage in the vitreous fluid filling the back of the eye.

Are the vascular changes the result of separate genetic defects which affect the vessels of the eye in a diabetic patient or do they occur as a complication of the diabetic process? Experiments using dogs and monkeys with chemically induced diabetes have clearly demonstrated that the vascular changes are complications of the abnormal metabolism and are markedly diminished if the animals are carefully controlled with insulin therapy. The mural cells which surround the retinal capillaries are the first cells to be affected; their viability and reproduction patterns are greatly changed. The pattern of blood flow is changed and aneurysms appear.[37]

The microaneurysms are discrete saccular dilatations of retinal-choroidal capillaries which appear through the ophthalmoscope as small red dots. Areas of exudate appear yellow and waxy (see Fig. 10-5). Angiography is used to locate and examine lesions of retinopathy; this procedure may be done on an ambulatory basis and includes intravenous injection of fluorescein. Although the cause of these lesions is uncertain, the view that they represent aneurysmal dilatations at focal points of weakening due to degeneration of the mural cells (pericytes) is favored. Presumably these cells are injured or destroyed when they become trapped in the reduplicated layers of basal membrane. About one-half the patients with retinal microaneurysms also have nodular glomerulosclerosis (which was discussed previously). Patients who have nodular glomerulosclerosis are almost certain to have retinal microaneurysms.[38]

Another question has been raised as to whether the vitreous humor contains too much of a vasoproliferative factor, which is found in some neoplastic lesions, or does not contain an inhibitor to such a substance.[39]

Aldose reductase, the enzyme responsible for the formation of sorbitol from glucose, has been found in the retina as well as in the lens of the eye. The sorbitol pathway is currently accepted as the cause of diabetic cataracts. Within the lens, the increased levels of sorbitol cause increased levels of water in the cell and lenticular swelling. Along with the influx of water is an influx of sodium and an efflux of potassium ions, along with the disruption of the amino acid concentrating mechanism. Free intracellular myoinositol is lost in proportion to sugar alcohol accumulations, and the ATP level drops along with the loss of osmotic integrity.[40]

Besides retinopathy, other structural and physiological changes contribute to the high incidence of visual impairment: cataracts, glaucoma, and optic nerve atrophy. Diabetic changes can affect the iris and ciliary body and the

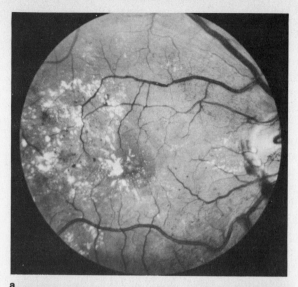

a

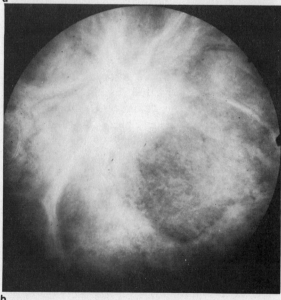

b

Figure 10-5   (a) Diabetic retinopathy. An ophthalmoscopic view of the retina showing exudates. (b) Diabetic retinopathy, with devascularized fibrous proliferative tissue. Visual acuity is
usually reduced at this stage. *(Photographs courtesy of T. W. Lieberman, M.D., from Jones,
Dunbar, and Jirovec, "Medical Surgical Nursing: A Conceptual Approach," New York,
McGraw-Hill, 1978, p. 681.)*

regulatory nerves to these structures and to the muscles controlling movement
of the eyeball and eyelid. Abnormal pupillary responses to light and accommo-
dation, ptosis of the eyelid, and limitation in oculomotor movements may
result.

Assessment Factors

One common problem for the diabetic during periods of poor control of blood glucose concentration is blurring of vision of near objects. If the patient perceives a daily pattern of changing visual acuity, she or he often adjusts those activities requiring close sight accordingly. The patient may need the assistance of others or she or he may change the timing of urine testing or insulin preparation. As better control of blood glucose is achieved, this symptom subsides. Because of the changes in refraction, examinations for corrective lenses are delayed until better control of blood glucose is achieved.

Any change in visual function reported by the patient should be thoroughly investigated. Careful questioning should follow a patient report of blurred vision. "Misty vision" or "looking through water" may accompany the report of "halos around lights" in the patient with glaucoma. Intraorbital pain and redness of the eye are always significant. "Floaters" indicate vitreous debris, and a "shade pulled down over my sight" indicates retinal detachment. Self-care ability should be evaluated in relation to the change in vision.

Examination of the eye and testing of visual acuity and the visual fields are part of the surveillance care for the diabetic patient. Direct ophthalmoscopy is used by the primary care provider; a more extensive examination is done by the ophthalmologist at regularly scheduled intervals and whenever abnormalities are judged significant by the primary care provider.

In proliferative retinopathy, viewing the retina (and the vision of the patient) may be hindered by the abnormal growth of blood vessels and glial tissue that overlie the retina or by blood in the vitreous chamber. Because the new blood vessels are friable, they rupture easily and may bleed into the vitreous chamber or behind the retina, dissecting it away from the choroid. A tractional retinal detachment and/or tears in the retina may occur as retinal-vitreous adhesions shrink and pull the retina away from the underlying choroid. Retinal detachment may be of varying size—a pinpoint area or one that extends throughout the retinal surface. The location of retinal detachment may be in the periphery of the fundus or involve the macula and the disk.

Therapeutic Measures

Surgical removal of cataracts, drainage procedures for glaucoma, and scleral implants and buckling procedures for retinal detachment are some of the intraocular surgical methods of treating eye disease in the diabetic. The reader should refer to specialized references for the care of the patient with eye surgery. Instructions after discharge should indicate clearly the length of time the patient is to avoid activities that increase intraocular pressure: bending, lifting, straining by Valsalva's test, eye medications, and the use of patches.

Systemic measures have been used in attempts to interfere with the processes of retinopathy. These include adrenalectomy, pituitary ablation, various antilipid compounds, calcium dobesilate (an agent to reduce capillary leakage), fat-restricted diets, PAS, salicylates, and androgens.[41] Kohner suggests that pituitary ablation be reserved for florid proliferative retinopathy, a rare and rapidly advancing retinopathy.[42] Patients who have been hypophysectomized need daily replacement of cortisol and thyroid hormones; in stress, additional cortisol replacement must be administered to prevent adrenal crisis.

Photocoagulation

Photocoagulation, the use of thermal energy to coagulate single or multiple areas of the retinal capillary bed, is used to "seal" areas of capillary leakage, thrombose actively bleeding vessels, destroy abnormal capillary growth, and disperse large blood clots. Photocoagulation may be used to treat local lesions or to reduce the stimulus for vascularization by "scatter" photocoagulation, causing up to 1500 "burns" of 1-mm diameter.[43] Argon and xenon are two sources of energy used. This treatment is often done on an ambulatory care basis.

Photocoagulation may be used to treat the retina after a vitrectomy, the removal of the vitreous humor that has been infiltrated by hemorrhage and scar tissue. The vitreous is replaced by a space-filling physiologic fluid.

A study sponsored by the National Institute of Health demonstrated a beneficial role of photocoagulation in proliferative retinopathy as well as in retinal edema and exudative formation. Blindness developed at a much lower incidence in treated eyes than in untreated eyes (the other eye of each individual served as the control). At the end of 2 years, 16.3 percent of untreated eyes and 6.4 percent of treated eyes showed severe visual loss; the *risk* of blindness was reduced in treated eyes when compared with that of the control eyes.[44]

Rehabilitation

Legal blindness is defined by two criteria of visual acuity, either of which constitutes legal blindness. The first criterion is stated thus: The central vision in the better eye is less than 20/200. The legally blind person therefore can see less at 20 ft than the person with normal sight can see at 200 ft (even with corrective lenses). The other criterion refers to a loss of perception of visual fields: The visual field is 30° or less.*

The establishment of legal blindness is important to the diabetic for economic reasons; financial assistance from several sources may be obtained for the legally blind (income tax deductions, applications for financial assistance under Social Security, and support for vocational education programs).

Whether sudden blindness occurs or there is gradual loss of vision, at some point the diabetic can benefit from rehabilitation services that are offered through community agencies. While working with the patient on diabetes self-care activities, the nurse may identify other patient needs for assistance in mobility, recreation, and vocational reeducation. Plans for working with the visually handicapped diabetic should be considered in the context of the total

* Normal degrees of visual fields are 60° nasally, 50° upward, 90° temporally, and 70° downward.

plan of rehabilitation, with attention given to the time and energy involved in each area.

Self-care activities related to diabetes should be considered within the context of other daily activities, levels of independence, and plans for rehabilitation. Investigation of community resources may reveal ongoing programs of training for the blind in mobility, braille, vocations, and other areas. Information about resources in a particular community may be found by consulting the local society for the blind, diabetes association, state, county, or city public health offices, or two national associations interested in the well-being of the blind: The American Foundation for the Blind, 15 West 16th Street, New York, New York 10011, and the National Society for the Blind, 79 Madison Avenue, New York, New York 10016.

Local libraries have information about materials for the blind. Thirty-four libraries throughout the United States distribute books (in braille or on records), which are provided by the Division for the Blind and Physically Handicapped, Washington, D.C. 20540. Recording for the Blind, Incorporated, at 215 East 58th Street, New York, New York 10022, may be contacted for records or tapes of educational materials including textbooks.

The Cleveland Society for the Blind has over 125 "low-vision aids" that may help the visually handicapped read, watch television, read street signs, bus, and house numbers, or perform job and recreational activities. Refer to Fig. 10-6 for illustrations of some low-vision aids. Some of these will be useful to the visually handicapped diabetic in reading diabetic materials and in carrying out activities related to insulin, foot care, and urine testing.

A brochure from the agency lists the following suggestions when offering services to the blind.[45]

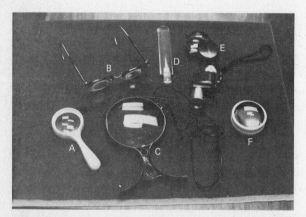

Figure 10-6 Magnifying aids. There are many aids to help visually impaired people carry out daily activities. Magnifying lenses may be combined with handles (A) or glasses (B). The Visolett Stand Magnifier may also be worn suspended from the neck so that the hands are free (C). The bar magnifier is useful for reading on flat surfaces (D). The Selsi Monocular Telescope is particularly useful for identifying signs and house numbers (E). Also illustrated is a carrying case for a magnifying glass (F). (*Photograph courtesy of Susan Jones.*)

Identify yourself and let them know you're talking to them (they won't know if you don't) and ask if they want some help.

If so, offer your arm—don't pull or push. Walk a step ahead and they will follow the motion of your body.

If you give directions, be specific and accurate. Pointing will not help.

Speak when you enter a blind person's room. Identify yourself and let them know when you're leaving. Don't leave them stranded and talking to air.

Speak directly to them, using a normal tone of voice. They won't mind words like "see" or "blind," so you needn't censor your conversation.

Avoid the temptation to pet a dog guide. The dog is responsible for leading a person who cannot see—and must not be distracted.

Speak directly to a blind person—not through another party.

If you have a money transaction with a person who is blind, identify each bill so that it may be folded accordingly to the person's own method.

When you dine with blind people, guide hands to the chair; advise them (unobtrusively) about the table setting and the location of the food on the plate.

If you take them to a car or bus, guide hands to the door handle. They'll manage the rest of the way.

When you do meet a blind person—common sense and sensitivity too are most important of all.

Location of food servings may be described as clock positions.

Diabetic Self-Care Activities

There are many aspects of diabetic self-care that are considered when working with the visually impaired diabetic. Ability to locate and take glucose in the event of hypoglycemia, dialing an emergency number, planning meals, shopping for and preparing of food, and proper foot care are examples. In all these activities, modifications can be made so that the individual's potential for independence may be reached.

In working with a patient who has some vision, the environment should be well lighted. Syringes should be chosen that have the darkest markings and widest spacings of calibrations. Equipment should be placed in the same position each time. White backgrounds seem more effective than dark.

Urine Testing   A test for urine sugar can be done by the blind diabetic during absences of family members or more regularly. Equipment includes a test tube, yeast, water, and a finger cot. Twelve milliliters of urine and ¼ tsp of yeast are mixed in a test tube, and the finger cot is securely fastened over the top of the tube. If glucose is present, gas will form. After 10 to 20 min, if there is bulging and tautness of the finger cot, the patient records this as strongly positive. A "mushy" feeling is recorded as moderately positive, and a relaxed, soft indentation as negative.[46]

Insulin Administration   In working with the blind diabetic, several options can be outlined to assist the patient in deciding how independent he or she can be. Systems can be set up to match the degree of independence with the degree of assistance desired or necessary. For example, the diabetic can become completely independent within the home, or a family member or visiting nurse might prepare a week's supply of prefilled syringes so that that patient can obtain one from the refrigerator* and inject it on a daily basis. Some patients with very severe illnesses have wanted to continue injecting insulin, even though family members were willing and able to do this. Other patients may want to be (or need to be) completely dependent on family members, neighbors, or others for insulin administration.

A major problem exists for the visually handicapped person in withdrawing insulin—not air—from the vial (see Fig. 10-7). To resolve this problem, modification of technique is necessary, or another person can check at regular intervals to verify that sufficient insulin is left in the vial and can transfer small amounts of insulin into other vials. In the next section various sensory aids to assist the diabetic in preparing insulin are illustrated and described.

Several nurses have reported their work with more than 100 blind diabetics. They report that most blind diabetics become independent in insulin administration. They have offered several suggestions to assist the blind with administration of insulin. These include teaching the patient to

1   Devise a method to use in counting used doses and knowing the amount of insulin left in the vial (a marble moved from one container to another)

2   Withdraw and reinject the insulin into the vial three times while listening for bubbling in the insulin as it is expelled

3   Stabilize the hand by placing the little finger against the skin instead of using a dartlike movement[47,48]

Tactile sensation and manipulative dexterity are obvious assets to the blind diabetic who wishes to learn to manage insulin administration. Many of the aids require fine sensitivity and agile fingers. Those people familiar with insulin administration prior to visual impairment often learn modifications easily, although changes due to neuropathy may decrease their sensitivity and dexterity.

Sensory Aids†

The existence of reliable devices that enable blind diabetics to measure and administer all types and combinations of insulin safely is not as widely known as it should be. These products, in conjunction with instruction and training in their usage, assist many blind people in achieving optimal independence in controlling their diabetes. The selection and suitability of a particular device must, of course, be based on the special needs, idiosyncrasies, and circumstances of the individual diabetic. Descriptions of products that a number of

---

* Although refrigeration of insulin is not necessary, no studies have been found that report levels of bacterial growth in prefilled syringes in the home or change in potency from adsorption of insulin into the syringe when syringes are prefilled.

† This section is adapted from American Foundation for the Blind, Sensory aids, *Visual Impairment and Blindness,* February 1977, pp. 78–81. Permission for publication has been granted.

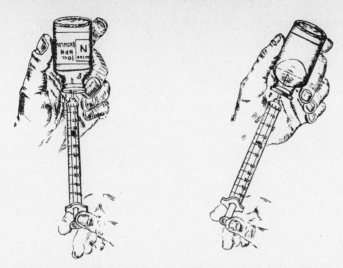

Figure 10-7 When the insulin vial is held on a slant, the needle is more likely to be above the level of insulin. Air, not insulin, is then drawn into the syringe. The blind person can be taught to prevent the withdrawal of air (see text).

visually impaired diabetics have found suitable and manageable are illustrated and described below.

Syringes Figure 10-8 illustrates several diabetic syringes. The B-D Cornwall syringe with metal pipetting holder (Fig. 10-8A), made by Becton-Dickinson and Company, is comprised of a 1-mL replaceable B-D Cornwall glass syringe that fits inside a metal pipetting holder equipped with a positive adjustable stop. The diabetic's physician or nurse presets the length of the column of insulin within the syringe so that the plunger, when released, draws the correct volume of solution from the vial. Disassembly is accomplished without disturbing the setting. Careful instruction in the assembly and disassembly

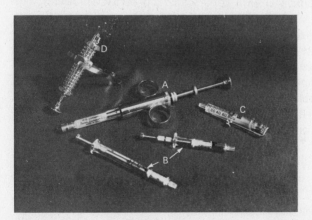

Figure 10-8 Syringes for visually impaired diabetics. (*Photograph courtesy of Susan Jones.*)

of its several components is imperative. The syringe is not to be used for mixed doses of insulin. Available in U-80 and U-100 scales, it is sent only to the individual's physician or registered nurse, who will set the syringe and teach the technique. It is sold by the American Foundation for the Blind, 15 West 16th Street, New York, New York 10011. Price: $14.50 (catalog no. MES166).

The Hill accurate-dosage insulin syringe (Fig. 10-8B) is a high-quality 1-mL glass syringe with an adjustable plunger that "clicks in" at the point where the desired dosage has been preset by the physician or registered nurse. It can be easily disassembled for cleaning and sterilization without disturbing the dosage setting. The syringe is filled by deflecting the plunger rod firmly to one side against the barrel as the plunger is being drawn out. A distinct "click" can be felt and heard when the correct setting has been reached. Calibration is in the U-80 scale only. Detailed instructions are included with each syringe. A mixed dose cannot be measured nor can the dosage be changed except by a sighted person. Sold by American Foundation for the Blind, 15 West 16th Street, New York, New York 10011. Price: $6.95 (catalog no. MES169).

Insulin syringe with "Tru-set" control (Fig. 10-8C) is a standard 1-mL glass syringe of the short type for U-100 use only and is fitted with a metal "Tru-set" syringe control that must be set by a physician or registered nurse to permit insulin measurement without sight. When used as instructed by the manufacturer, it helps ensure that the exact dose of insulin prescribed will be drawn into the syringe and tends to simplify preparation for the injection. Plunger can be removed for cleaning and sterilizing the syringe without changing the setting of the control or detaching it from the syringe. However, care should be exercised to prevent the screw from loosening. Distributed by Eisele and Company, Incorporated, Nashville, Tennessee 37210. Price: $9.00.

Insulin syringe MES260 (Fig. 10-8D) is a precision device developed in Holland and manufactured in West Germany. It consists of a standard 2-mL replaceable glass barrel fitted within a 3½-in-long metal casing on which a large nut is threaded. As this nut is rotated, "clicks" can be felt and heard. Each "click" represents $1/20$ mL or 4 U on a U-80 scale (2 U on a U-40 scale). For example, if a diabetic needs 20 U for U-80 insulin, he or she must rotate the nut five "clicks." Complete directions are included with each syringe. Although well-engineered and simple in concept, the weight, bulk, and manipulative requirements of this syringe are considered excessive by some. Others assert that its several component parts pose difficulties for tactually impaired patients in disassembly and assembly for sterilization purposes. Not available in the U-100 scale, it is sold by American Foundation for the Blind, 15 West 16th Street, New York, New York 10011. Price: $19.95 (catalog no. MES260).

Syringe Gauges and Filling Devices   The Insulgage Loading Gauge (Fig. 10-9) is a simple yet precise loading gauge for B-D long or Jelco disposable syringes that enables blind and visually impaired diabetics to load an insulin syringe safely and accurately, as well as vary their doses and measure mixed dosages. It is considered by many as the most versatile form of insulin self-

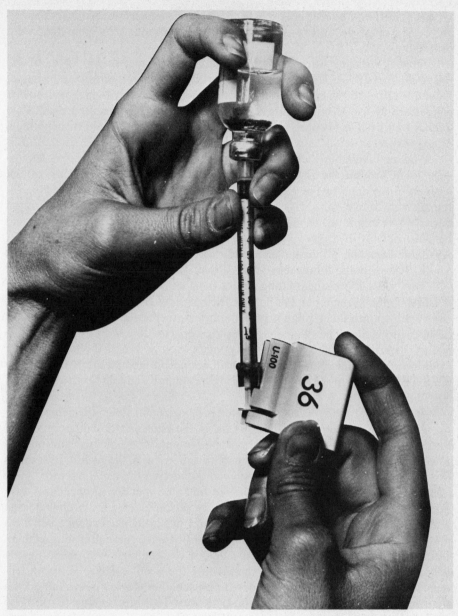

Figure 10-9 Insulgage loading gauge. (*Photograph courtesy of C. Mellor.*)

measurement. Made of durable plastic, this device is a precalibrated volume regulator available in a wide range of dosage sizes for U-40, U-80, and U-100 preparations. The gauges are assembled in sets to meet individual requirements. Specific, color-coded models are made for the B-D Plastipak, long type (no. 8409 for U-100; no. 8406 for U-80; no. 8401 for U-40). Also, the Jelco long type (no. 1022 for U-100; no. 1023 for U-40). The gauges are not interchangeable; they must be used only with the specific brand for which they were ordered.

Special versions have dosages identified by braille or by large, black, raised numbers. User selects gauge sizes with the help of a physician or nurse. Directions for use, warranty, and a receipt are included with each order. The gauges are available by mail directly from Meditec, Incorporated, 9485 East Orchard Drive, Englewood, Colorado 80110. (They are not sold through local drugstores.)

Another available loading device is made of copper tubing cut lengthwise to fit around the plunger of an individual syringe. The length of the sleeve corresponds to the exact measurement of a specific insulin dose. Although easy to use, this device is not interchangeable among different syringes nor can it be employed to measure a mixed dosage or to vary a dose. It should be used only with a glass syringe or B-D disposable with attached needle. Available from the Minneapolis Society for the Blind, 1936 Lyndale Avenue South, Minneapolis, Minnesota 55403. Price: $2.00.

The "dos-aid" syringe filling device is an adjustable volume regulator for positioning the syringe plunger so that the length of the column of insulin that can be drawn into the syringe is predetermined, thereby governing the number of units of insulin. The device is of plastic construction and designed for use mainly with disposable type U-100 syringes such as the B-D Plastipak long (⅝-in needle), or Jelco long. (Note: It will not accommodate the B-D Lo-Dose 0.5-mL disposable insulin syringe nor is it considered suitable for the Monoject 501.)

In use, a disposable syringe is placed in a horizontal slot in the center of the device and the plunger pulled back as far as the plunger stop will permit. The insulin vial is then positioned at the opposite end of the device and pushed toward the syringe. As the vial approaches the syringe, the needle penetrates the rubber stopper so that the syringe can be filled in the usual manner. After filling, the syringe and vial are removed and the injection proceeds as prescribed by the physician, who must initially set the device for proper dosage and syringe width and then lock the settings firmly in place. Once set for a particular brand of syringe, this device should be used thereafter only with an identical brand type of syringe. However, it is unpopular with some people because it is difficult to avoid contaminating the needle. There is also a tendency for settings of previous models to loosen. The device is available from the American Foundation for the Blind, 15 West 16th Street, New York, New York 10011. Price: $8.95 (catalog no. MES563).

The Andros IDM (insulin dosage monitor) is an elongated plastic strip that the nurse or physician snips off at the point on its scale that corresponds to the desired insulin dosage. The monitor is designed to be used with the Becton-Dickinson 8409 Plastipak U-100 disposable syringe only and is not to be used for mixed doses. To self-inject, the user pushes the U-100 syringe lip into the slot and draws the plunger back until it snaps past the snipped-off edge.

Shipped only to the physician, registered nurse, or other health professional managing the diabetic's condition. Sold by Andros, Incorporated, 2332 4th Street, Berkeley, California 94710. Price: $35.00, box of 100.

Other practical aids have been developed to aid the diabetic in placing the needle into the insulin vial. The Insulin Vial Guide helps the user place the syringe needle directly into the rubber stopper of the insulin bottle. Made of white enameled wood and measuring 5 by 1½ by ⅜ in, it has an extended arm against which the vial is positioned, plus a groove into which the syringe is placed. As the syringe is slid laterally along the groove, the needle penetrates the vial stopper. The guide is customarily used in conjunction with the SS62 Insulin Needle Guide, described below. Price: $2.00. From the Minneapolis Society for the Blind, 1936 Lyndale Avenue South, Minneapolis, Minnesota 55403.

The Insulin Needle Guide illustrated in Fig. 10-10 is designed to fit over the top of Eli Lilly insulin bottles. This lightweight aluminum device has a concave, funnel-shaped opening that guides the syringe needle directly into the rubber stopper. It can be used effectively with the Insulin Vial Guide described above and is sold by the American Foundation for the Blind, 15 West 16th Street, New York, New York 10011. Price: $1.50 (catalog no. MES168).

The AFB Insulin Needle Guide is a custom-made device that consists of an aluminum trough, at one end of which is a V-shaped notch. In use, the V end of the trough is first sterilized and the insulin vial placed at the opposite end with its stopper toward the V. The syringe needle is then laid in the V and the vial pushed toward it, allowing the needle to penetrate the rubber stopper. Because vial sizes vary, an empty one must accompany the order so that a guide can be

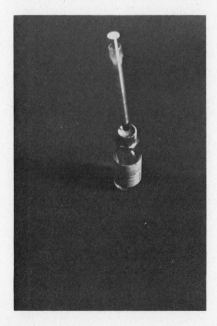

Figure 10-10 Insulin needle guide. (*Photograph courtesy of Susan Jones.*)

specially made to fit. Weight is 10 oz. This guide is sold by the American Foundation for the Blind, 15 West 16th Street, New York, New York 10011. Price: $4.50 (catalog no. MES165).

The "C-Better" Syringe Magnifier, is a simple, snap-on magnifier for diabetics, doctors, nurses, and others administering medicine by syringe where calibrations are difficult to read. Made of clear plastic, the device magnifies 2 times without distortion. It can be boiled in water, soaked in alcohol, or washed in soap and water, and it does not come into contact with needles. Snap-on wires can be bent to fit different-sized syringe barrels. The magnifier is available from Tri-County Rehabilitation Center, Incorporated, 4461 S.E. Federal Highway, Stuart, Florida 33494. Price: $3.00 postpaid.

REFERENCES

1 Garcia, M. J., et al. Diabetics in the Framingham population; sixteen year follow-up study, *Diabetes,* **23:**105–111, 1974.
2 U.S. Department of Health, Education and Welfare. *Report of the National Commission on Diabetes,* vol. III, part 1, Scope and Impact of Diabetes, Washington, D.C., 1975, p. 219.
3 Entmacher, P., et al. Longevity of diabetic patients in recent years, *Diabetes,* **13:**373, 1964.
4 Cahill, G., and Lacy, P. *Report to the Committee on the Etiology and Pathology of Diabetes to the National Commission on Diabetes,* vol. III, part 3, DHEW Publication NIH-76-1023, Washington, D.C., 1975.
5 Salinas-Madrigal, L., et al. Glomerular and vascular "insudative" lesions of diabetic neuropathy: electron microscopic observations, *Am. J. Pathol.,* **59:**369, 1970.
6 Borhani, N. O., et al. The control of elevated blood pressure in the community—an epidemiological perspective, *Heart and Lung,* **3:**478, 1974.
7 Gold, R., et al. High blood pressure and hospitals, *J.A.H.A.,* **48:**57, 1974.
8 Pell, S., and D'Alonzo, C. A. Some aspects of hypertension in diabetes mellitus, *J.A.M.A.,* **202:**10, 1967.
9 Veterans Administration Cooperative Study Group on Antihypertensive Agents. Effects on morbidity and hypertension. II. Results in patients with diastolic blood pressure averaging 90 through 114 mmHg, *J.A.M.A.,* **213:**1143, 1970.
10 Griffith, E. W., and Madero, B. Primary hypertension: patient's learning needs, *Am. J. Nur.,* **73:**624–627, 1973.
11 Bierman, E. Therapy of hyperlipidemia in the diabetic patient, in *Diabetes in Review: Clinical Conference, 1976* (New York: American Diabetes Association and the New England Affiliate, 1976), p. 92.
12 Krall, L. P., and Joslin, A. P. General plan of treatment and dietary regulation, in A. Marble (ed.), *Diabetes Mellitus* (Philadelphia: Lea and Febiger, 1971), pp. 27, 255–256.
13 Montgomery R., et al. *Biochemistry: A Case-Oriented Approach,* 2d ed. (St. Louis: Mosby, 1977).
14 Guyton, A. *Basic Human Physiology: Normal Function and Mechanisms of Disease,* 2d ed. (Philadelphia: Saunders, 1977).
15 Bray, G. *The Obese Patient* (Philadelphia: Saunders, 1976).
16 Rabinowitz, D., and Zierler, K. Forearm metabolism in obesity and its response to

intra-arterial insulin: characteristics of insulin, resistance and evidence for adaptive hyperinsulinism, *J. Clin. Invest.,* **41**:2173, 1962.

17 Bagdade, J. D., et al. The significance of basal insulin levels in the evaluation of the insulin response to glucose in diabetics and non-diabetic subjects, *J. Clin. Invest.,* **46**:1549, 1967.

18 Sims, E., et al. Endocrine and metabolic effects of experimental obesity in man, *Prog. Horm. Res.,* **29**:457, 1973.

19 Felig, P., et al. Plasma amino acid levels and insulin secretion in obesity, *N. Engl. J. Med.,* **281**:811, 1969.

20 Rabinowitz, D. Hormonal profile and forearm metabolism in human obesity, *Am. J. Clin. Nutr.,* **21**:1438, 1968.

21 Rabinowitz, D. Insulin secretion in acromegaly, *J. Clin. Endocr.,* **30**:288, 1970.

22 Sims et al. Loc. cit.

23 Salinas-Madrigal et al. Loc. cit.

24 Amatruda, J., et al. Insulin receptors: role in the resistance of human obesity to insulin, *Science,* **188**:264, 1975.

25 Datey, K. K., and Nanda, N. C. Hyperglycemia after acute myocardial infarction, *N. Engl. J. Med.,* **276**:262, 1967.

26 Kotler, M. N., et al. Hypoglycemia precipitated by propanolol, *Lancet,* **2**:1389, 1966.

27 Rifkin, H., and Berkman, J. Diabetes and the kidney, in M. Ellenberg and H. Rifkin (eds.), *Diabetes Mellitus: Theory and Practice* (New York: McGraw-Hill, 1972), p. 862.

28 Spiro, R. Biochemistry of the renal glomerular basement membrane and its alterations in diabetes mellitus, *N. Engl. J. Med.,* **288**:1337, 1973.

29 Robbins, S., and Angell, M. *Basic Pathology,* 2d ed. (Philadelphia: Saunders, 1976).

30 Ibid.

31 Kimmelstiel, P. Diabetic nephropathy, in E. Mostofi, and D. Smith (eds.), *The Kidney* (Baltimore: Williams & Wilkins, 1966).

32 Britt, M. R., et al. Value of catheter care challenged, *Hospital Infection Control,* **3**:146, 1976.

33 Bell, E. T. A post mortem study of vascular disease in diabetes, *Arch. Pathol.,* **53**:444–455, 1952.

34 Rhodes, B. A., et al. Assessment of peripheral vascular disease in patients with diabetes, *Diabetes,* **25**:307, 1976.

35 U.S. Department of Health, Education, and Welfare. *Report of the National Commission on Diabetes,* vol. III, p. 16.

36 Patz, A. Diabetic retinopathy: an overview, *Dimensions in Diabetes,* **6**:Winter 1977.

37 Cahill and Lacy. Loc. cit.

38 Robbins and Angell. Loc. cit.

39 Cahill and Lacey. Loc. cit.

40 Gabbay, K. The sorbitol pathway and the complications of diabetes, *N. Engl. J. Med.,* **288**:831, 1973.

41 Leopold, I., and Lieberman, T. W. The eye and diabetes mellitus in M. Ellenberg and H. Rifkin (eds.), *Diabetes Mellitus: Theory and Practice* (New York: McGraw-Hill, 1972), p. 813.

42 Kohner, E. M., et al. Florid diabetic retinopathy and its response to treatment by photocoagulation or pituitary ablation, *Diabetes,* **25**:104–110, 1976.

43 L'Esperance, F. A. The management of diabetic retinopathy, in *Diabetes in Review:*

Clinical Conference, 1976 (New York: American Diabetes Association and the New England Affiliate, 1976), p. 110.

44 The Diabetic Retinopathy Study Research Group. Preliminary report on effects of photocoagulation therapy, *Am. J. Ophthalmol.* **81:**383–1700, 1976.

45 Cleveland Society for the Blind. "When You Meet Blind Persons," brochure.

46 Shultz, J. M., and Williams, M. Encouragement breeds independence in the blind diabetic, *Nursing,* **76:**19–22, 1976.

47 Fulton, M., et al. Helping diabetics adapt to failing vision, *Am. J. Nurs.,* **19:**54–57, 1974.

48 Shultz. Op. cit., p. 20.

Chapter 11

The Child or Adolescent Who Is Diabetic

Ellen H. King

This chapter will discuss working with the family who has a child with diabetes. The person who is knowledgeable, enjoys close relationships with clients, and values teaching/learning as a tool of preventive health care can find great rewards working with families with diabetic children. The diagnosis of diabetes is viewed by families as a life crisis. During crises, family members often pull together and exhibit their best selves. Health professionals have the opportunity to witness the family grow and develop in ways never thought possible as they help the child and the family deal with the altered life-style a diagnosis of diabetes necessitates.

The diabetic child as a member of the family is the person around whom the altered life-style revolves. In addition to normal developmental tasks, the child must learn the skills and attitudes necessary for healthy living and incorporate them into his or her pattern of living and self-concept. Children do work hard to incorporate this health problem and its requirements into their life-styles. They deserve the best that health professionals have to offer.

The purpose of this chapter is to point out many of the factors which health professionals must consider when individualized plans of care are developed for children with diabetes. One of the principal factors which make plans for care for children different from those of adults is the extent to which the family must be considered. The parent or primary caretaker is responsible for seeing that the treatment is carried out when a child has a chronic illness.* In planning home care, the health professional will be dealing with at least two people, the primary caretaker and the child. They must function together for treatment to be effective. A philosophy of family-centered care is essential if compliance with a treatment regimen is the goal. Family-centered care can be defined operationally as occurring when the primary caretaker is considered as a member of the health team and the role relationships within the family that functioned prior to the child's illness are supported. The area of expertise of the primary caretaker is defining and meeting the child's needs on a day-to-day basis.

The primary caretaker can facilitate those actions which are consistent with approaches used at home. At the same time the primary caretaker can learn the skills and attitudes necessary for home care. Family-centered care is possible to the extent that the structure and role relationships within the family are intact, support systems are available, at least one member of the family has skills in decision making, and members of the health team value and work toward family-centered care.

Theory regarding adaptation to chronic illness and childhood diabetes is mostly descriptive and far from ready for direct clinical application. The approaches suggested in this chapter are a combination of attitudes gained from clinical experience and reviews of the literature. As knowledge about diabetes and its effects on the child and family increases, health professionals will be able to be more conclusive about approaches to care. Until that time, however, the approaches suggested in this chapter should be considered as suggestions.

Certain general factors will need assessment with any diabetic child. The first section of this chapter will deal with these factors:

1 The child's physical status, particularly regarding the disease process
2 The child's developmental status
3 The status of the family, particularly the primary caretaker

Later sections will deal with three special situations:

1 The child who is newly diagnosed
2 The child who is receiving outpatient follow-up
3 The child who is out of control

This chapter focuses on children with insulin-dependent diabetes, which is the usual type of diabetes in the young.

---

* The terms *parent* and *primary caretaker* will be used synonymously in this chapter.

ASSESSMENT FACTORS FOR DIABETIC CHILDREN

The needs of a diabetic child are assessed in terms of physical status, developmental status, particular family and social situation, and management of the disease process. The nurse will be working with other health professionals as the care of the child evolves. This group of people may be a formally designated team with well-defined functions or a loose aggregate of people. These people come together to meet the needs of a particular child.

The nurse has other functions as well as working with the diabetic child. The nurse will be concerned with evaluating the child's health status and teaching the family to do the same. Plans of care must be congruent with the physician's plan of care and also relevant to the needs of the particular child and family. The nurse will teach the family the skills and attitudes necessary for caring for the child at home. The nurse will evaluate the family's adaptation to the treatment regimen and plan modifications in keeping with the physician's goals for management and the family's values.

The team can function more effectively and efficiently in terms of the total child and his or her family if all the health professionals take part in mutual goal setting with the family and each member of the health team knows what the others are doing.

The overall goal which all health professionals are working toward is to meet the health needs of the child. When goals for care are inexplicitly defined, needs often go unmet. One must accept the notion that there is not yet consensus among physicians as to what constitutes good or high-level control in diabetic patients. The physician's concept of pattern of control influences his or her decisions about both goals for medical management and treatment regimens. Nurses tend to be reticent in making goals for care explicit and written. The patient and family suffer from the resulting conflict of information and approaches. Those health professionals working with the child and his or her family must work toward mutual goal setting, particularly where functions overlap. The primary caretaker and the child, when he or she is older, are members of the health team and need to be a part of the mutual goal setting if care is to be individualized.

Long-Term Goals

The physician will define specific goals for management of blood glucose and the means by which this level of management will be realized and evaluated. Long-term goals can be summarized as follows:

1 The disease process is controlled within the limits prescribed by the physician.

2 The child and one other member of the family can demonstrate consistently good technique with urine testing; insulin administration; and record keeping with regard to insulin administration, diet, urine testing, activity, and infection.

3 The child chooses his or her diet wisely in terms of the limits set by the physician.

4 Everyone in the family can explain the signs and symptoms of hyperglycemia and hypoglycemia.

5 The child and at least one other person in the family takes appropriate action when the child exhibits signs and symptoms of hyperglycemia and hypoglycemia.

6 The child and at least one other member of the family can state factors which precipitate hyperglycemia and hypoglycemia.

7 The child and one other member of the family can modify the treatment regimen within the limits prescribed by the physician to adapt to changes in activity and changes due to mild-to-moderate illness.

8 The child's growth and development are within normal limits.

9 The treatment regimen is integrated into the family life-style and is not perceived of as an undue hardship or a dominating worry by any member of the family.

10 Members of the health team, including the child and parent, are in agreement with regard to the child's strength and limitations.

The health team is dealing with a constantly changing set of factors which affect the realization of these goals. The rate of progression of the disease process is changing. The child is a rapidly developing human being whose developmental attributes are changing. The child's physical growth, which occurs in spurts rather than at a steady rate, makes greater and lesser demands on the pancreas. The child is changing developmentally, carrying out all or parts of treatment regimens of greater or lesser importance. How well these goals will be realized will vary depending on many factors such as other life crises and stresses, presence or absence of a support system, and the ability to grow and develop. As a member of the health team, the nurse must have a thorough understanding of the disease process in order to assess the child's physical status.

The Child's Physical Status

The child's physical status relates to progression of the child's disease. Hornback identified the following three phases in the development of diabetes which prove useful in structuring discussion: (1) the inactive phase, (2) the prodromal phase, and (3) the active phase.[1]

The *inactive phase* is present when there is an ab....ce of any abnormalities which can be identified with present-day tests. This category gives recognition to the genetic predisposition of the disease, while allowing practitioners to work toward identifying high-risk populations. The *prodromal phase* occurs when subclinical findings may suggest diabetes but no overt symptoms are present. The *active phase* occurs when signs and symptoms are overt and lead to diagnosis. A child may not demonstrate all these phases or may demonstrate them only briefly. The onset of childhood diabetes is very rapid, and often the child presents with ketoacidosis. The child who is in the prodromal phase may show a blunted insulin secretory response, but no abnormalities in blood glucose or urine excretion of glucose can be demonstrated.[2]

Screening   Screening programs have been used by communities to detect diabetes before the onset of ketoacidosis. There is controversy about the effectiveness of these tests. Urine testing for glucose and acetone is often the only screening test that is economically feasible. McFarlane identified the weakness of such screening programs as follows:

1   The rapidity of the onset of symptoms would necessitate weekly screening to be totally effective.
2   Negative readings on the screening tests give teachers, health professionals, and parents a false sense of security.
3   The expense of weekly screening rapidly becomes prohibitive.[3]

Diagnosis   The onset of active-phase symptoms in the child is rapid. The most common age of onset is 8 to 12 years. The parent and child report symptoms of weakness and fatigue occurring over 3 to 4 weeks. The child often appears undernourished, and weight loss may be documented prior to the onset of glucosuria and ketoacidosis.

The onset of these more overt signs is often associated with stress. The stressor can be a growth spurt, menarche in girls, or an infection. Stress precipitates an acute insulin deficiency with fasting hyperglycemia and glycosuria. The parent and child report a large appetite, large intake of water, and a large output of urine; often enuresis is reported.

During the early stages of the disease, biologically inactive insulin seems to be produced. The pancreas is capable of responding to hyperglycemia, but gradually the beta cells become exhausted.[4] With the hyperglycemia there is an increased loss of water and electrolytes through urination, with concurrent thirst. Cellular metabolism in insulin-dependent cells slows as the body mobilizes and uses fat as a source of intracellular glucose. Intermediate metabolites of fatty acid metabolism, ketone bodies, accumulate in blood. Glucose and ketone bodies accumulate in the body and are then excreted in urine as they reach the renal threshold. The body begins to compensate for the increased organic acid in the blood by increasing carbon dioxide excretion by the lungs. Respiration becomes deep and rapid. Dehydration, the result of diuresis and electrolytic imbalance, will progress until there is loss of consciousness, coma, and death unless treatment intervenes.

Parents usually recognize that something has gone wrong and obtain health care prior to the time the child loses consciousness. At diagnosis the child's ability to produce insulin is at least partially overwhelmed. The first treatment of ketoacidosis usually includes dosages of exogenous insulin. As the child is treated, his or her pancreas usually recovers and produces some insulin. When this occurs, there is a rapid drop in the amount of exogenous insulin needed. In time, complete atrophy of islet cells will take place. The period of time from onset of symptoms to atrophy ranges from 3 months to 5 years. The average length of time is 15 months.

The period during which the islet cells are making some insulin is called the "honeymoon" period or period of recovery. During this time, the child's body is able to respond to unexpected elevations of blood sugar with secretion of additional insulin; therefore, control of the disease process is relatively easy. In some children the disease process is halted and the child can be controlled without exogenous insulin. Physicians generally agree that small amounts of insulin should continue to be given during the honeymoon period. These small amounts of insulin may protect the pancreas in future stress situations and may extend the period of recovery. Many professionals feel that starting children with changes in life-style when control is easy may facilitate establishing habits that will be essential as control becomes more difficult. This recovery period is characterized by stability and can often be maintained until there is alteration in the growth rate, emotional upheaval in the family, infection, or the child begins to test the limits of the disease.

As time passes, control usually becomes more difficult. The factors which must be regulated in order to control the disease process are insulin, diet, and activity. Illness, especially infectious illness, changes the relationship of these measures. During periods of rapid growth, insulin and dietary needs can change quickly, necessitating continuing surveillance of the child and adjustments in his or her food and insulin requirements. Since activity is not predictable in children, attacks of hypoglycemia are a common problem. Children cannot always discriminate between hypoglycemia and hunger or verbalize what they are experiencing. The primary caretaker is required to watch the child's behavior for the first signs of hyperglycemia or hypoglycemia. This can be difficult until parents become comfortable with the "normal" behavior of their child. Infections in children with diabetes tend to be frequent and severe. Added energy requirements during infection alter the nutritional and insulin needs, making control difficult.

The Child's Developmental Status

A child's age or developmental status affects the particular health needs which are present at a given time. Some developmental problems are common to specific age groups. The level of functioning may or may not relate to chronological age. Approaches must address the level of functioning, not the chronological age. Stress, whether it be the result of life crises, illness, or hospitalization, is associated with regression. Regression need not be supported as the crisis is resolving, yet sometimes regression with withdrawal is the only defense mechanism a small child has to deal with stress. A child may not have all characteristics of a particular age group, or may have characteristics of several age groups at once. Since development is a process, a developmental trait may be present to a greater or lesser extent at any one point in time. This portion of the chapter will discuss developmental needs of children as they relate to control of the disease process.

Infancy Few children develop diabetes in infancy. When diabetes occurs in infants, one assumes that the disease and its treatment affect the child's development. It is generally believed that the later in life a chronic illness develops and the longer the child has lived as a "normal" child, the less impact the illness will have on psychosocial development.[5] During infancy, the foundations of psychosocial development are laid down. A most important foundation is the infant's relationship to his or her parents. The effect that diabetes and its treatment are having on parent bonding and the child's development of trust is a most important area of evaluation. There is ample evidence to suggest that separation of parents and the child in the newborn period can inhibit the forming of a nurturant attitude among them.[6] While the effects of chronic illness occurring later in the infancy period are less clearly defined, it is assumed that the illness does affect the ability of the parents to give care in a nurturant way. Many tools have been developed to assess parent-child interaction during the infancy period.[7] The child is developing a sense of trust in the environment. Consistency of routine and consistency in the satisfaction of his or her basic needs are essential if the child is to develop a sense of trust. The child is developing basic skills that will be needed for motor and cognitive development. Auditory stimuli, from music boxes and radios, tactile stimuli, provided by stuffed toys or human touch, and visual stimuli, from television or mobiles, are important components of a child's environment if these motor and cognitive skills are to be learned.

Developmentally the child learns that he or she can manipulate the environment with variations in behavior. When the child cries, mother comes. When the child smiles and coos, people talk and smile. These associations must be consistently reinforced if they are to be learned. Each child needs systematic evaluation in terms of whether or not the environment is capable of providing these growth-producing experiences. Tools now exist for evaluating these facets of development and can be used in either the home or outpatient settings.

The following situations are considered by health teams as danger signals that psychosocial development requires more extensive evaluation:

1 A parent is avoiding becoming attached to an ill child.
2 Both parents are unable to give support to the child after painful and intrusive procedures.
3 The child is showing signs of maternal deprivation.
4 The child is not meeting his or her developmental landmarks.

Parents of these children may be having problems with their parenting skills, and parents who are having problems with their parenting skills require much support themselves. A teaching/learning approach will be effective if lack of knowledge is the reason for the situation. Two approaches which may be effective in changing parental behavior are praise and modeling. Verbal praise can be offered for the positive components of parenting, and nursing personnel can serve as role models for affectionate behavior toward the child.

Certain aspects of diabetes treatment are difficult to carry out with infants.

Injection of infants is a particular challenge. Parents and nurses must learn
to restrain and inject insulin at the same time. Learning to support the infant
after injections is just as important as the skill itself. Urine testing on an ''un-
potty-trained'' child can be a problem. Double voiding is impossible until urinary continence is well established. Generally, urinary continence is physiologically possible after the child can walk well, sometime after 18 months of age.
Until this time, parents are asked to test a specific number of urine specimens
each day. Parents choose those voidings which are closest to feeding times.
Tes-Tape can be used on a saturated diaper. Three cotton balls well placed in
the diaper can catch enough urine for Clinitest and Acetest determinations. The
cotton balls saturated with urine are squeezed into a test tube or other appropriate container. Some parents are reluctant to touch excrement and prefer to
use plastic gloves.

Toddlerhood   Toddlerhood produces many crises in child rearing which
can be exacerbated by diabetes. Three changes in eating behavior may occur.
First, the child may begin to refuse to comply with requests, and eating habits
can become erratic and manipulative as self-feeding is begun. A child learns
that he or she can cause quite a reaction in his or her parents by refusing to eat.
The second problem may be ''food jags.'' Food jags are considered normal in the
toddler, but a diet of all french fried potatoes for a week can cause the conscien-
tious parent much concern. Hopefully the child will be in the honeymoon phase
of the disease and can tolerate breaches in dietary management. Generally it is
wise for parents not to make an issue of food and eating if it is not absolutely
necessary for management. The third change is that the toddler will be eating less
because he or she is not growing as fast as during infancy. Parents can be
reassured that this decrease in appetite is normal. Plotting the child's measurements on a growth grid often convinces parents that the child is growing
normally.

Toilet training is another area of conflict between child and parent. Withholding urine and putting urine in the wrong place at the wrong time are other
sources of conflict. Generally it is best to wait for psychological readiness
before attempting to toilet train the child. The child will demonstrate his or her
readiness when he or she can stay dry for 2 to 4 h, walk *well,* and express
interest in things going on in the bathroom. When parents attempt toilet training
before the child is ready, resistance may be encountered. Examples of resistance are refusing to sit on the ''potty,'' and voiding right after being removed.
If resistance is encountered, it is best to wait about 6 weeks before trying again.
It is generally best to wait until urinary continence is well established before
attempting to teach double voiding.

Temper tantrums are another source of parental conflict with the toddler.
At the beginning of the toddler period, temper tantrums are generally the result
of not having words or actions to express anger and frustration. Often tantrums
are the direct result of overstimulation and can be halted by removing the child
to a less stimulating environment. Toward the end of the toddler period, temper

tantrums may be manipulative in nature, an attempt to gain something from the caretaker. This type of tantrum may be corrected by removing the source of pleasure. It is important for parents to know that irritability is a sign of hypoglycemia. If the child is at a point of peak insulin action, or if he or she has had an increase in exercise, food rather than punishment may be the remedy. If *freshly formed* urine can be obtained and is positive for glucose, parents can easily discern the difference between a hypoglycemic reaction and a manipulative tantrum. (A negative test for glucose, however, does not *necessarily* mean the child is hypoglycemic.)

In summary, it is particularly important to avoid making issues of food and toilet training. Long-term goals are directed toward healthy attitudes concerning food and urine testing which will always be a part of the child's healthy life. Small losses in control have to be weighed against the risk of developing negative attitudes toward the treatment regimen. Parents also need support as they attempt to maintain the fine line between control of the disease process and encouragement of healthy psychosocial development.

Preschool Age Preschool-age children are becoming verbal. They continue to have difficulty separating things that happen in their imagination from things that happen in their environment. Their attention span is increasing. Usually preschoolers have experiences with people other than the immediate family. Hopefully, they begin having perceptual motor experiences such as coloring, cutting, etc., which will prepare them for school. Parental overprotection at this point may severely retard a child's later development, making her or him fearful of venturing alone out into the environment and limiting the amount and kind of experiences which prepare her or him for later life.

There are several reasons for parental overprotection. Parents may be unable to resolve their feelings of guilt with regard to their responsibility for the child's illness. Parents may fear small breaches in treatment regimen and their results. Schools, other parents, and adults may avoid assuming responsibility for the diabetic child for even short periods of time. The result is social isolation for the child and the family and limitation with regard to growth-producing experiences. If the child is in the honeymoon period, problems of control should be minor in nature. All adults involved may be reassured of that fact. If control is already difficult, the health team and family will need to be creative in planning experiences for the child which will be growth-producing.

School Age School-age children begin to go into the community increasingly on their own. They are more active, and they generally enjoy learning to do new things. Skill in sports may become increasingly important. Since physical activities are the center of many social activities, it is unwise to limit physical activity unless it is absolutely necessary for control. Activity in school-age children may occur at irregular intervals and necessitate changes in treatment regimen. The school-age child can be taught to handle increases in activity by using food sources. At school children come into contact with values and expectations that are different from those at home. These are the values of the teacher and the peer group. Parents exert less control over their child's life after the child starts school.

Problems the diabetic school-age child might have can be discussed in the following three categories: learning of self-care skills, problems with the peer group, and problems with the school system.

There is a controversy as to which age is the most appropriate time for learning the skills involved in diabetic management. If the child can give his or her own insulin, regulate his or her own diet, and do his or her own urine testing, he or she will be able to participate in many more normal activities. Overnights away from home will be limited if the child is unable to give his or her own insulin and do the urine testing.

One rapidly becomes aware of the role food plays in the social life of school-age children. Soft drinks and potato chips after school or the Scout "wienie" roast must be dealt with. The child needs both experiences with peers and control of the disease process. During the school age the child must begin to deal with peers. The diabetic child must do different things, and the reasons for the differences may be unclear since diabetes is not a disease that is readily observable. Knowledge concerning the inner workings of the human body is limited in the school-age child. All these factors make diabetes a difficult disease to understand—much less explain to peers.

Health team members can help the child deal with his or her peers by making sure that the child understands the disease. An analogy that has been useful in explaining diabetes to school-age children is the analogy of the car: The car engine is like a cell. The car needs energy to work; the cell needs energy to work. The car engine uses gasoline for energy; the cell uses glucose which is a kind of sugar for energy. The service station attendant puts gasoline in the car to make energy. Insulin is like the service station attendant. Insulin puts glucose in the cell to make the cell work to make energy.

The school-age child needs to understand what food, urine, and insulin (things he or she can see) have to do with glucose, ketones, and the pancreas (things he or she cannot see). The school-age child needs to begin to have an understanding of glucose in the blood and insulin in the blood if he or she is to venture into society with more independence. Using one set of terms consistently is important for understanding. The author prefers the terms "hyperglycemia" or "too much sugar" and "hypoglycemia" or "too little sugar." Using these terms in this way requires the child to deal with only one concept, that of blood sugar. Eventually the child will need to learn the interrelationship of sugar and insulin level. The next step is to relate these words to the child's feelings as she or he experiences both hyperglycemia and hypoglycemia. The last step of this process is for the child to be able to take appropriate action as he or she experiences either hyperglycemia or hypoglycemia. The actions need to become automatic because the decision-making ability of the child is affected with both hyperglycemia and hypoglycemia.

As the child begins to understand the disease and manage it with increasing independence, he or she begins to develop a realistic, hopefully positive self-concept. This, of course, assumes that parents perceive the child positively and offer support as the child begins to handle the disease. Such a child can handle the questions of peers. However, the shy child who has had limited experience with age mates may have difficulty and need adult support. Adults can help the child with his or her explanations and support and encourage the child's strengths. Adults should think about emphasizing areas of sameness rather than areas of differentness. Eventually, the child will need to deal with his or her peers without adult intervention. Inability to affiliate with a peer group should be considered a danger signal and evidence of a need for further assessment.

The health team must have good communication with people in the school system. Indeed, the teacher as well as the school nurse may be included as members of the health team. People in the school system may have valuable information concerning the problems a child is experiencing which may affect control. Many school information forms have been developed. (See Fig. 11-1 for a sample form that includes information about diabetes and a guide for information to be obtained from parents.) Direct communication with the child's teacher may allay many problems related to lack of understanding about diabetes and its treatment by teachers and school officials. Many problems may be solved by communication and correction of misconceptions. Ames Laboratory has developed a guidebook of general information which teachers find useful.[8]

Hypoglycemia is the most common problem of control in children. The child needs to be sent to school with a source of readily available glucose and money to purchase more. Although candy has quickly absorbed glucose, it may be too big a temptation for the school-age diabetic child and his or her friends—the candy will be eaten before it is needed. Candy may be more acceptable to the child for use in the view of peers, while Instant Glucose or going to the school nurse may add to the feelings of differentness. The most important point is that the child must have some glucose to take if symptoms of hypoglycemia occur. Should control become a problem, with attacks of hypoglycemia and hyperglycemia occurring frequently, the plan of action can be spelled out specifically and concretely to the child's teacher. Teachers should be informed about the relationship between hypoglycemia and irritable behavior so that they will understand when to feed and when to discipline.

Adolescence Some developmental characteristics of adolescents may affect the management of their disease. The adolescent gains more independence from parents and becomes more responsible for management of her or his health status. Toward the end of adolescence the diabetic will need to be totally responsible for carrying out the treatment regimen. There are three factors which together make control difficult for many adolescents with diabetes. Puberty and the adolescent growth spurt combine to make energy needs for the diabetic somewhat irregular. The adolescent tends to have emotional highs and lows, making glucose utilization irregular. The adolescent tests his or her limits

WARNING SIGNS OF INSULIN REACTIONS

Excessive Hunger	Blurred Vision	Poor Coordination
Perspiration	Irritability	Abdominal Pain
Pallor	Crying	or Nausea
Headache	Confusion	Inappropriate
Dizziness	Inability to Concentrate	Actions/Responses
Nervousness or Trembling	Drowsiness or Fatigue	

TREATMENT

At the first sign of any of the above warning signs:

Give sugar immediately in one of the following forms:

    a. Sugar—5 small cubes, 2 packets, or 2 teaspoons
    b. Fruit juice—1/2 to 2/3's cup
    c. Carbonated beverage—*(Not diet or sugarless soda pop)*—6 ounces
    d. Candy—1/4 to 1/3 candy bar

THE FOLLOWING INFORMATION SHOULD BE OBTAINED FROM PARENTS WHEN CONFERENCE IS HELD AT THE BEGINNING OF THE SCHOOL TERM.

Child's Name _____ Date _____

Parent's Name _____ Address _____ Phone _____

Alternate person to call in emergency _____ Relationship _____ Phone _____

Physician's Name _____ Address _____ Phone _____

Signs and symptoms the child usually exhibits preceding insulin reaction: _____
_____

Time of day reaction most likely to occur: _____

Most effective treatment (sweets most readily accepted): _____

Kind of morning or afternoon snack: _____
_____

Suggested "treats" for in-school parties: _____

SUBSTITUTE AND/OR SPECIAL TEACHERS SHOULD HAVE ACCESS TO THE ABOVE INFORMATION.

This material may be reprinted for the child's cumulative school record.

Figure 11-1 School information form. In addition to what is shown here, the form provides brief descriptions of diabetes, insulin reactions and their treatment, and urine testing and offers general advice to teachers. (*American Diabetes Association, 1 West 48th Street, New York, New York 10020.*)

and abilities in many areas. Most diabetic adolescents seem to test the limits of their disease to see how much they can control their body and how much their body controls them. The process of testing may necessitate several hospitalizations and many conferences with health professionals to work through the problem of control. Parents may have varying amounts of difficulty relinquishing control over the treatment schedule. Relinquishing control is particularly difficult when parents see their child making errors in judgment that result in costly hospitalization. Parents may need support to maintain that thin line between guidance and control in relation to growth.

Health professionals should be *very* careful with their assessment when problems of control occur with the adolescent. Noncompliance is only one cause of poor control. Other factors that may cause poor control are:

1 Change in activity—particularly an increase in activity at peak action of insulin dosage
2 Change in dietary habits, often an unknowing increase in carbohydrate source
3 Growth spurt or puberty
4 Emotional crisis
5 Infection
6 Error in understanding of some aspect of the disease

Peer groups are increasingly important. Adolescents fear being different and not being in control of themselves. The adolescent will have to deal with his or her identity as a diabetic, a person who has different physical needs and who does some special self-care activities. The adolescent diabetic begins to establish sexual relationships. As these relationships develop, the issue of childbearing may be raised. The health professional must be prepared to discuss the genetic aspects of diabetes and the benefit versus risk of childbearing for the diabetic individual. Decisions about childbearing may not be made during the adolescent period, but the health professional should be there to explain the options available and to facilitate discussion. Refer to Chapter 3.

Assessment of Attitudes—A Tool A tool for assessing the adolescent's attitude toward his or her disease has been developed by the nursing staff at Rainbow Babies' and Children's Hospital.* The tool, a *Discovery Booklet*, utilizes several projective techniques and is comprised of six pages. The pages can be given in any order depending on the characteristics of the adolescent. Except for five open-ended questions designed for the adolescent who has lived with diabetes for a period of time, the tool can be used with any diabetic. Parental approval is secured, but the information is shared with parent only as need arises. The adolescent completes the tool alone. The beginning of the *Discovery Booklet* states:

Every day, all over the world, people are learning new ideas, developing new ways of making them work, and sharing these "discoveries" with others. DISCOVERY

* University Hospitals, Cleveland, Ohio.

comes in all sizes, kinds, and people. It can be something learned about one's self or about one's world; it can be kept inside as one's private thoughts or expressed "outside" and shared with another person. Sometimes, by sharing, one's thoughts are more easily understood.

People with diabetes have many new feelings about themselves. This book was made for YOU . . . to help you learn more about yourself, and to help you let those feelings outside, into the open. The thoughts you write down in this book will be shared only by those involved in your care. By knowing that YOU think and feel, others who want to help you will be able to do a better job.

On the first page the adolescent is asked to make a pictorial representation: "Draw a picture that shows how you feel about diabetes." Figure 11-2 presents a response that communicates that the person felt left out or different. Many of the responses received communicate this basic feeling. A second thing to note about the picture is its primitive nature. The figures are stick figures and only very essential detail is included. This fact generally indicates that the subject matter may be anxiety-provoking. Again the pictures received are often primitive. The third point which should be noted is the sad expression on the face of the diabetic person, while the people in the group are smiling.

The person discussing this response could begin by stating what the picture says to them, e.g., "It must be sad to feel different." The person would have an opportunity to validate this impression. The discussion could focus on the feeling expressed.

The second page consists of a list of seven open-ended questions concerning the diagnosis and treatment of diabetes. See Fig. 11-3 for the responses of one diabetic adolescent to the questions. The major theme of these answers appears to be fear. The answers themselves denote this in their content, but the short answers imply the same thing. Approaching fear directly may increase the anxiety. Generalizing the opening approach sometimes makes things easier, e.g., "Some people think diabetes is scary." Allow time for an answer. "I wonder what they think will happen?" When some of the questions are unanswered—as in questions 5 and 6 in the sample—they can be verbally asked; one should take care not to increase the threat.

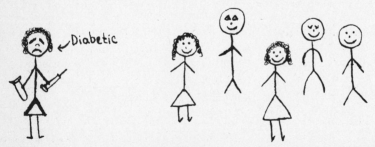

Figure 11-2 Response of one adolescent to the direction "Draw a picture that shows how you feel about diabetes." (*"Discovery Booklet,"* p. 1.)

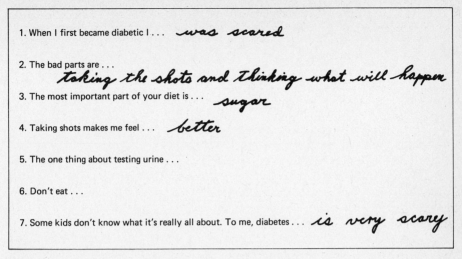

1. When I first became diabetic I . . . *was scared*

2. The bad parts are . . . *taking the shots and thinking what will happen*

3. The most important part of your diet is . . . *sugar*

4. Taking shots makes me feel . . . *better*

5. The one thing about testing urine . . .

6. Don't eat . . .

7. Some kids don't know what it's really all about. To me, diabetes . . . *is very scary*

Figure 11-3 Open-ended questions elicited these responses concerning the diagnosis and treatment of diabetes. (*"Discovery Booklet,"* p. 2.)

The third page consists of five more open-ended questions concerning living with diabetes. An example of responses appears in Fig. 11-4: "Life is no different but he feels strange and other kids are lucky." There are many inconsistencies in the answers on this page. The approach to discussion would be the same as explained previously. Given the answer to question 8, it would be advisable to explore the statement about what the parents think in some detail. Parental support of the treatment regimen is essential as a healthy life-style is being learned.

The fourth and fifth pages have abstract drawings (see Fig. 11-5). The comments are used as a basis for discussion in the same way that the comments to the open-ended questions are used. One point that could be explored with

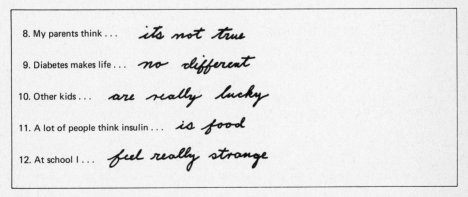

8. My parents think . . . *its not true*

9. Diabetes makes life . . . *no different*

10. Other kids . . . *are really lucky*

11. A lot of people think insulin . . . *is food*

12. At school I . . . *feel really strange*

Figure 11-4 These questions from the *Discovery Booklet* are designed for the adolescent who has lived with diabetes for some time. Inconsistencies in responses are seen. (*"Discovery Booklet,"* p. 3.)

Below are some roughly sketched figures. Write down what you think about or feel next to each figure. If you have trouble thinking of something to put down, try thinking back to other days in the hospital or doctor's office.

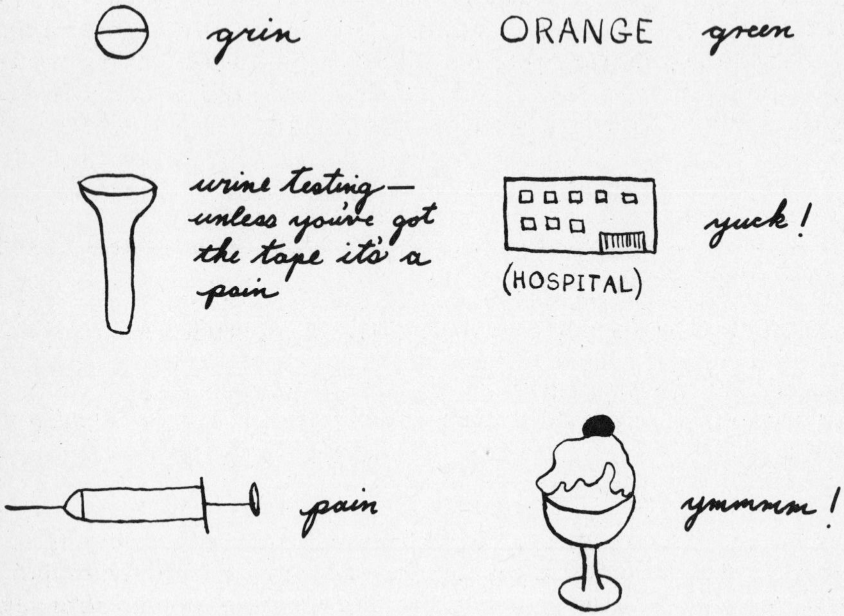

Figure 11-5 Interpretations of pictures by one adolescent with diabetes. (*"Discovery Booklet," pp. 4, 5.*)

the sample shown in Fig. 11-5 is the use of the word "pain," e.g., "Is all of this a pain?" The first figure is supposed to represent a Clinitest or Acetest tablet or a pill of some sort. The professional could explore further the "grin" in the client's statement.

The sixth page asks for a description of what the client would tell a friend. "Suppose your best friend just found out that he has diabetes. What would you tell your friend to help him?" The professional looks for consistencies and negative feelings which have not been expressed previously or incorrect information. Expressions of negative feelings are not bad. The client does not have to express all positive feelings about his or her life to be considered emotionally healthy or adjusted. The *Discovery Booklet* provides an opportunity for the expression of both positive and negative feelings.

Nursing personnel using this tool have expressed surprise at the number of serious concerns expressed by diabetic adolescents who were considered to be "well-adjusted" to their disease and its treatment. The fact that more concerns were picked up than expected implies that assessment at consistent intervals is needed to determine how the adolescent's attitude and concerns are changing over time.

The Status of the Family

The socioeconomic position and the health status of the family affect whether or not goals of treatment will be realized. The primary caretaker will function by making sure the treatment regimen will be followed and by being a member of the health team until such time as the child is capable of assuming those functions. The following factors influence a parent's ability to carry out treatment:

1 The degree to which one's life-style must be altered
2 The amount of support that can be gained by the parent/child from the family and community
3 The value the family places on preventive health care
4 The amount of resistance to the treatment regimen which the child demonstrates
5 Primary caretaker comfort and ability with the parenting
6 The emotional, financial, and other stresses which the disease will place on the family unit
7 Other family stresses

All these factors need continuing reevaluation, particularly if noncompliance is a suspected reason for poor control. The family who values a loose, "free" life-style where people eat, sleep, and exercise at irregular intervals may find the orderly life the diabetic child requires difficult. The parent who is unable to delay immediate gratification for long-term benefit may find parenting the diabetic child difficult. Often this parent will not be able to help the child conform to the health regimen, which calls for giving up short-term pleasures for a longer, healthier life.

Socially isolated families often have a great deal of difficulty during stressful periods because they lack support systems. Family members often find it comforting to hear from other families with similar problems that bad things get better and negative feelings about the disease and its treatment are common. If they have been identified, support systems can be utilized by the family for care of other children during periods of stress.

Carrying out the treatment regimen for diabetes takes motivation on the part of the primary caretaker. This person must value preventive health care, since many of the effects of poor control may not become evident for years. Having values that are in direct opposition to the plan of care may be a reason for noncompliance.

When a child resists all or part of the treatment regimen, the primary caretaker needs more energy to deal with the situation. It is interesting to note that the child who resists treatment is often the child of a parent who is insecure with parenting skills. Parents who are secure in their role as parents can deal with the conflict between development and control of the disease process. They can allow both themselves and their children to make mistakes, learn from them, and go on with life. Less secure parents may be so afraid that mistakes will be made that they have difficulty learning and implementing the treatment regimen. These parents may become excessively dependent on the health team for decisions about care.

The amount of energy a family brings to diabetic management is related to how much stress the family is experiencing. Additional stresses such as economic problems or another ill child limit the amount of energy that can be used to meet the needs of the child with diabetes.

Assessing Sources of Support Information concerning the community within which the family resides may be a factor that influences the health team, for this information can be useful in defining support systems. The lay referral system may be used for a variety of positive ends if it has been identified. Social isolation can be a problem to many people engaged in rearing a chronically ill child; therefore, information regarding the amount and nature of isolation may be important. The fact that the diabetic child is left for periods of time with another person, freeing the primary caretaker for other activities, implies that the family is not totally isolated. Questions and comments concerning the amount of time spent in community activities or leisure-time activities with other people give other clues to the amount of social isolation present. The family's knowledge of and ability to use community resources are important. Families of diabetic patients often discover community resources before the health team does.

The abilities and disabilities of the individual members of the family are factors that change over time and influence the functioning of a particular treatment regimen. Emphasis is generally placed on the adult members of the household and the diabetic child. The adult members of the household are evaluated with regard to physical, emotional, educational, and interpersonal attitudes. Any physical limitations that cause added stress or necessitate modification of treatment regimen will need particularly careful assessment. The parents' emotional status particularly with regard to chronic illness, children, and child rearing need evaluation.

Since diabetes does have a genetic etiology, parents may have had experience of diabetes with another family member. If these experiences were negative with regard to treatment and prognosis, this negative attitude may be reflected in the treatment of the child. Changing negative misconceptions may take time. Parents who value "free" children or feel unduly guilty or regard themselves as responsible for their child's illness tend to have difficulty setting and enforcing limits. They may have difficulty maintaining a treatment regimen. Attitudes of long standing take time to change.

Parental educational skills need continuing reevaluation. Parents are growing and developing too. Often parents go to great lengths to learn about diabetes or become involved in activities of the diabetic association where they gain a lot of knowledge. Sometimes, however, parents, as well as children, may use words before their full meaning is understood or the idea expressed is put into practice. The health professional's explanations should be matched to the level of understanding of the parents or the ideas will not be understood. Worse, partial understanding may cause parents to make dangerous treatment errors. If discussions are too elementary, the parents may begin to lose faith in the ability of the health team to meet their needs.

Signals to Modify Care   One of the first signs of difficulty within a family is behavior problems in the children. When children have unmet emotional needs, they may develop behavior problems in an attempt to get these needs met. Examples of the kinds of problems that occur are stealing, bullying, or a drop in school grades. Children who withdraw may also have unmet needs. The behavior should be interpreted by the health team as an appeal for help. The child with diabetes has a disease process that can be used to call attention to unmet needs. The child's use of symptoms to gain attention can range from manipulative to self-destructive.

There are seven major problems which signal danger and imply that the plan of care needs modification. These problems are as follows:

1   An intellectual deficit on the part of either the primary caretaker or the child has been identified.

2   Psychological factors which inhibit learning—excessively long period of denial, excessively compulsive or phobic behavior about one or more aspects of treatment, and documented self-destructive behavior on the part of the child—have been identified.

3   Stresses in the family are so great that energy cannot be mobilized to meet the physical needs of the child.

4   There are consistent behavior problems in the child or siblings.

5   The family does not value preventive measures with regard to health.

6   The primary caretaker has excessive difficulty delaying immediate gratification for long-term benefit.

7   There is excessive dependence on the health team.

THE CHILD WHO IS NEWLY DIAGNOSED

The factors discussed in the previous section cannot be ignored as one discusses the newly diagnosed diabetic. However, the newly diagnosed diabetic does present the health team with particular problems. In many communities there is a trend toward shorter hospitalization for newly diagnosed diabetic patients. Some institutions are experimenting with teaching diabetic self-care on an outpatient basis if ketoacidosis is not a problem. Where short hospitalizations are the rule, children may be discharged from the hospital before their disease has been fully regulated. Some diabetic children will have had no experience in inpatient settings.

The Hospitalized Child

Nurses who have responsibility for diabetic teaching have little time to waste. Assessments must be made systematically and objectives defined clearly so that plans can be implemented efficiently. The nurse who enjoys a leisurely approach to patient teaching and feels frustrated by the rapidity with which goals must be met must realize that the child will not be fully regulated until she or he is in a normal environment, with the usual patterns of eating and activity. Hospitalization is expensive and may excessively drain family resources.

The nurse should assess client response to this rapid approach to teaching self-care. When questions arise about a client's ability to carry out the required treatment and few community support systems are available, the date of discharge should be delayed.

Physical Needs of the Child with Ketoacidosis   The child who enters the hospital with newly diagnosed diabetes may be in one of various states of health depending on the progression of his or her disease. If the child is in severe ketoacidosis, he or she may be nonresponsive and have severe fluid and electrolytic disturbances. During this acute period, the physical needs of the child will assume priority. The child will be in shock and severely dehydrated. Vital signs will be monitored frequently; urine will be monitored for sugar and acetone frequently; and blood will be drawn frequently for glucose, ketone, and electrolyte tests. If a Foley catheter has been inserted, urine determination will be as frequent as every hour. If there is no Foley catheter, all voidings must be tested. Intake and output by all routes will be monitored strictly. Most children will be receiving insulin and parenteral fluids to correct dehydration, expand circulating blood volume, and correct electrolytic imbalance. Once good urine flow has been established, potassium replacement may be added, and monitoring of output continues to be important (see Chapter 8). One should note that a child can go from acidosis to hypoglycemia without regaining consciousness. This fact makes regular and frequent assessment particularly important. Attention to respiratory status is important, particularly if the child has a concurrent respiratory infection. Attention to turning, coughing, and deep breathing will be an important component of care.

Nurse-Family Relationships   On admission, both the parents and the child tend to be very fearful. A calm approach may help allay some anxiety. Parents must feel that their child is being cared for by experts. A calm, organized approach to care communicates more than words. The source of parental anxiety is generally expressed as fear that the child will die, fear that the child will have a permanent injury, and guilt. The guilt is evidenced from two sources. Parents have feelings of guilt concerning their genetic responsibility for this disease, or they may blame themselves for not having recognized the symptoms earlier. In addition, parents often express relief that they no longer have total responsibility for care of the child. Many parents need to see that their child is settled and being cared for, then they may need to be away for a while to relax and remobilize their coping mechanisms.

As parents are able to take in more of their environment, they will need an orientation to the hospital division. The goals for nursing care at this point are to establish a relationship of trust with the family, to begin to assess the strengths and limitations of both the child and family, and to devise a plan for teaching. Nurses then may begin to concentrate on taking a health history and discovering those factors which will help in the design of a teaching plan. At the same time, the nurse will be offering support and encouragement as the parents talk about the circumstances which led to the hospitalization. In so doing, the nurse can begin to build a relationship that will facilitate teaching. Answering parents' questions simply will establish the nurse as a person the parents can go to for assistance. The nurse will usually be able to discern valuable information about family methods for dealing with stress and the kinds of assistance coming from the lay referral system.

The data collected are used in defining the objectives for care. The objectives that must be met before discharge from the hospital are as follows:

1 One family member can demonstrate the correct technique for administration of insulin.

2 One family member can demonstrate the correct technique for urine testing.

3 The primary caretaker can explain the diet plan chosen.

4 One family member can explain the signs and symptoms of high and low blood sugar and the actions to be taken in the event of each.

5 One family member can demonstrate accurate record keeping.

Other objectives can be attempted if time permits:

1 Two members of the family, one person being the child, can demonstrate the following: urine testing, insulin administration, and record keeping.

2 The child can explain the diet plan chosen.

3 The child can explain the signs and symptoms of high and low blood sugar and the actions to be taken in the event of each.

4 The child and one family member can explain the relationship between insulin, diet, exercise, and illness.

Needs of the Recovering Child As the child regains consciousness, his or her physical status improves and a period of repletion occurs, so named because the child is replenishing lost nutritional stores. The child will be receiving insulin therapy and caloric intake to replace these stores. The physical problems which occur at this time usually involve diet or insulin administration. If solid foods are pushed while the child is still encountering nausea, he or she may vomit the solid food. The child may be cut back to a liquid diet at about the same time his or her appetite is increasing. A second problem can occur when the child's caloric prescription is too low. When the child's appetite peaks, he or she begins to scavenge for food. This can be an unfortunate precedent for future dietary habits.

As the child becomes aware of the hospital environment, nursing personnel can allay anxiety by making the environment consistent and predictable. The child needs to be oriented to the hospital and consistently prepared, given his or her developmental level, for painful and intrusive procedures. Systematic assessment of the child's perception of the situation, his or her strengths and limitations, begins as the child regains consciousness. As the child begins taking part in normal childhood activities, the priorities of care change from physical care to discharge planning. The family must learn to care for the child at home. Signs of readiness for learning on the part of either the child or the parents may include questions about procedures or what is taking place or just careful observation as the nurse administers a procedure. Nurses can attempt to stimulate interest by bringing insulin to the bedside to draw it up, by explaining the procedure as they do it, or by taking a family member with them to do a urine test.

Teaching Urine Testing   The skills are begun, one at a time, starting with the least stressful one, urine testing. Children who are of school age tend to enjoy urine testing unless they are reluctant to touch their own urine. They become proficient rapidly. The points to be stressed in urine testing are

1   The correct technique for the method of analysis chosen
2   The correct reading of the results of the test
3   The recording of the results
4   The meaning of the test results

The parents should be warned to store Acetest and Clinitest out of the reach of small children and unknowing adults. These tablets can cause severe esophageal burns if taken internally. Children can get further involved in the care by making a book to record the information they are learning to collect. The information to be recorded will vary with the physician, but generally it includes the date, time, insulin given and site of injection, urine testing results, and general comments. Any small spiral notebook can be used. Commercially prepared record books can be purchased and used if desired. Some have reported success with matching colored crayons with the color of test results.[9] This practitioner has been unable to repeat this success.

Insulin Administration   The second skill to be learned is insulin administration. Injection of insulin into oneself or another person tends to produce some stress initially. The first step is to decide which adult member of the family will learn the skill. While it is hoped that all members of the family will learn these skills in time, initial efforts should be concentrated on one adult family member. An adolescent patient may be the first member of the family to learn the skill. If the child is not ready to learn the technique, he or she can be involved in the technique to the extent of his or her ability. Some aspects of insulin administration such as charting of injection sites, keeping track of the rotation of the sites, or swabbing the area before injection can be the child's responsibility.

Parents often need much support to be able to give their child an injection. The first injection by the parent tends to be an anxiety-provoking experience for all involved. Once this major hurdle is passed, parents can move on to considering other facets of care. On the last day in the hospital the person giving the injections should be confident enough to draw up and give the insulin with just family members in the room. If this point has not been reached, the family may need nursing follow-up in the home. If disposable equipment is used, safe disposal of needles and syringes should be covered in discussion. A taped shoe box kept out of the reach of small children is one simple means. The syringes and needles of diabetics have been known to be used by drug addicts. It is wise therefore to counsel parents to dispose of needles and syringes in a container sealed with tape immediately before a garbage pickup.

Teaching about Diet   The specifics of dietary teaching will depend on the type of diet chosen by the physician. All members of the health team should be thoroughly familiar with the diets prescribed by physicians with whom they work. They should be familiar enough with the prescribed diet and specific goals of control to answer the following questions:

1 "Can I have pizza?"
2 "Can I have ice cream and cake at birthday parties?"
3 "What happens if supper has to be late?"
4 "Can I skip breakfast?"
5 "What do I do if I am hungry and I'm not supposed to eat?"

Parents and children can practice dietary management if selection menus are used in the hospital. The nurse or dietitian can give guidance for appropriate selection, and misconceptions can be picked up. Parents can take the menus home to use as guides. A real test of knowledge and its application can be given by taking the child and her or his family to a cafeteria. In this way, children and parents demonstrate not only their knowledge of but also their attitudes toward the dietary prescription. The health team member accompanying the child should note the child's facial expressions as selections are made, and who makes the selections. Comparison of what is selected for the child versus what is selected for the parent may give the health team members an idea of how the dietary treatment will be handled at home.

Teaching Concepts of Diabetic Management   Learning about hyperglycemia and hypoglycemia and their relationship to insulin, diet, and exercise is often difficult. Information should be given in short sessions. Examples of topics for the sessions are

1 Hyperglycemia, its causes, signs, symptoms, and treatment
2 Hypoglycemia, its causes, signs, symptoms, and treatment
3 Insulin, the kinds, effects, and peak action times
4 Dietary carbohydrate and its effect on blood sugar
5 Exercise and its effect on blood sugar

Some school-age children and adolescents can participate in many of these discussions. School-age children will need something to do with their hands if they are to participate in discussions. A pool table in the empty play room or modeling clay keeps the hands busy while the mind is working.

Feedback about understanding of information is sought throughout the teaching process. Questions should be asked in such a way that understanding rather than recall is evaluated. Attitude as well as knowledge may be evaluated by asking the parent and the child to problem solve situations that will occur when they return home. Questions that may elicit problem-solving discussions are

1 "What will you tell your friends when you get home?"
2 "Suppose you feel shaky, weak, and hungry and you are in the middle of class, what will you do?"

Examples of problems the parent may need to solve are

1 "What are you going to do about your child's diet in relation to the needs of the rest of the family?"
2 "What are you going to tell your other children about your diabetic child?"

Remember, these questions have no right and wrong answers. They are designed to elicit attitudes and feelings to help family members begin to picture themselves in their community environment. Be careful not to attempt to force the family into some "adjusted" attitude before they have worked with the problems of living with diabetes.

The problems listed above help the family begin thinking about the post-discharge period. It is also helpful to prepare both the parent and the child for some of the feelings they may have. Relief that the child's physical condition has improved and intensive education and support measures often combine to give the parent and child a sense of well-being, an emotional "high." At home, without the direct support of the health team, the family may later become anxious and angry. The family must begin to deal with the frustration that a change in life-style usually precipitates. The family and the child need to grieve for the loss of normality. Feelings of depression are common in both parents and child. A system of daily telephone contact arranged prior to discharge can give the parents and the child a mechanism for communicating these feelings to the health team. The daily telephone calls should last at least until the first return visit.

Discharge is not completed until the nurse makes sure that the following have been accomplished:

1 The family has all the equipment that they need: syringe; sterilizing equipment, if needed; cotton balls with alcohol; urine-testing equipment.
2 The family has the prescription for the insulin needed, money to purchase it, and access to a pharmacy.
3 The family knows whom to call for questions.

The Child Who Is Receiving Outpatient Follow-up

The major goals for the honeymoon phase are to have the treatment regimen well integrated into the life-style of the child and her or his family, to have the child accomplish the developmental tasks appropriately, and to have two members of the family, one of whom is the child, be able to carry out the treatment regimen. In addition to treatment of the diabetes, the child must have her or his other health needs met.

Well-Child Care A commonly neglected aspect of care for chronically ill children is well-child care. These children need regular physical examinations, immunizations, health counseling, and health teaching just as other children do. Some mechanism should be established to take care of these health needs. A visit to the outpatient facility or pediatrician's office for well-child care may give the family the extra support needed. Visiting nurses, public health nurses, or nurse-practitioners can be used in many communities for well-child care.

Assessment in the Ambulatory Setting During visits to the outpatient setting, evaluation along the preceding lines will be continuous. Questions that elicit information in these areas can be asked of both the parents and the child. It is important to note the dynamics between parents and child, particularly when the child is answering questions. If problems in parent-child interaction are suspected, it is sometimes wise to interview the two separately, particularly if the child is an adolescent.

Questions which may give information about integration of treatment into the life-style include the following:

1 "Describe a typical day."
2 "What is the best thing that has happened since the last visit?"
3 "What is the worst thing that has happened since the last visit?"
4 "Is it hard to do what we are asking you to do?"

It is important to ask whether there are any problems in carrying out treatments and to review the record the child or family is keeping. This will provide information concerning potential problems and will also reveal the level of knowledge being used by both the child and the family. If the information has not already been elicited, question the parent present about the spouse's participation in the child's care. Note also the parent's skill in setting and enforcing limits. This is particularly pertinent if some areas of treatment are not being carried out.

In assessing the effect diabetes is having on development, questions should be appropriate to the age of the child. For patients younger than school age, the parent can answer questions pertaining to developmental behavior of the child. The Denver Developmental Screening Tool can be used effectively to assess the child's developmental status. The school-age child can be asked some of the following questions:

1 "What kind of grades are you making in school?"
2 "Who is your best friend?"
3 "Do you have a girl/boy friend?"

Problems may be suspected if there is a change in school performance or the child cannot tell you about friends or after-school activities.

The adolescent may have problems of social isolation. He or she may also have problems of body image and feel inordinately different. The health team may need to evaluate movement toward adult role taking in the adolescent. Questions about career plans, college or vocational plans, and plans about marriage and family may elicit this information. Remember that many adolescents feel alone, different, and friendless during some portion of this developmental period. These feelings are a problem only if they continue for a long period of time or cause the adolescent to exclude herself or himself from social experiences.

Defined Goals Problems will be identified and short-term goals can be established by parents, child, and health team members. Review of information or skills will take place as indicated. It is important that the child and parents be given an opportunity to define the plan for meeting the goals. This approach allows the health team to support the parents' and child's growing competence and confidence. These families often develop many creative ideas that can be passed on to other families. Evaluation of movement toward goals takes place at each visit, with both the parents and the child participating in the evaluation.

THE CHILD WHO IS OUT OF CONTROL

When control of the child becomes difficult for the family, the family usually experiences another crisis. Diabetes and its treatment become a major part of family life. Prior to this time, the child may have been able to "get by" with minor breaches in treatment regimen and few problems with control. Now breaches present problems of control. Some children will have problems of control even when the treatment regimen has been strictly adhered to. The crisis situation usually precipitates a reaction within the family, especially if noncompliance is suspected. Feelings of anger and guilt can run high. The fact that problems of control occur often during adolescence has been alluded to. The stereotype of the rebellious adolescent is accepted as the norm by many. Many adolescents do test the limits of their disease in some way. It should be stressed again, however, that there are other reasons for lack of control, and these reasons should be considered equally in the assessment. Reasons for lack of control can be summarized:

1 Change in the character of the disease
2 Increase in stress
3 Change in life-style
4 Noncompliance

The character of the disease does change as the child moves from the honeymoon phase to complete atrophy of the beta cells; i.e., the child is less able to deal physiologically with changes in glucose level. Insulin resistance is considered to be a relatively uncommon reason for lack of control; however, it has been known to occur at both school age and adolescence. Added stress can come from three major sources: emotional stress, growth spurt, and disease. Chronic stress can be both environmental and self-imposed, or a combination of both. The emotionally stressed child will have periods of hypoglycemia followed rapidly by periods of glycosuria. Changes in treatment regimen may prove ineffective without decreasing the stressors. Counseling or direct psychiatric intervention may be needed to modify the stressors. Changes in life-style occur which affect control of the disease process; common ones in children will be either dietary or activity changes. The health team can pick up these changes if a 24-h history including diet is taken. The parents and the child can be unaware that the change can affect control. Family teaching in relation to lack of understanding would be the appropriate action.

Noncompliant behavior that is willful and knowing is a difficult behavior to modify. Noncompliant behavior can occur in the parent or in the child as he or she becomes more independent. Noncompliant behavior is often a maladaptive way of dealing with anger. The goal of care is to obtain the best control that can be integrated into a life-style. The realization of this goal often takes the combined efforts of the health team. Modification in both the treatment regimen and the life-style can be made. Essential information to be assessed will be the child and parents' perceptions of the situation and the reasons for noncompliance. Many people do not know the reason for their noncompliance or its effects. It is important to identify those people who are overtly self-destructive, for these people need psychiatric help.

The first step of the plan will center around the child's and parents' becoming aware of the reasons for noncompliance. The second step will involve modifying attitudes, treatment regimen, or life-style in such a way that control is possible. Realistic mutual goal setting is essential, for the child and parents must be committed to participating in changing behavior. If parent-child conflict is suspected as a reason for noncompliance, the health team may need to work directly with the child to help him or her become responsible for his or her own behavior.

SUMMARY

This chapter has dealt with some of the problems inherent in working with the diabetic child and her or his family. The discussion has been organized around the types of patient problems exhibited. The newly diagnosed diabetic child has physical problems of health status and problems which are related to learning self-care. The child in the honeymoon period has problems related to integrating the treatment into the life-style in such a way that growth and development can proceed normally and control is possible. The diabetic who has lost control must reestablish control of the disease process.

This chapter has discussed the child with diabetes as he or she is treated currently. Today 50 percent of children with juvenile-onset diabetes will die of renal disease within 25 years of diagnosis.[10] Diabetics are more prone to blindness, gangrene, and heart disease. Experimentation with transplanting of islet cells and synthesis of artificial beta cells is well under way,[11] and the outlook for the child with diabetes is increasingly hopeful. Good control, which allows for movement toward adult role taking, will enable the child with diabetes to benefit from new knowledge as it develops.

REFERENCES

1 Hornback, M. Diabetes mellitus—the nurse's role, *Nurs. Clin. North Am.,* **5:**5–6, 1970.
2 Ehrlich, R. M. Diabetes mellitus in childhood, *Pediatr. Clin. North Am.,* **21:**871, 1974.
3 McFarlane, J. Children with diabetes: special needs during growth years, *Am. J Nurs.* **73:**1360, 1973.
4 Guthrie, D. W., and Guthrie, R. A. *The Child with Diabetes: A Monograph for Nurses.* Univ. of Missouri Department of Pediatrics. Compiled in cooperation with the Univ. of Missouri School of Nursing and Division of Health of Missouri Bureau of Maternal and Child Health, Bureau of Public Health Nursing, Bureau of Nutrition, 1970, p. 6.
5 Kessler, J. W. The impact of physical disability on the child, *Phys. Ther.,* **46:**153, 1966.
6 Kennell, J. H., and Klaus, M. H. Caring for parents of premature or sick infants, in M. H. Klaus and J. H. Kennell (eds.), *Maternal-Infant Bonding* (St. Louis: Mosby, 1976), pp. 99–166.
7 Erickson, M. L. *Assessment and Management of Developmental Changes in Children* (St. Louis: Mosby, 1976).
8 *Care of the Child with Diabetes: Guidebook for Parents and Teachers,* Ames Company, Division of Miles Laboratories, Inc., Elkhart, Indiana, 1977.
9 Traisman, H. S. *Management of Juvenile Diabetes Mellitus,* 2d ed. (St. Louis: Mosby, 1971), p. 64.
10 Crofford, O. Commission report: full scale attack on diabetes, *Dimensions in Diabetes,* Winter 1976:4.
11 Lacy, P. E. Research highlight: present status, future hopes, *Dimensions in Diabetes,* Winter 1976:8.

BIBLIOGRAPHY

Crain, A. J., et al. Effects of a diabetic child on marital integration and related measures of family functioning, *J. Health Soc. Behav.* **7:**122–127, 1966.
Fenske, M. The endocrine system, in G. M. Scipien et al. (eds.), *Comprehensive Pediatric Nursing.* New York: McGraw-Hill, 1975, pp. 754–783.
Guthrie, D. W., and R. A. Guthrie. Diabetic children: special needs, diet, drugs and difficulties, *Nursing,* **73**(3):10, 1973.

Litman, T. The family as a basic unit in health and medical care: a social-behavioral overview, *Soc. Sci. Med.*, **8**:495–519, 1974.

McFarlane, J. Children with diabetes: special needs during growth years, *Am. J. Nurs.*, **8**:1360–1365, 1973.

Petrillo, M., and S. Sanger. *Emotional Care of Hospitalized Children: An Environmental Approach*. Philadelphia: Lippincott, 1972.

Schwartz, R. Diabetic ketoacidosis and coma, in C. A. Smith (ed.), *The Critically Ill Child, Diagnosis and Management*. Philadelphia: Saunders, 1977, pp. 230–243.

Steele, S. Nursing care of the child with juvenile diabetes, in S. Steele (ed.), *Nursing Care of the Child with Long Term Illness*, 2d ed. New York: Appleton-Century-Crofts, 1977, pp. 443–471.

Traisman, H. S. *Management of Juvenile Diabetes Mellitus*, 2d ed. St. Louis: Mosby, 1971.

Voy Sey, M. Impression management by parents with disabled children, *J. Health Soc. Behav.*, **13**:80–89, 1972.

Waechtner, E. H., and F. G. Blake, *Nursing Care of Children*. New York: Lippincott, 1976, chap. 32, pp. 702–708.

Diabetes Mellitus and the Elderly

Betsy A. Schenk

Mary Anne Caston

Mary Adams

Although diabetes is not a disease unique to the elderly, statistics show that in no other age group is it as prevalent. The incidence of diabetes increases with age and reaches its peak between the ages of 65 and 74, with 64.4 per 1000 tested found to have the disease. After age 75 the incidence of newly diagnosed diabetes levels off to 57.9 per 1000.[1] Among those over the age of 65, diabetes ranks as the seventh leading cause of death.[2]

A major factor that must be considered in discussing diabetes and the elderly is the tremendous impact of complications of the disease on many older people. Many aged diabetics who were diagnosed earlier in life develop varied complications as they age. Before the advent of improved medical care and the increased capacity to save people with severe metabolic disorders, infection, and cardiovascular disease, many insulin-dependent diabetics would not have survived to reach 65.

It is not uncommon for the older person to come to the physician or clinic not with the signs and symptoms of hyperglycemia, but with manifestations of one or more complications. Some aged who are newly diagnosed as diabetics may present at the same time with advanced complications that may have been attributed to other causes. Many aged diabetics never experience the classic signs and symptoms of hyperglycemia that usually occur in the younger person.

The impact of complications of diabetes on the life of the elderly diabetic becomes even more significant when it is realized that often these complications are superimposed on already present chronic diseases such as arthritis, hypertension, cardiac disease, or sensory problems such as deafness, cataracts, or glaucoma.

DIAGNOSIS

The elderly diabetic patient usually develops the adult-onset or mature type of diabetes, which evolves gradually and follows a relatively stable, benign course. The definition of diabetes must remain flexible in the elderly patient, and blood sugar levels alone cannot be used to make the diagnosis.

In the elderly, diabetes is the result of a diabetic defect that may not produce active disease unless superimposed exogenous factors such as illness, infection, hyperthyroidism, surgery, or obesity are present.[3] Psychological stress has also been shown to precipitate hyperglycemia, as has prolonged inactivity or immobilization. A severe carbohydrate restriction may decrease glucose tolerance in the aged person. Finally, certain drugs may decrease the glucose tolerance and increase blood sugar levels, e.g., nicotinic acid, diuretics, and cortisone.[4]

Some increase in blood glucose is normal in the elderly; as age advances there is a corresponding decreased glucose tolerance until the age of 75 or 80. After this age, further decrease in glucose tolerance does not occur. Interpretation of blood glucose levels in the elderly requires consideration of this aging effect on fasting, postprandial, and particularly postglucose determinations of blood glucose levels. For example, the average 2-h postglucose serum glucose is 30 mg per 100 mL higher for a 75-year-old than that of a 25-year-old.[5] On page 106 is listed one set of age-modified normal blood glucose levels for glucose tolerance testing.

It is unwise to make the diagnosis of diabetes mellitus on the basis of one laboratory value or one hyperglycemic episode. If the older person was in a particularly stressful period at the time the first elevated blood glucose was found, repeated tests are delayed until 3 to 4 weeks after recovery from the physiological or psychological stress. The elderly person should be followed closely after a suspicious test result, but the final diagnosis is reserved until at least two or three repeated tests can be made.

The elderly person who has been told that he or she is "prediabetic" or possibly diabetic often will be anxious and puzzled. He or she may question why no medication has been prescribed or why a wait-and-see attitude is being followed. The nurse working with this person can do much to help alleviate the anxiety and educate the person about the program of care. Feelings about the disease can be explored and misconceptions corrected. Many of these patients with obesity will have been prescribed a reducing diet or diet restricted in carbohydrates. The nurse can help the older person understand the restrictions and plan accordingly.

COMPLICATIONS OF DIABETES

Although it is not within the scope of this chapter to completely discuss the complications of diabetes in the elderly, it is the premise of these authors that the nurse must have at least a basic understanding of the complications in order to effectively teach the patient or client (see Chapter 10).

In discussing the complications of diabetes in the elderly patient, several points must be considered. First is the fact that many elderly people present at the time of diagnosis with already established complications that are irreversible, even with good control of the blood sugars. The second point is that more and more people are living to the older ages and so are experiencing complications of diabetes and the difficulties associated with aging. The elderly person often has apprehension and concerns that are related to loneliness, increasingly restricted resources, changes in living arrangements, and aging itself. These factors relate to the person's self-care ability, learning potential, and general health status.

Metabolic Complications

In most aged people with diabetes, acidosis is not the problem that it is in the younger diabetic. In most it may never occur. However, in a small group of insulin-dependent aged diabetics, ketoacidosis develops as a result of emotional or physical stress or after omission of insulin. This acidosis has a much greater impact on the homeostasis of the older patient; it may therefore require greater effort to realign the blood sugars to desirable levels because of the tendency to swing from acidosis to hypoglycemia. The elderly person may be controlled at a relatively higher postprandial blood sugar than the younger person. The aim of treatment often is to control symptoms that can be related to hyperglycemia and to keep the patient free of acetone and hypoglycemia.[6]

Hypoglycemia   Hypoglycemia by far poses the more serious threat to the aged person, especially to one taking either insulin or one of the oral hypoglycemic agents. The onset of severe and even fatal hypoglycemia may be unheralded by the usual symptoms, and the elderly person may even become unconscious without warning. Falling blood sugar levels can cause vasoconstriction, tachycardia, and a tendency for ectopic tachyarrhythmias. Cerebral vascular accidents or myocardial infarctions have followed hypoglycemic episodes in the elderly. In the aged, signs of acute brain syndrome such as episodes of bizarre or psychotic behavior, slurring of speech, convulsive seizures, confusion, disorientation, and sleepiness may actually be a result of low blood sugar. The aged diabetic who has experienced a more chronic form of hypoglycemia may have been mistakenly diagnosed as having chronic brain syndrome. With proper treatment of the diabetic condition, the chronic brain disorder often miraculously disappears.

The magnitude of the problem of hypoglycemia and the elderly diabetic is indeed great when one considers the number of elderly people who may be taking hypoglycemic agents without proper medical follow-up. The nurse working with the elderly diabetic in any setting should regard any of the following symptoms with a great deal of suspicion: nocturnal headaches, nightmares, crying out during sleep, unusual sleep postures, and somnolence.[7]

Nonketotic Hyperosmolar Coma   This metabolic disorder most often occurs in elderly diabetics rather than younger ones. Metabolic acidosis from excessive ketone formation is not present. Severe hyperglycemia exists, and often in the history there is a decrease in oral intake, secondary to a superimposed illness or disability. Severe dehydration, hyperosmolar fluid shifts and resultant decrease in mental status, cardiovascular adequacy, and renal function occur. Symptoms develop insidiously.

Monitoring the adequacy of fluid intake in the elderly diabetic and the effect of illness on the person's ability to respond to thirst are important nursing assessments that can lead to earlier detection of this serious disorder. Treatment includes hospitalization, insulin, and hydration.

Chronic Complications

The elderly diabetic may present with a variety of chronic diseases including diabetic complications. It has been estimated that approximately 5 to 15 percent of the elderly diabetic population experience some type of neuropathy and that the incidence increases with the age of the person and the duration of the disease.[8] Probably the most distressing and common neuropathy is the mild peripheral type with impaired peripheral circulation, absent tendon reflexes, muscular wasting, and peripheral sensory loss. A loss of vibratory sense is relatively common, as is the occurrence of pain, tingling, and a burning sensation in the feet. This peripheral neuropathy can also affect the upper extremities and is usually irreversible. Diabetic amyotrophy is a more defined neuropathy in which there is progressive weakness, wasting of muscles, and pain in the pelvic girdle and thighs; it is often treatable, however, with good diabetic control.

The neuropathies may also attack the autonomic nervous system. With this involvement the elderly person may present with complaints of orthostatic hypotension and vasomotor instability. The gastrointestinal system may be affected, associated with anorexia, vomiting, and diarrhea.

Diabetes in the aged is characterized by a high incidence and severity of complications involving the large and middle-sized blood vessels. Atherosclerosis, while not specific to diabetes, occurs earlier and may be more severe in the diabetic. The chief vessels affected are the arteries supplying the lower extremities, the kidney, the heart, and the brain. In one study, 25 percent of all hospitalized diabetic patients were found to have peripheral vascular disease, as indicated by intermittent claudication, reduced or absent arterial pulses, postural color changes, and asymmetrical coldness. The same author found that of 135 patients with diagnosed coronary artery disease, 64 percent had a glucose abnormality, whereas of 54 patients with documented normal coronary arteries, 18 percent had a glucose abnormality.[9]

Renal disease in the elderly diabetic involves small-vessel disease of the kidney in addition to problems in the arterial supply. In those who develop renal disease, asymptomatic and progressive proteinuria may be present, leading to azotemia, edema, and kidney failure. Accompanying complications include severe hypertension and cardiac failure. Even in those aged diabetics who have no evidence of renal disease, kidney or bladder infections may be a problem, and frequent urine testing, including culture and sensitivities, should be done. As aging occurs, there is an increased renal threshold for glucose, so that hyperglycemia may be present in the absence of glycosuria.

Visual complications can include any of the following in the elderly: glaucoma, infection or inflammation of the eyelids or orbit, cataracts, ulceration of the cornea, conjunctivitis, and retinopathy.[10] Retinopathy is estimated to affect 35 to 45 percent of diabetics over the age of 60, and in many of these, visual impairment is sufficient to cause difficulty in employment.[11]

The elderly diabetic patient may be especially prone to certain skin conditions (diabetic dermopathies) that are further emphasized because of the normal aging changes in the skin. These skin conditions include generalized itching, thin and delicate skin, and atrophy of subcutaneous tissues. The skin of the aged diabetic is also more prone to bacterial and fungal infections. A specific cutaneous lesion called *diabetic dermopathy* is present in many long-term diabetics. The plaques are small, oval or round, and measure 0.5 to 1.0 cm in diameter. The edges are well defined and crusts may form on the skin between the plaques. The most frequent location of these lesions is the lateral and anterior aspects of the lower extremities, but they also have been observed on the forearms. These cutaneous lesions result in round or oval pigmented scars.[12]

CARRYING OUT THE NURSING PROCESS

The nurse working with the aged diabetic patient, especially the newly diagnosed patient, must begin with an assessment of where the patient is in terms of knowledge and misconceptions about the disease. The patient's only education up to this point may have been well-intended advice from friends or relatives, and his or her memory of diabetes-affected individuals may extend to the preinsulin era.

At the same time that this information is being gathered, the nurse can assess the older person's mental status and ability to learn and remember facts and routines. This is not to say that all older people have mental slowing, but instead that each person must be judged individually. Language barriers should also be assessed. As the nurse or other health professional continues to work with the older person, he or she must constantly reassess the person's mental state. If confusion and disorientation are present because of the diabetes itself (or hypoglycemia), definitive treatment may reverse the condition. A language barrier or a hearing deficit can also alter the elderly person's ability to learn about diabetes. The nursing assessment should also include the aged person's health history, including past life routines and dietary patterns. Certain questions need to be answered. These include, but are certainly not limited to, the following:

1 Living arrangements
2 Financial resources
3 Support services that could provide reliable assistance
4 Presence of a care giver
5 Past exercise patterns

In addition to this information, the physical status of the aged person must be assessed. Included should be whether the person's vision, sensory perception, and agility are adequate for self-care activities. Any neuropathy or arthritis that is present in the hands and fingers that might influence manual skills should be considered. Other concomitant chronic diseases that are present and use of medications that might influence the course of the diabetes or make control more difficult should be recognized and included in the total plan of care. Chapters 8 and 9 discussed further details of assessment that apply to the elderly.

Planning and Giving Care

After the nurse has assessed the patient, she or he must, with the patient's assistance, set goals and plan how to accomplish these goals. As one author stated, "Education is an integral part of therapy and the diabetic who is given up-to-date information and careful instruction can become an active participant in his own care."[13]

Certain areas are considered very important in the care of the diabetic. These will be considered below. The nurse covering these areas will do well to remember that education about diabetes cannot be given in one afternoon. The best instructions are those which are communicated over a period of time and can be repeated as needed. Any patient can tolerate only certain amounts of teaching before saturation points are reached. This is particularly true of the elderly.

Up to this point, this chapter has addressed the questions of assisting the elderly person in understanding and setting goals to control his or her diabetes. It cannot be forgotten, however, that some elderly will not be able to manage at home without a responsible care giver and/or support services. About 90 percent of all elderly are found in their own homes or living with relatives. This figure would include the majority of diabetics also. It is obvious, then, that great emphasis should be placed on the home care of the elderly diabetic. The nurse must work with the elderly person or care giver to promote health, monitor complications, maintain function, and explore compensatory services. Community supports are often available, but those available should be sorted out by the nurse. The care giver of the elderly diabetic often needs education and support to deal with the complexities of home care. The public health nurse or visiting nurse can often make the difference in determining whether an older person can stay in his or her own home environment or must be institutionalized.

Diet

One of the most difficult areas to consider while dealing with the elderly diabetic, especially the newly diagnosed patient, is diet. Many diabetics with adult-onset disease can be controlled by manipulation of diet alone, but this is easier said than done, since in the aged person food intake habits are an accumulation of years of ethnic and social patterns. Finances also are a factor to be considered, for many elderly people live on fixed incomes that never seem to stretch enough to cover everything. As a result, many use their food budgets to buy the cheaper foods, often containing many carbohydrates and fats. Protein foods are often prohibitive in cost, as are fresh fruits and vegetables. The older patient may also be on a restricted diet because of other problems, such as hypertension or cardiac disease. Because of the complexity of these problems, as well as the difficulty many older people have in adjusting to the many limitations, it is extremely wise to get input from a dietician (refer to Chapter 7 for discussion of dietary management of diabetes mellitus). In the elderly, it is very important to incorporate set patterns of food and fluid intake into plans. For those diabetics with unstable disease who are treated with insulin and/or hypoglycemic agents, regularly spacing food throughout the day is important for management of hyperglycemia and prevention of hypoglycemia. For those diabetics with stable and mild disease who are obese, reduction of caloric intake becomes the priority goal.

The patient's understanding of the diet should not be assumed. The diet should be reviewed with the patient in a way that is not seen as judgmental and does not make the person fearful of presenting problems and areas where there is difficulty in compliance.

Many of the elderly have difficulty with food that is rough in consistency or requires chewing because of the lack of teeth or poor condition of gums and/or teeth. Some should have extractions done and dentures made. For some the dentures may have been fitted years before and no longer fit well or may need repair. The nurse who investigates these problems and helps arrange for treatment may be solving a great many of the diet problems of these people.

A final factor that must be considered in planning a diet for the aged diabetic is the home situation. If the elderly person lives alone, it is often found that cooking or other food preparation is kept to a minimum. Human beings are social creatures and therefore do not like to eat alone. Nor do many people who live alone feel like taking the time to prepare meals for their consumption alone. If the elderly diabetic is affected by visual complications, this may also limit safe food preparation.

Many communities are now offering Meals-on-Wheels programs for a nominal charge. Some senior citizen centers also offer hot meals at lunchtime. These should be investigated as alternatives for the elderly diabetic.

Medication

Not all elderly diabetics will be started on either insulin or oral hypoglycemics at the time of diagnosis. Many can be managed by diet alone. The decision to prescribe insulin or oral hypoglycemics is one that deserves careful attention. It has recently been reported in at least one study, the University Group Diabetes Program, that patients on oral hypoglycemics had more deaths from cardiovascular incidents than occurred in control patients having similar cardiovascular episodes.[14] Oral hypoglycemics, however, may well allow the patient to live independently rather than having to accept institutionalization or outside help if unable to administer his or her own insulin.

Even with oral hypoglycemics, the nurse may have to assist the elderly patient to set up a system of remembering when to take the drug. An empty egg carton labeled with days of the week and hours of the day has been successfully used by many. Confusion about medication may reflect the many medications that are prescribed for the elderly. It has been the experience of these authors that it is not uncommon to find elderly patients who are on five or six different medications every day, some several times a day.

The two classes of oral hypoglycemic agents now prescribed are the sulfonylureas and the biguanides. These drugs have a variety of possible side effects, which were discussed in Chapter 7. The nurse must remember and teach the patient that the action of these drugs is potentiated by the simultaneous use of other drugs such as aspirin, phenylbutazone, coumarin, MAO inhibitors, sulfasoxazole, and probenecid. The use of alcohol is also discouraged with the use of the biguanides because of the danger of lactic acidosis.[15] Chapter 7 discusses other drug-drug and drug-disease interactions common to the elderly.

It is important that the elderly person realize that insulin or oral hypoglycemic agents should not be taken more often than prescribed; they are not to be used like aspirin for a feeling of "not being well." The health professional must also remember that at times of stress, either psychological or physiological, the aged person may have to have the medical regimen adjusted for a period of time.

As described earlier in this chapter, one of the real dangers to the elderly in the use of either the oral hypoglycemics or insulin is hypoglycemia. This should always remain in the mind of the health professional. Ways of assisting the disabled diabetic in the preparation and safe administration of insulin are described in Chapter 10. Initial plans should include actions to be taken in the event of insulin reaction.

Exercise

The aged person should be encouraged to exercise, since increased activity on a regular basis in the stable diabetic has been found to reduce blood glucose levels. Walking is an excellent exercise for the aged, unless arthritis or some other chronic disease or disability makes it too difficult to walk for any distance. If the patient also has arterial occlusive disease and/or neuropathy, walking may increase the discomfort. Other exercises that some of the aged have begun to use are bicycle riding (stationary or moving) and swimming. Some senior citizen centers provide exercise periods. Again the nurse must remember that lack of finances or fear of being out alone may inhibit the exercising. Also, it may not be easy to motivate someone who has never taken part in regular exercise to begin at such an advanced age.

Foot Care

The diminished peripheral blood flow of the lower extremities plus accompanying peripheral neuropathy in the diabetic makes him or her a perfect candidate for tissue necrosis, infection, and gangrene. These problems can occur even after the most trivial injury. The diabetic patient (or caretaker) should be taught to inspect the feet daily for lesions, to bathe them in warm water, to dry them well without chafing, to wear clean socks daily, and to wear shoes that fit well and have a smooth lining. Commercial corn plasters or medications should not be used, and toenails should be trimmed neatly across and even with the toes. It is important to emphasize that temperature extremes, going barefoot, and wearing restrictive clothing should be avoided. Smoking is discouraged because it may further decrease circulation to the feet. The health professional should examine the feet carefully at each visit, and if possible, a podiatrist should regularly provide foot care. This is especially important in the aged diabetic patient because many no longer have the flexibility and manual dexterity as well as vision necessary to reach and safely and effectively care for their feet.

Urine Testing

The elderly diabetic should be taught how to test urine for glucose and acetone. Testing for glucose once or twice a day is usually adequate for the stable diabetic. All insulin-dependent diabetics should also test their urine routinely for acetone; others should test for acetone when glycosuria increases or when illness occurs. The double-void method of collecting the urine should be explained, and the patient should be asked to perform the procedure under supervision.

Debate exists as to what is the preferred method of urine testing of the stable patient. Most agree, however, that only with an insulin-dependent diabetic is it necessary to use Clinitest tablets, preferably the two-drop method, because higher glycosuria levels can be determined. With those patients who are being controlled by diet alone or diet plus oral hypoglycemic agents, a simpler method can be used. Most important, the elderly diabetic or caretaker should understand when the nurse or physician is to be called. In addition, they should be taught the importance of recording daily urine results. (See pages 234–239.)

Other Health Precautions

All elderly diabetic patients should be taught the importance of good hygiene in general. The elderly person should frequently look for skin infections or other lesions on all parts of the body. A good time to do this is when the person is bathing or showering. The female diabetic should understand the importance of cleansing herself from front to back after voiding or elimination because of the frequency of urinary tract infections in the aged diabetic. Patients should also be alerted to the fact that their physician probably will want urine samples at intervals to detect any asymptomatic infection of the urine.

Because of the visual problems in the aged diabetic, it is important to have regular checkups by the ophthalmologist. In this way early problems can be picked up and treated before they can cause permanent damage.

The nurse should review safety precautions with the elderly person and attempt to make the person's home as safe as possible. This includes removing throw rugs, making sure stairways are well lighted and have banisters, adding grab bars in the bathroom, and making sure any radiators have protective coverings to prevent burns. The older person who realizes the potential dangers will be much more cooperative in correcting problems and practicing safety precautions.

The older diabetic patient should know the warning signals of both acidosis and hypoglycemia and the appropriate actions to take in either situation. It is helpful for the aged person to wear an identification tag and carry a card that indicates that he or she is a diabetic, the medication he or she is on, and where he or she receives care.

The nurse should be sure that the diabetic understands the follow-up plan of care in terms of teaching and visits to the clinic or physician. Ideally, the nurse should make frequent visits until there is no doubt that the elderly person has the knowledge to safely control the treatment regimen. In reality this may not be possible, so the nurse should take advantage of every opportunity to teach and receive feedback.

SUMMARY

With the aged diabetic there are certain aspects of control and treatment that need to be considered in the plan for self-care. Complications are more prevalent in the elderly and may cause great reordering of daily routines, especially when superimposed on already present diseases or disabilities. The nurse who understands the disease, its complications, and the stresses of aging is well prepared to assess the person's ability to learn new tasks. With the cooperation of the older person or care giver, the nurse can set goals and devise plans to teach what is necessary and evaluate progress. The nurse can assume a most important place in helping the elderly diabetic or the care giver assume control of the disease.

REFERENCES

1 *Diabetes Source Book,* U.S. Public Health Service, Publication no. 1168, Washington, D.C., 1968.
2 *Epidemiology of Aging,* U.S. Department of Health, Education and Welfare, Publication no. 77-711, Washington, D.C.

3 Cowdry, E. V., and Steinberg, F. *The Care of the Geriatric Patient* (St. Louis: Mosby, 1971).

4 Rossman, I. *Clinical Geriatrics* (Philadelphia: Lippincott, 1971).

5 DeLaurentis, D. A. How to evaluate and treat lower extremity ischemia in the diabetic, *Geriatrics,* **31**:83–91, 1976.

6 Shagan, B. P. Diabetes in the elderly patient, *Med. Clin. North Am.,* **60**:1191–1208, 1976.

7 Rossman. Op. cit., p. 402.

8 Cowdry. Op. cit., p. 76.

9 Ibid.

10 Morse, P. H. Ocular symptoms and signs of diabetes, *Geriatrics,* **31**:56–63, 1976.

11 Rossman. Op. cit., pp. 393–394.

12 Ibid.

13 Duncan, T. Teaching common sense health care habits to diabetic patients, *Geriatrics,* **31**:93–96, 1976.

14 University Group Diabetes Program. Effects of hypoglycemic agents on vascular complications in patients with adult-onset diabetes. III. Clinical implications of UGDP results, *J.A.M.A.,* **218**:1400–1410, 1971.

15 Shagan. Op. cit., p. 1204.

Chapter 13

Pregnancy and the Diabetic Woman

Karen Budd
Shirley O. Wood

Pregnancy is considered to be a normal developmental stage in the maturation of a woman. In most instances the fetal physical outcome is good, the mother navigates the developmental crisis successfully, and the mother-infant unit embarks on the next developmental stage of womanhood: mothering. However, for a diabetic woman, the course is not as smooth, and perhaps can't be navigated at all. Before the insulin era it was rare for a diabetic woman to conceive, and when she did, maternal as well as infant mortality was high. Now, with insulin, pregnancy itself does not appear to significantly alter the course of diabetes, although maternal morbidity and perinatal mortality continue to be problems. In 1974, perinatal mortality remained at about 10 percent at the Joslin Clinic, and presumably would be higher in less sophisticated settings.[1]

White devised a classification of maternal diabetes to provide guidelines for study and management of diabetes mellitus and pregnancy.[2] In general, the classes are based on differences in age of onset, duration of disease, use of insulin or oral agents, and presence of vascular disease, all of which affect the relative risk to the fetus. In addition, four factors that increase perinatal loss were reported by Pederson and Pederson.[3] These were pyelonephritis, keto-acidosis, toxemia, and neglect of appropriate care. Mounting evidence indicates the need for close control of maternal blood glucose during pregnancy. The implications for nursing of one regimen for close control will be discussed.

METABOLISM OF CARBOHYDRATES DURING PREGNANCY

Pregnancy effects changes in carbohydrate metabolism in all women. In order to provide glucose in the amounts needed by the growing fetus, the body transports glucose by facilitated diffusion through the placenta, leading to fasting glucose levels that are 15 to 20 mg/dL lower during pregnancy than postpartum. During the first half of pregnancy, fasting insulin concentrations are reduced proportionately, so basal uptake of glucose is reduced. In order to meet the energy needs, the woman increases use of free fatty acids and ketone bodies. In other words, her response is an acceleration of the normal response to starvation. During the second half of pregnancy, the placenta manufactures increasing amounts of human chorionic somatomammotropin (HCS), a growth hormone that increases the availability of amino acid and glucose to the fetus.

HCS is a potent insulin antagonist and diminishes the effectiveness of insulin in translocating glucose into cells. Consequently, in late pregnancy, plasma insulin concentrations increase to where insulin/glucose ratios are nearly twice those of early pregnancy, but the end result is a constant plasma glucose concentration of below 100 mg/dL (5.6 mm/L) except for the first hour following a meal. This provides the fetus with a constant glucose environment.[4]

CONTROL OF HYPERGLYCEMIA

Increased attention is being given to the strict control of maternal hyperglycemia in all classes of diabetes. The stress of pregnancy may "uncover" an underlying deficit in carbohydrate metabolism in the mother. *Gestational diabetes* is the name given to the onset of hyperglycemia during pregnancy; the hyperglycemia often subsides after delivery. It is generally agreed that management by diet (and insulin if necessary) is important in reducing risks to the infant. (Refer to pages 149 to 151 for discussion of diet management in pregnancy.)

THE INFANT OF THE DIABETIC MOTHER

It is a fact that infants of diabetic women (including those labeled prediabetic, latent, or subclinical) tend to be longer, heavier at birth, and *less mature* than those of nondiabetic mothers. Some of the higher morbidity and mortality rates of infants of diabetic mothers stem from prematurity, respiratory distress syndrome, and immature mechanisms for regulation of bilirubin, glucose, and calcium. The occurrences of congenital abnormalities and stillbirths are higher in diabetic mothers than in nondiabetic mothers. Table 13-1 lists effects on the infant (and the fetus in utero) of maternal hyperglycemia, ketosis or ketoacidosis, and hypoglycemia.

Table 13-1 Effects of Maternal Diabetes on the Infant

Maternal condition	Effect on infant	
	In utero	Neonatal
Hyperglycemia	Beta-cell hypertrophy and hyperinsulinism	Hypoglycemia
	Fat and glycogen deposits Decrease in some contrainsulin hormones:	Macrosomia (large infant)
	Epinephrine	Catecholamine depletion at delivery in some infants
	Cortisol	Lack of cortisol has been implicated in lung tissue immaturity
Ketosis and/or ketoacidosis	Dehydration and acidosis; central nervous system damage	Dehydrated and acidotic infant; central nervous system damage
Hypoglycemia	Central nervous system damage	Central nervous system damage

Gillmer et al. demonstrated that during pregnancy, insulin-dependent diabetics who were thought to be in optimal control had higher mean hourly glucose concentrations with a tendency to nocturnal hypoglycemia.[5] The gestational diabetics demonstrated a consistently higher mean hourly blood glucose concentration. The significance of this study in terms of questionable fetal outcome for the pregnant diabetic can be seen clearly when a study by Karlsson and Kjellmar is considered. This study reports a direct correlation of perinatal mortality rates to mean blood glucose concentrations. A fetal mortality rate of 3.8 percent was associated with mean concentrations of less than 100 mg/dL, a rate of 15.3 percent with concentrations of between 101 and 150 mg/dL, and a rate of 23.6 percent with concentrations above 150 mg/dL.[6] Mortality rates improved as the normal changes of pregnancy were approximated.

Pregnancy Management in Diabetics

The management of pregnancy in diabetics proposed by Rodman et al. has as its chief objective the control of fasting blood glucose concentrations to under 100 mg/dL, and postprandial levels to under 120 mg/dL.[7] The periods of pregnancy needing particular attention are the first trimester, when there is need to decrease insulin dosages, and after 24 weeks, when there is need to drastically increase the amount of insulin. Dangers in these periods are hypoglycemic reactions in the first trimester and ketoacidosis in the third trimester with associated fetal loss. To support the philosophy of management, liberal hospitalization is used to supplement the ambulatory management.

During these hospitalizations, preprandial blood glucose concentrations are measured at 8 A.M., 11 A.M., 4 P.M., and 9 P.M. To attain a level of between

70 and 120 mg/dL, split doses of short- and intermediate-acting insulins are given before the morning and evening meals. Gestational diabetics may be maintained on a 2000- to 2400-cal ADA diet only, unless their blood glucose levels are above the optimal range, and then they too are put on insulin (this generally occurs in the third trimester). Monitoring the fetal status includes tests of maturation and stress, which are important in deciding the optimal time of delivery. These include

1   Ultrasonography in midtrimester to document fetal age
2   Biweekly plasma estriol determinants after week 30 if ambulatory
3   Daily urinary estriol levels during hospitalization
4   Periodic contraction stress tests (electronic monitoring of the fetal heart and Braxton Hicks uterine contraction).
5   Weekly amniocentesis to determine fetal pulmonary maturation, usually starting at 36 weeks[8],*

HYPOGLYCEMIA POSTDELIVERY

The mode of delivery (as well as the time of delivery) often is not determined until late. Regardless of the mode, both the insulin-treated mother and the infant are subject to hypoglycemia postdelivery. The maternal blood glucose drops as placental hormones no longer exert antiinsulin effects; reduction of insulin dosage and the use of intravenous glucose maintain adequate blood glucose levels. The infant has existed in utero with hyperglycemia and resultant fetal hyperinsulinism; after delivery, the hyperinsulinism persists. The infant is usually given care in an intensive care unit. Administration of glucose by oral or intravenous routes is discontinued gradually with the initiation of milk feedings.

IMPLICATIONS FOR NURSING

Helping a patient follow a therapeutic regimen as described above holds several implications for nursing. Whether the woman is newly diagnosed as having gestational diabetes or she has known about her diabetes for a period of time, hospitalization during pregnancy can assume crisis proportions. For now, in addition to resolving the developmental crisis of pregnancy in an environment that does not provide her usual support systems, she must deal with the fact of the hospitalization.

Pregnancy: A Developmental Crisis

In pregnancy, the diabetic state and its diagnostic and therapeutic procedures are superimposed upon a developmental process. Pregnancy is considered one of the normative crisis points in life. When a woman is considered "well," her adjustment to this physical and emotional event is considerable. Reordering the

---

* One test is the L/S (lecithin/sphingomyelin) ratio which indicates the maturity of the fetal lung: a ratio near 1:1 indicates immaturity, 2:1 indicates transition, and 3:1 maturity.

priorities of her life, adjusting her role relationships within her family and society, and accommodating the physical and emotional aspects of a pregnancy comprise major areas to consider in providing nursing care.

Rarely does a pregnancy occur at the "right" time under the "right" circumstances: the house isn't finished, the finances could be better, the children aren't spaced in age as one had planned, etc. Even though this is the usual story accompanying the announcement "You're pregnant," women *can* accommodate this unplanned event. Many modes and models are used to accomplish this work: the woman may try to readjust her life by spending hours reading, conversing with friends, or using professionals as sounding boards to "sort out" the impact of the pregnancy on her and her family. She will carefully observe other pregnant women to see how they have negotiated the work she now senses must be done.

Frequently, this "work" of accommodating never becomes an intellectually cognitive event until the professional caring for the woman helps her put into words those tasks completed and those yet to be completed. The nurse can assist the patient in her adjustment by helping her identify guidelines. Careful listening will often detect subtle changes in priorities and in role relationships.

How are these changes noted? One begins to hear a woman expressing less turmoil about restrictions and alterations in goals and activities and more interest and investment in plans for the new member of the family. The past tense may be used to indicate a change in orientation: "When I worked," for example, even though she may still be working outside the family. If this is a second baby, she will tell you how she and her family will adjust to this new baby. She begins to "work through" what it is like to mother two children rather than only one. She may seek out friends who have two children to observe how they "spread themselves out" as mothers. Women spend a lot of time in thought when they are pregnant. They may even appear to be daydreaming a lot, but they are hard at work doing mental gymnastics as they contemplate the huge task at hand.

Pregnancy and Chronic Illness

When a pregnancy is negotiated in conjunction with a chronic illness, there are many complicating factors which influence the course of the pregnancy and a woman's adjustment to it. If, for example, the woman believes she is healthy but develops gestational diabetes, she may need time with the nurse to discuss her feelings as well as to learn about diabetes. Uncertainty about the outcome of pregnancy is a major stress with which she must deal. Some questions that may help to ferret out the woman's feelings follow. They may need to be modified according to the client's age, ethnic background, or educational level:

1 "Tell me your feelings when you were told you were a gestational diabetic."
2 "Does the word *diabetes* make you think of anything in particular?"
3 "Has anyone close to you had diabetes?"

4 "You were probably told about your condition by the doctor. What did the doctor tell you about how these findings would affect you and your baby?"

Not knowing when delivery will occur is verbalized universally as stressful. Patients need to have as much information as possible about the status of their pregnancy and the measures used to determine the most optimal time of delivery. Even though this doesn't give them definite dates, it does assist them in coping better with an uncharted course.

Impact of Hospitalization

Any hospitalization episode carries with it the expectation that the patient will modify his or her pattern of daily activities to one where compliant and dependent behavior is expected.[9] In order to help the woman adjust to the hospital, the nurse should try to help her understand the rationale and the need for hospitalization by teaching and supporting.

The nurse should explain to the gestational diabetic the nature of diabetes, the effects of pregnancy and diabetes on each other, and the procedures for fractional urine examinations and insulin injections. For patients with other classes of diabetes, the nurse should reinforce previous teachings concerning the nature of diabetes and correct any misunderstandings. Diversional therapy may need to be planned with the patient. This may take the form of walks through the hospital and its grounds, participation in crafts, or perhaps consultation with a physical therapist. The latter may provide the patient with an exercise plan that will simulate energy expenditure at home.

Pregnant women with diabetes often experience frustration in their inability to supervise or manage their disease and in the expectation that they will be totally in the hands of their obstetrician. They must submit to the discomfort of possible insulin reactions as insulin dosages are adjusted and to venipuncture four times a day. They need a supportive nurse who will listen and help reduce the frustrations.

The patient/client should participate as much as possible in her health care. She will have many concerns and stresses which come with separation from family, hospitalization, and the tasks of pregnancy. Frequently, the nurse will identify strengths or deficits within the family relationships, and these may become a major area for nursing intervention. Cooperation and clear communication among all members of the health team, including the patient and her family, are vital. Anxieties over the condition of the infant and feelings of guilt and inadequacies are common. Factual information, given in a nonjudgmental manner, and support for expressions of feelings and concerns can assist both parents to mobilize their own resources, confront reality, and act in a productive manner.

SUMMARY

Pregnancy is a developmental crisis point in the life of all women; for the diabetic woman it is more difficult because of chronic illness, its therapy, and the threat to fetal well-being. Gestational diabetic women need to deal with both the pregnancy and the impact of diabetes. One program of management with implications for nursing has been described.

REFERENCES

1 White, P. Diabetes mellitus in pregnancy, *Clin. Perinatol.*, **1**:331, 1974.
2 White, P. Infants of diabetic mothers, *Am. J. Med.*, **7**:609, 1949.
3 Pederson, J., and Pederson, L. M. Prognosis of the outcome of pregnancy in diabetics. A new classification, *Endocrinol. (Kbh.)*, **50**:70, 1965.
4 Rodman, H. M., et al. The diabetic pregnancy as a model for modern perinatal care, in *Diabetes and the Endocrine Disorders during Pregnancy and in the Newborn* (New York: Liss, 1976), pp. 13–32.
5 Gillmer, M. D. G., et al. Carbohydrate metabolism in pregnancy. Plasma glucose profile in normal and diabetic women, *Br. Med. J.*, **3**:399, 1975.
6 Karlsson, K., and Kjellmar, I. The outcome of diabetic pregnancies in relation to the mother's blood sugar level, *Am. J. Obstet. Gynecol.*, **112**:213, 1972
7 Rodman et al. Loc. cit.
8 Gyves, M. T., et al. A modern approach to management of pregnant diabetics. A two year analysis of perinatal outcomes. *Amer. J. Obstet. Gynecol.* (in press).
9 King, J. H. *Perceptions of Illness and Medical Practice* (New York: Russell Sage, 1962).

BIBLIOGRAPHY

Blair, C. L., and E. M. Salerno. *The Expanding Family: Childbearing.* Boston: Little, Brown, 1976.
Budd, K. Behavioral tasks of the high-risk maternity patient, in N. A. Lytle (ed.), *Nursing of Women in the Age of Liberation.* Dubuque, Iowa: Brown, 1977.
Rubin, R. Tasks of pregnancy, in *A.N.A. Clinical Sessions.* New York: Appleton-Century-Crofts, 1974.

Index

Index